IMMUNOLOGICAL APPROACHES TO THE DIAGNOSIS AND THERAPY OF BREAST CANCER

IMMUNOLOGICAL APPROACHES TO THE DIAGNOSIS AND THERAPY OF BREAST CANCER

Edited by
Roberto L. Ceriani
John Muir Cancer and Aging Research Institute
Walnut Creek, California

PLENUM PRESS • NEW YORK AND LONDON

Library of Congress Cataloging in Publication Data

International Workshop on Monoclonal Antibodies and Breast Cancer (2nd: 1986: San Francisco, Calif.)
Immunological approaches to the diagnosis and therapy of breast cancer.

"Proceedings of the Second International Workshop on Monoclonal Antibodies and Breast Cancer, held November 20-21, 1986, in San Francisco, California"—T.p. verso.
Includes bibliographies and index.
1. Breast—Cancer—Immunological aspects—Congresses. 2. Antibodies, Monoclonal—Diagnostic use—Congresses. 3. Antibodies, Monoclonal—Therapeutic use—Congresses. 4. Breast—Cancer—Immunotherapy—Congresses. 5. Immunodiagnosis—Congresses. I. Ceriani, Roberto L. II. Title. [DNLM: 1. Antibodies, Monoclonal—immunology—congresses. 2. Breast Neoplasms—immunology—congresses. W3 IN93266 2nd 1986i / WP 879 I61 1986i]
RC280.B8I58 1986 616.99′449075 87-15373
ISBN 0-306-42601-3

Proceedings of the Second International Workshop on Monoclonal Antibodies and Breast Cancer, held November 20–21, 1986, in San Francisco, California

Printed in the United States of America

2ND INTERNATIONAL WORKSHOP ON MONOCLONAL ANTIBODIES AND BREAST CANCER

San Francisco, California

November 20-21, 1986

Organized by the John Muir Cancer & Aging Research Institute, with the cooperation of the International Association for Breast Cancer Research.

CHAIRPERSON Dr. Roberto L. Ceriani
John Muir Cancer & Aging Research Institute

ORGANIZING COMMITTEE

Chairpersons: Dr. Roberto L. Ceriani
Dr. Jean Hager-Rich (AMC Cancer Research Center, Denver, Colorado)

Members:
Ms. Shannon Jackson
Dr. Bernard Larner
Dr. Howard Maccabee
Dr. Jerry A. Peterson
Ms. Kelly Travers
Ms. Patricia Woycheese

PROGRAM COMMITTEE

Chairperson: Dr. Roberto L. Ceriani

Members:
Dr. Robert Cardiff
Dr. Arthur Frankel
Dr. Kenneth McCarty, Jr.
Dr. William L. McGuire
Dr. Ricardo Mesa-Tejada
Dr. Luciano Ozzello
Dr. Jeffrey Schlom

ACKNOWLEDGEMENTS

The Organizing Committee for the 2nd International Workshop on Monoclonal Antibodies and Breast Cancer, together with the John Muir Cancer & Aging Research Institute, gratefully acknowledge the support of the following in making the Workshop possible:

SPONSORS

COULTER IMMUNOLOGY, HIALEAH, FLORIDA
TRITON BIOSCIENCES, INC., ALAMEDA, CALIFORNIA
Abbott Laboratories, North Chicago, Illinois
Cambridge Research Laboratory, Cambridge, Massachusetts
Cetus Corporation, Emeryville, California
Medi+Physics, Inc., Emeryville, California
Stuart Pharmaceuticals, Wilmington, Delaware
Bio-Rad Laboratories, Richmond, California
Bristol-Myers Company, New York, New York
Eli Lilly and Company, Indianapolis, Indiana
Genelabs Incorporated, San Carlos, California

CONTRIBUTORS

The Christian Brothers Winery, FM Productions, Hyclone, Micco Office Equipment, Polysciences, Inc., Zymed Laboratories, Inc.

PREFACE

Once again we have gathered to discover and evaluate advances made in our ability to understand, diagnose and possibly treat breast cancer with the new reagents provided by monoclonal antibody techniques.

In the last two years since our first International Workshop on Monoclonal Antibodies and Breast Cancer there has been an enormous surge in the number and quality of applications for these new reagents. Solid achievements have been made in identification and quantitation of estrogen and progesterone receptors, in histopathological diagnostic procedures, in serum diagnosis, and we are witnessing now the first attempts to treat breast cancer with immunoconjugates.

Cytosolic estrogen receptors can now be quantitated with monoclonal antibodies, and also their cellular distribution can be directly assessed histologically. In addition, monoclonal antibodies to progesterone receptors have been generated that show promise in having similar uses as those to the estrogen receptor.

In the field of diagnosis, the use of monoclonal antibodies has permitted the development of serological approaches for early diagnosis by identifying and measuring breast epithelial antigens in serum, and of histological approaches for establishing criteria for breast cancer dissemination and prognosis.

With great expectations we are all following developments in the area of breast cancer treatment using conjugates of anti-breast epithelial monoclonal antibodies which are now confirming earlier reports in affecting breast tumor control. The recent creation of newer monoclonal antibodies and conjugates await experimentation and clinical trials to determine their value.

As a whole, we are at the threshold of an explosive development in uses of these reagents and the many contributions to this 2nd International Workshop attest to this fact. The enthusiasm and investment of many laboratories worldwide in these new techniques and approaches stems also no doubt from the steady progress made in basic aspects of the field for which we have evident proof here.

This 2nd Workshop was made possible by the generosity of our Sponsors, the commitment of the members of the Program and

Organizing Committee, and the strong dedication of the John Muir Cancer & Aging Research Institute staff. A special mention should be made of the effort and care put into the preparation of this volume by Ms. Shannon Jackson.

Evidence of the progress made is presented in this volume and the excitement generated by these accomplishments make us believe in the important role to be played by reagents produced with monoclonal antibodies in breast cancer diagnosis and treatment in the near future.

Roberto L. Ceriani

CONTENTS

SESSIONS I AND II

SESSION III

SESSION IV

SESSIONS I AND II

CHARACTERIZATION OF CROSS-RELATED ANTIGENS OF HUMAN MILK FAT GLOBULE MEMBRANE AND BREAST TUMORS DETECTED BY A NEW MONOCLONAL ANTIBODY PANEL

Arnold S. Dion, Pierre P. Major*, and Masao Ishida*

Institute of Molecular Genetics
Center for Molecular Medicine and Immunology
One Bruce Street
Newark, NJ 07103 USA

*McGill Cancer Centre
McIntyre Medical Sciences Building
3655 Drummond
Montreal, PQ H3G IY6 Canada

INTRODUCTION

The initial impetus for the generation of antisera versus milk fat globule membranes (MFGM) was to provide immunological reagents for the identification of differentiation markers specific for breast epithelial cells.[1] In view of the paucity of such reagents and their potential for defining normal ontogenic processes comprising mammary gland development and function, this was a logical approach. What was perhaps less obvious at the inception of this strategy, however, were the observations by Ceriani et al.[1] and others, as cited later, that mammary tumor cells and MFGM expressed common antigens associated with highly differentiated functions. Not unexpectedly, therefore, antibodies prepared against breast tumor cells or subcellular components were likewise found to frequently react with MFGM preparations (vide infra).

Recently, a panel of ten monoclonal antibodies was prepared and selected for reactivity against membrane fractions of a moderately differentiated breast tumor as well as poorly differentiated breast tumors metastatic to liver, and eight of these preparations were found to also react, in various degrees, with MFGM components.[2] A primary goal of these and subsequent studies was to define various biological and biochemical parameters of these cross-related tumor and MFGM antigens vis-a-vis analogous observations of others. In particular, the present investigations were focused on determining cell and organ-type antigen distributions, physicochemical characteristics, and the nature of immunoreactive determinants shared by these tumor and MFGM antigens.

PREPARATION AND INITIAL CHARACTERIZATION OF MONOCLONAL ANTIBODY PANEL

Immunogens for the generation of monoclonal antibodies consisted of cellular membrane components[3] of either primary or metastatic breast tumors, resulting in a total of 1,938 hybridomas derived from 33 fusions.[2] As summarized in Table 1, 10 of these hybridomas were selected for further study by the criteria of: a. reactivity with the cognate immunogen and at least one additional tumor membrane preparation; b. greater reactivity with membranes from tumors than normal breast tissues (reduction mammoplasties); and c. lack of reactivity with normal liver cells or membranes, bile ducts, vascular endothelium, lymphocytes or granulocytes.

As reviewed later, the finding of cross-related antigens that are shared by both breast tumors and MFGM has been frequently noted. Because of this phenomenon and for the purpose of immunoreactivity ordering, antibody-binding to equivalent amounts of primary (PT3) and metastatic breast tumor membranes (MB5 and MB6), as well as MFGM, was evaluated by the enzyme-linked immunosorbent assay (ELISA) and by dot blotting. For both assay techniques, similar results were obtained and a representative dot blot assay is shown in Figure 1. Cumulatively, the ELISA[2] and dot blot techniques demonstrated that the monoclonal antibody panel (MA1 to 10) could be grouped according to their reactivities with these four test antigens (Table 2), and corresponded to reactivities with distinct antigenic molecular weight species, as discussed later.

BIOLOGICAL AND BIOCHEMICAL CHARACTERISTICS OF THE MILK FAT GLOBULE MEMBRANE

The lipid-rich fractions of all milks are typically composed of milk fat globules (1 to 10 microns in diameter) which share similar ultrastructural features.[4] The structural model initially advanced by

Table 1. Immunogens and Monoclonal Antibody Isotypes

Immunogen	Mouse Strain	Antibody Designation	Isotypes
Primary Breast Tumor	A	MA1*	IgG1 k
Primary Breast Tumor	A	MA2*	IgG1 k
Primary Breast Tumor	Balb/c	MA3	IgG3 k
Metastatic Breast Tumor 1	A	MA4+	IgG1 k
Metastatic Breast Tumor 1	A	MA5+	IgG1 k
Metastatic Breast Tumor 1	Balb/c	MA6	IgG1 k
Metastatic Breast Tumor 1	Balb/c	MA7	IgG1 k
Metastatic Breast Tumor 5	A	MA8'	IgG1 k
Metastatic Breast Tumor 5	A	MA9'	IgG1 k
Metastatic Breast Tumor 5	A	MA10'	IgM k

For immunization, membrane preparations from either a primary breast tumor (moderately differentiated) or breast tumor metastasis (poorly differentiated) were used as immunogens.

*,+,'; Antibodies derived from the same fusion.

Bargmann and Knoop[5] proposed that milk fat droplets were progressively enveloped by the cellular plasma membrane. This model has been generally verified by current evidence, reviewed by Anderson and Cawston [6] and Patton and Keenan,[4] that milk triacylglycerols are secreted from mammary epithelial cells as discrete droplets surrounded by a surface membrane, termed the milk fat globule membrane (MFGM), which is derived from the apical pole of secretory alveolar cells.[7] Consistent with this scheme, bovine MFGM is enriched with components typical of the plasma membrane, viz. sphingomyelin, 5'-nucleotidase, phosphodiesterase and alkaline phosphatase.[8] Human MFGM, as well, contains enzymes characteristic of plasma membranes of the Golgi apparatus and endoplasmic reticulum.[9] SDS-polyacrylamide gel electrophoretic (SDS-PAGE) analyses of the MFGM's isolated from the milks of several species have indicated the presence of 8 to 10 major protein/glycoproteins, as reviewed by Patton and Keenan.[4] Two components, xanthine oxidase and butyrophilin, account for 50% of the total proteins/glycoproteins stainable with Coomassie blue.[7,10,11] Xanthine oxidase, although present in the cytoplasm of secretory epithelial cells, occurs in higher concentrations in the cellular apical

Table 2. Relative Antibody Reactivities Versus Four Test Antigen Preparations

Group	Antibody	Relative Reactivity
I	MA1	PT3 > MB6 > MB5 > MFGM*
II	MA2	PT3 = MFGM > MB5 = MB6
III	MA3 to 6	MFGM > MB5 = PT3 > MB6
IV	MA7	MFGM > MB5 = PT3 > MB6
V	MA8 and 9	MB5 > PT3 = MFGM > MB6
VI	MA10	MB5 > PT3 = MB6 = MFGM

*Underlining indicates an ELISA value <0.05 optical density units and is scored as non-reactive.

pole.[11] Therefore, xanthine oxidase exists in both soluble and membrane-bound forms of isolated MFGM's.[11-13] In contrast, butyrophilin is found primarily in the apical plasma membrane and is firmly bound to the MFGM.[7,10]

With specific reference to human MFMG, more than 35 protein/glycoprotein components have been observed following two-dimensional separations.[14] However, there is no general agreement as to the number of molecular weight species of proteins/glycoproteins associated with human MFMG. [Undoubtedly, these varied conclusions are the result of different MFGM-preparation procedures, amounts analyzed by SDS-PAGE, differences in electrophoresis conditions, and detection

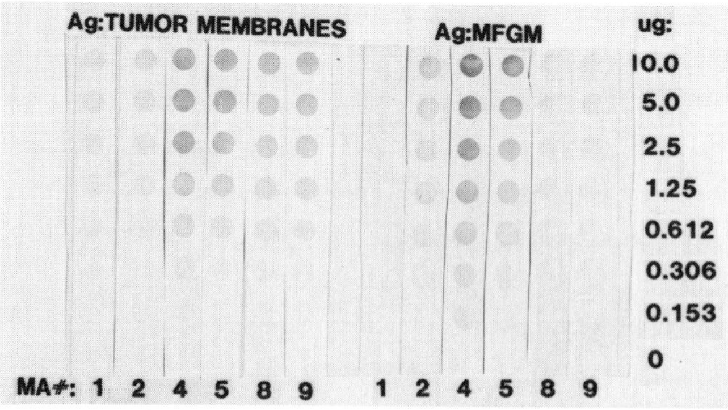

Figure 1. Monoclonal antibody (MA) binding to dot blotted membrane preparations derived from a metastatic breast tumor (MB5) and milk fat globule (MFGM).

sensitivities. This situation is further complicated by the fact that Coomassie blue often does not stain, or poorly stains, membrane glycoproteins.][15] The initial studies of Martel et al.[16] demonstrated the association of at least six major Coomassie blue-staining bands within the molecular weight range of approximately 160 and 15.5 kd; the 160 and 84 kd bands were identified as glycoproteins on the basis of periodic acid Schiff (PAS)-staining. Sasaki et al.,[17] in contrast, reported that human MFGM consisted of four major molecular weight species of 150, 75, 60, and 48 kd, and the 60 and 48 kd components were PAS-positive.

The finding that 8 of the 10 monoclonal antibodies produced against tumor membranes also reacted with MFGM (Table 2) prompted us to investigate the protein/glycoprotein complexity of the latter. Initial results (not shown) employing disc gel electrophoresis and detection of protein and glycoprotein species by Coomassie blue and PAS-staining, respectively, revealed a relatively simple profile of proteins/glycoproteins as previously described.[16,17] However, the use of more sensitive techniques involving slab gel electrophoresis,[18] blotting to nitrocellulose,[19] and visualization by india ink staining [20] and reaction with <u>Lens culinaris</u> hemagglutinin (LcH) revealed a more complex pattern, as illustrated in Figure 2. Also, these data demonstrate that components of MFGM isolated from milks of 4 separate individuals are relatively constant. Most of the variable components are lower molecular weight

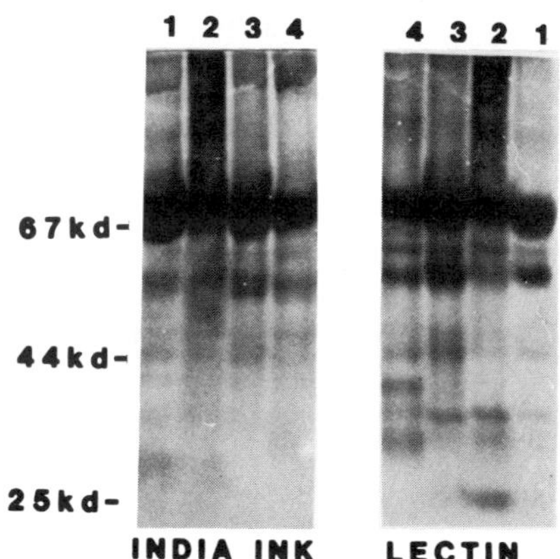

Figure 2. SDS-PAGE analysis of proteins/glycoproteins of MFGM's prepared from the milks of four separate individuals by the technique of Ceriani et al.[1] Following electrophoresis, separated components were transferred to nitrocellulose by two-dimensional diffusion, resulting in mirror images, and stained with india ink and lectin (<u>Lens culinaris</u> hemagglutinin, LcH).

species that are glycosylated, i.e. bind LcH, and probably represent variable contamination with skim milk components or possible breakdown products. As noted by Imam et al.,[21] the predominant glycoprotein constituent of human MFGM possesses an apparent molecular weight of 70 kd (gp70). In addition to LcH-binding, we should note that concanavalin A (ConA), wheat germ agglutinin (WGA), Ricinus communis agglutinin-I (RCA-I), and peanut agglutinin (PNA) bound to multiple human MFGM constituents, and will be reported elsewhere.

BIOLOGICAL AND BIOCHEMICAL CHARACTERISTICS OF RECOGNIZED ANTIGENS

With regard to mammary epithelial cells, previous studies[2] of this antibody panel established that recognized antigens were, in general, distinguishable by the criteria of membrane polarity and intensity. Specifically, recognized antigens were moderately expressed and confined to the apical surface of normal breast cells, whereas secretory breast epithelial cells displayed increased expression at the apical surface of most acini and ducts. In distinct contrast, antigen expression was most intense for tumor cells, associated with a diffuse cytoplasmic localization for most tumors while others displayed accentuation of peripheral staining.

Previous studies[2] also established cell- and organ-type antigen distributions. In brief, antigens recognized by this antibody panel were not expressed in connective tissue, smooth or striated muscle, endocrine tissues, or lymphoid or hematopoietic tissues. However, these antigens were generally expressed, at lower levels than those of normal breast epithelial cells, in other secretory epithelia as well as in other epithelial tissues. From this survey,[2] only sebaceous and sweat glands possessed a level of expression commensurate with that found for normal breast epithelium.

Diffuse cytoplasmic expression or peripheral localization of recognized determinants for tumor cells, as compared to polarized surface expression in normal cells, suggested the possibility of aberrant biosynthesis and/or processing of these antigens as a function of malignancy. Therefore, Western blot analyses were performed to address this question and to provide preliminary characterization of recognized antigens. From the results given in Figure 3A, antibody reactions versus breast tumor membrane antigens revealed that MA1 (Group I, see Table 2) and MA2 (Group II) recognized a single component (MW = 300kd), whereas MA3

Table 3. Group Designations of Monoclonal Antibodies According to Origin and Molecular Weights of Immunoreactive Antigens (Determined by Immunoblotting) and Reactivity with MCF-7 Cells.

Antigen Source:	Molecular Weight:	Antibody Group:* I	II	III	IV	V	VI
Milk Fat Globule Membrane	330,000	-	+	+	ND	+	-
Metastatic Breast Tumors	300,000	+	+	+	-	+	-
	280,000	-	-	+	-	+	-
Primary Breast Tumor	300,000	+	+	+	-	+	-
	280,000	-	-	+	-	+	-
MCF-7 Immunofluorescence:							
	Treatment						
	Before Trypsin	-	+	+	+	+	+
	After Trypsin	+	+	+	+	+	-

* Antibody Groups Include: I (MA1), II (MA2), III (MA3-6), IV (MA7), V (MA8&9), VI (MA10).

and MA5 (Group III) and MA9 (Group V) reacted with two bands (MW's = 300 and 280 kd); MA7 (Group IV) demonstrated reactivity with at least three bands (MW range = 230 to 300 kd).

Similar analyses were employed to assess whether cross-related antigens in tumor and milk fat globule membranes differed with regard to molecular weights. As shown in Figure 3B, MA3 (Group III) reactions with tumor or MFGM preparations differed significantly, i.e. two bands with MW's of 300 and 280 kd were detected in the tumor preparation while a single band of 330 kd was detectable in the MFGM. Cumulatively, group designations, originally assigned on the basis of antibody-binding to various tumor and milk fat globule membranes (Table 2), could be further refined on the basis of immunoreactivities with specific antigens and MCF-7 cells with and without prior trypsin treatment (Table 3). Furthermore, these results suggest that this panel of 10 antibodies recognizes at least 6 distinct epitopes.

The finding of related epitopes on antigens displaying molecular weight heterogeneity suggested the possibility that differences in post-translational glycosylation could, at least in part, be responsible for this phenomenon. To clarify this point, studies were initiated to obtain preliminary characterizations of the carbohydrate moieties. This was accomplished by in situ lectin-binding to electroblotted glycoproteins of tumor membranes and MFGM following SDS-PAGE, and by lectin affinity chromatography.[24] Both of these techniques yielded similar results, viz. immunologically related antigens from both tumor and MFGM have low affinities for ConA and high affinities for WGA; however, differential binding to PNA and RCA-I was observed. Specifically, PNA affinity for the 280 and 300 kd tumor antigens was clearly less than that observed for the 330 kd MFGM antigen, and enhanced affinity resulted from sialic acid removal. For binding to RCA-I, only the 280 kd antigen failed to bind significantly and this also was enhanced by the removal of sialyl residues. From these results and the known structural requirements for lectin-binding,[25] we have tentatively assigned the oligosaccharide structures given in Figure 4 to each of these antigens.

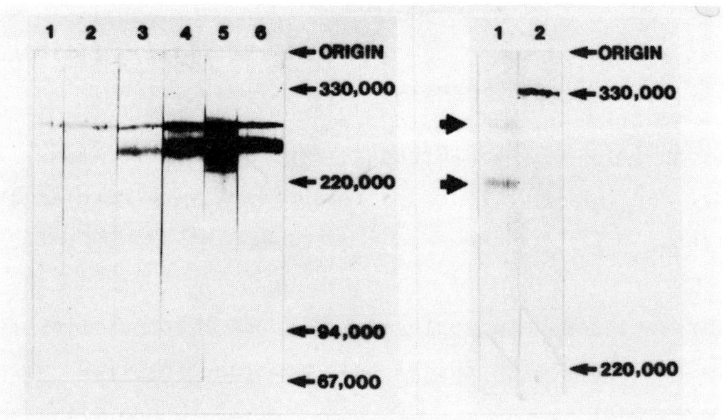

Figure 3. Molecular weight determinations for antigens recognized by monoclonal antibodies. Left Panel: Tumor antigen (MB5) was electrophoresed on a 4 to 20% SDS-polyacrylamide gel containing 4M urea under reducing conditions and electroblotted to nitrocellulose.[22] Nitrocellulose strips were then reacted with MA1 (lane 1), MA2 (lane 2), MA3 (lane 3), MA5 (lane 4), MA7 (lane 5), and MA9 (lane 6). Right Panel: Immunoblot reactivity of MA3 with 100 ug of tumor preparation MB5 (lane 1) or MFGM (lane 2). Thick arrows denote bands of 280 and 300 kd in lane 1, whereas only one band of 330 kd is stained in lane 2. Thin arrows indicate molecular weight standards (330 and 220 kd).

For the present, these assignments are consistent with the lack of binding affinity to ConA, i.e., N-asparaginyl-linked oligosaccharides with at least a triantennary structure. These terminal structures are also compatible with increased sialylation of the N- and O-linked carbohydrate moieties of the tumor-associated antigens, resulting in an increased affinity for PNA and RCA-I following desialylation. In this regard, we have observed decreased electrophoretic mobilities of the 280 and 300 kd antigens following neuraminidase treatment.[24] The lower apparent molecular weights of these antigens, as compared to the normal (330 kd) antigen, therefore, are likely explainable in whole or in part by increased sialylation of the former.

N-GLYCOSIDIC LINKAGES:

330kd (milk):	(NANA) 2-6 Gal-GlcNac-
	(NANA) 2-6 Gal-GlcNac-
	(NANA) 2-6 Gal-GlcNac-
300kd (tumor):	(NANA) 2-6 Gal-GlcNac-
	(NANA) 2-6 Gal-GlcNac-
	NANA 2-3 Gal-GlcNac-
280kd (tumor):	NANA 2-3 Gal-GLcNac-
	NANA 2-3 Gal-GLcNac-
	NANA 2-3 Gal-GLcNac-

O-GLYCOSIDIC LINKAGES:

330kd (milk):	Gal-GalNac-(Ser/Thr)
300kd (tumor):	(NANA)-Gal-GalNac-(Ser/Thr)
280kd (tumor):	NANA -Gal-GalNac-(Ser/Thr)

Figure 4. Tentative assignment of terminal oligosaccharide structures associated with recognized antigens. NANA, N-acetyl neuraminic acid; Gal, galactose; GlcNac, N-acetyl glucosamine; GalNac, N-acetyl galactosamine. Parentheses indicate the possible presence or absence of sialyl residues.

NATURE OF IMMUNOREACTIVE DETERMINANTS

The purpose of this phase of our studies was to broadly address the nature of the immunoreactive determinants, i.e., whether the recognized epitopes consisted of covalently attached carbohydrate moieties or peptide sequences. To accomplish this goal, we have of necessity employed several approaches, some of which are noted here. To obtain unequivocal answers, however, will require additional investigations which are in progress.

Our initial studies consisted of controlled periodate oxidation of carbohydrate structures, a technique which was recently devised specifically for application to glycoproteins blotted to nitrocellulose.[23] The results shown in Figure 5 demonstrate that dot blotted tumor membrane antigens extensively lose (>90%) the ability to bind peroxidase-conjugated LcH lectin following periodate treatment. In contrast, the binding of the indicated monoclonal antibodies was only slightly inhibited. Considering the fact that periodate treatment of antigens virtually eliminated antibody-binding in previous studies,[26-28] is evidence that our antibody panel recognizes primarily peptide determinants. Variability in the degree of sialylation (Fig. 4) and the lack of effect of neuraminidase treatment on antigenicity[2] similarly support this conclusion.

For MA5, three additional approaches have indicated that a peptidyl determinant is recognized. These include the findings that: 1. total human milk oligosaccharides (215 ug galactose equivalents/ml) do not

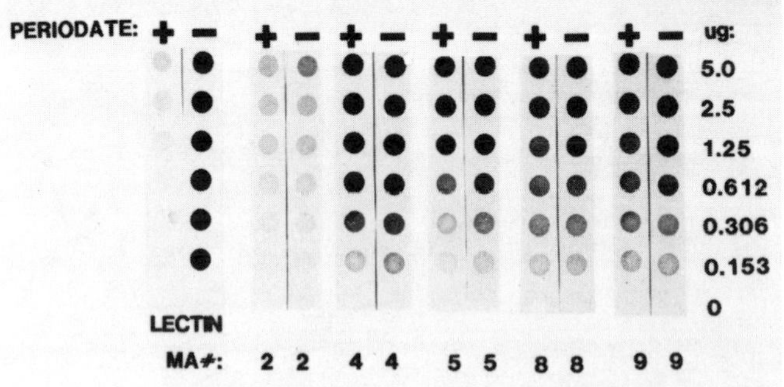

Figure 5. Antibody binding to antigen before (-) and after (+) carbohydrate modification by periodate oxidation. Extent of oligosaccharide destruction was monitored by lectin-binding (Lens culinaris hemagglutinin, LcH).

compete for antibody (4 ug/ml) reactivity for dot blotted MFGM; 2. prior reaction of dot blotted MFGM with WGA does not abrogate reactivity with antibody; 3. MA5 does not react with glycolipid extracts from human milk, and MA's 2,5 and 8 display similar reactivities to metastatic breast tumor membrane preparations with or without prior methanol extraction.[2]

CONCLUSIONS AND DISCUSSION

From results accumulated to date, the salient characteristics of this monoclonal antibody panel include: 1. recognition of at least six epitopes, most of which are shared by antigens common to both tumor cell membranes and MFGM; 2. preferential expression of recognized antigens is characteristic of secretory and malignant breast epithelial cells; however, low antigen expression was found for resting breast cells as well as for sebaceous and sweat glands; 3. expression of these antigens in other secretory epithelial cells occurred at trace levels;
4. cross-related antigens of normal secretory and malignant breast cells differ with regard to molecular weights which appears to be due, at least in part, to increased sialylation of tumor-expressed antigens;
5. intracellular processing of antigens is aberrant in tumor cells resulting in diffuse cytoplasmic or peripheral surface localization as compared to the asymmetrical surface expression on normal cells;
6. peptidyl determinants are primarily recognized.

Table 4 summarizes previous results with regard to antibody reagents which recognize antigens shared by breast tumor cells and MFGM. Consonant with the possibility that some of these antisera (Table 4) are specific for differentiation antigens, heterogeneity of antigen expression has been generally observed for both normal and malignant breast epithelial cells.[38] In addition, an asymmetric distribution of at least some MFGM-related antigens has been noted.[26,32,39] In general, differences in antigen expression between normal and malignant cells have also been found, i.e., a cytoplasmic localization in less well-differentiated tumor cells.[14,26,40,41] Also, Burchell et al.[42] and Abe and Kufe[40] observed that MFGM-related antigens differed with regard to molecular weights, i.e., of significantly lower mass in tumor cells as compared to MFGM. In this context, these biological and biochemical characteristics are consistent with data presented here and may be generally applicable for differentiation-specific antigens.

As summarized in Table 4, the nature of recognized epitopes, when determined, were invariably identified as carbohydrate moieties by lectin

Table 4. Some characteristics of antisera which recognize antigens shared by tumor cells and MFGM.

Immunogen	Antibody Designation	Type	Recognized Determinant	Reference
MFGM	α-HMEC	P[1]	ND[2]	1
MFGM	α-EMA	P	Carbohydrate	26,29
MFGM	HMFG-1 HMFG-2	M	Carbohydrate	30,31
MFGM	LICR-LON-M8 LICR-LON-M18 LICR-LON-M24	M	ND Carbohydrate Carbohydrate	32,33
Tumor membranes	MBr1	M	Carbohydrate	27
MFGM	Mc3/Mc5 McR2	M	ND	34
MFGM-gp70	α-MFGM-gp70	P	ND	14
Tumor membranes	DF3	M	Carbohydrate	35,37
MFGM	Various	M	Carbohydrate	28
MFGM	IIID5	M	ND	36

[1] P = polyclonal; M = monoclonal

[2] ND = not determined

competition assays,[31] periodate oxidation[26-28] or by blood group oligosaccharide binding or inhibition.[33] It is noteworthy, therefore, that antibodies generated versus cell surface antigens associated with embryogenesis, differentiation or oncogenesis often recognize carbohydrate structures of surface-expressed glycoproteins and/or glycolipids. Furthermore, Edwards[38] has suggested the possibility that almost all existing monoclonal antibodies to surface-expressed antigens of epithelial tumors may have carbohydrate specificities. As reviewed by Feizi,[43] this phenomenon may be intimately related to important roles of glycoconjugates in growth, development and neoplasia. From this perspective, our tentative conclusion that recognized epitopes consist primarily of peptide sequences clearly distinguishes these antibodies from those previously generated (Table 4), and offers the prospect of utilizing these reagents for DNA cloning protocols.

ACKNOWLEDGEMENTS

These studies were supported by funds from the National Cancer Institute of Canada, the Fonds de la Recherche en Sante du Quebec, the Cancer Research Society, the New Jersey State Cancer Commission and by PHS grant number R01 CA44628 awarded by the NCI, DHHS. The secretarial assistance of Danielle Jadkowski and Lois DePadova and the photographic assistance of John Hart, respectively, are also sincerely appreciated.

REFERENCES

1. R. L. Ceriani, K. Thompson, J. A. Peterson, and S. Abraham, Surface differentiation antigens of human mammary epithelial cells carried on the human milk fat globule, Proc. Nat. Acad. Sci. USA 74:582-586 (1977).

2. P. P. Major, P. E. Kovac, M. L. Lavalee, and E. G. Kovalik, Monoclonal antibodies to antigens abnormally expressed in breast cancer, J. Histochem. Cytochem. in press.

3. D. Colcher, P. Horan-Hand, Y. A. Teramoto, D. Wunderlich, and J. Schlom, Use of monoclonal antibodies to define the diversity of mammary tumor viral gene products in virions of mammary tumors of genus mus., Cancer Res. 41:1451-1459 (1981).

4. S. Patton, and T. W. Keenan, The milk fat globule membrane, Biochim. Biophys. Acta 415:273-309 (1975).

5. W. Bargmann, and A. Knoop, Uber die morphologie der milchsekretion. Licht und electronmikroscopische studien an der milchdruse der ratte, Z. Zellforsch. 49:344-388 (1959).

6. M. Anderson, and T. E. Cawston, The milk-fat globule membrane, J. Dairy Res. 42:459-483 (1975).

7. W. W. Franke, H. W. Heid, C. Grund, S. Winter, C. Freudenstein, E. Schmid, E. D. Jarasch, and T. W. Keenan, Antibodies to the major insoluble milk fat globule membrane-associated protein: Specific location in apical regions of lactating epithelial cells, J. Cell Biol. 89:485-494 (1981).

8. I. H. Mather, and T. W. Keenan, Function of endomembranes and the cell surface in the secretion of organic milk constituents, in: "Biochemistry of Lactation," T. B. Mepham, ed., Elsevier/North Holland Biomedical Press, Amsterdam (1983).

9. M. B. Martel-Pradal, and R. Got, Presence d'enzymes marqueurs des membranes plasmiques, de l'appareil de golgi et du reticulum endoplasmique dans les membranes des globules lipidiques de lait maternel, FEBS Letters 21:220-222 (1972).

10. H. W. Heid, S. Winter, G. Bruder, T. W. Keenan, and E. D. Jarasch, Butyrophilin, an apical plasma membrane-associated glycoprotein characteristic of lactating mammary glands of diverse species. Biochim. Biophys. Acta 728:228-238 (1983).

11. E. D. Jarasch, C. Grund, G. Bruder, H. W. Heid, T. W. Keenan, and W. W. Franke, Localization of xanthine oxidase in mammary gland epithelium and capillary endothelium, Cell 25;67-82 (1981).

12. I. H. Mather, C. H. Sullivan, and P. J. Madara, Detection of xanthine oxidase and immunologically related proteins in fractions from bovine mammary tissue and milk after electrophoresis in polyacrylamide gels containing sodium dodecyl sulphate, Biochem. J. 202:317-323 (1982).

13. G. Bruder, H. Heid, E. D. Jarasch, T. W. Keenan, and I. H. Mather, Characteristics of membrane-bound and soluble forms of xanthine oxidase from milk and endothelial cells of capillaries, Biochim. Biophys. Acta 701:357-369 (1982).

14. A. Imam, C. R. Taylor, and Z. A. Tokes, Immunohistochemical study of the expression of human milk fat globule membrane glycoprotein 70, Cancer Res. 44:2016-2022 (1984).

15. D. Kobylka, and K. L. Carraway, Proteins and glycoproteins of the milk fat globule membrane, Biochim. Biophys. Acta 288:282-295 (1972).

16. M. B. Martel, P. Dubois, and R. Got, Membranes des globules lipidiques du lait humain. Preparation, etude morphologique et composition chimique, Biochim. Biophys. Acta 311:565-575 (1973).

17. M. Sasaki, J. A. Peterson, and R. L. Ceriani, Quantitation of human mammary epithelial antigens in cells cultured from normal and cancerous breast tissues, In Vitro 17:150-158 (1981).

18. U. K. Laemmli, Cleavage of structural proteins during the assembly of the head of bacteriophage T4, Nature (London) 227:680-682 (1970).

19. B. Bowen, J. Steinberg, U. K. Laemmli, and H. Weintraub, The detection of DNA-binding proteins by protein blotting, Nucl. Acids Res. 8:1-20 (1980).

20. K. Hancock, and V. C. W. Tsang, India ink staining of proteins on nitrocellulose paper, Anal. Biochem., 133:157-162 (1983).

21. A. Imam, D. J. R. Laurence, and A. M. Neville, Isolation and characterization of a major glycoprotein from milk-fat-globule membrane of human breast milk, Biochem. J. 193:47-54 (1981).

22. H. Towbin, T. Staehelin, and J. Gordon, Electrophoretic transfer of proteins from polyacrylamide gels to nitrocellulose sheets: Procedure and some applications, Proc. Nat. Acad. Sci. USA, 76:4350-4354 (1979).

23. M. P. Woodward, W. W. Young, and R. A. Bloodgood, Detection of monoclonal antibodies specific for carbohydrate epitopes using periodate oxidation. J. Immunol. Meth. 78:143-153 (1985).

24. M. Ishida, P. P. Major, and A. S. Dion, Characterization and purification of a cell surface glycoprotein from normal and malignant breast cells, Submitted for publication.

25. N. Sharon and H. Lis, Lectins: Cell-agglutinating and sugar-specific proteins, Science 177:949-959 (1972).

26. M.G. Omerod, K. Steele, J.H. Westwood and M.N. Mazzini, Epithelial membrane antigens: Partial purification, assay and properties. Brit. J. Cancer 48: 533-541 (1983).

27. S. Canevani, G. Fossati, A. Balsari, S. Sonnino, and M.I. Colnaghi, Immunochemical analysis of the determinant recognized by monoclonal antibody (MBrl) which specifically binds to human mammary epithelial cells. Cancer Res. 43: 1301-1305 (1983).

28. J. Hilkens, F. Buijs, J. Hilgers, P. Hageman, J. Calafat, A. Sonnenberg and M. vander Valk, Monoclonal antibodies against human milk-fat globule membranes detecting differentiation antigens of the mammary gland and its tumors. Int. J. Cancer 34: 197-206 (1984).

29. E. Heyderman, K. Steele and M.G. Ormerod, A new antigen on the epithelial membrane: Its immunoperoxidase localisation in normal and neoplastic tissues. J. Clin. Pathol. 32: 35-39 (1979).

30. J. Taylor-Papadimitriou, J.A. Peterson, J. Arklie, J. Burchell, R. L. Ceriani, and W. F. Bodmer, Monoclonal antibodies to epithelium-specific components of the human milk fat globule membrane: Production and reaction with cells in culture. Int. J. Cancer 28: 17-21 (1981).

31. J. Burchell, H. Durbin and J. Taylor-Papadimitriou, Complexity of expression of antigenic determinants, recognized by monoclonal antibodies HMFG-1 and HMFG-2, in normal and malignant human mammary epithelial cells. J. Immunol. 131: 508-513 (1983).

32. C.S. Foster, P.A.W. Edwards, E.A. Dinsdale and A.M. Neville, Monoclonal antibodies to the human mammary gland I. Distribution of determinants in non-neoplastic mammary and extra-mammary tissues. Virchows Arch. [Pathol. Anat.] 394: 279-293 (1982).

33. H.C. Gooi, K. Uemura, P.A.W. Edwards, C.S. Foster, N. Pickering and T. Feizi, Two mouse hybridoma antibodies against human milk-fat globules recognise the I(MA) antigenic determinants B-D-Galp-(1→4)-B-D-GlcpNAc-(1→6). Carbohyd. Res. 120: 293-302 (1983).

34. R.L. Ceriani, J.A. Peterson, J.Y. Lee, R. Moncada and E.W. Blank, Characterization of cell surface antigens of human mammary epithelial cells with monoclonal antibodies prepared against human milk fat globule. Somatic Cell Genetics 9:415-427 (1983).

35. D. Kufe, G. Inghirami, M. Abe, D. Hayes, H. Justi-Wheeler and J. Schlom, Differential reactivity of a novel monoclonal antibody (DF3) with human malignant versus benign breast tumors. Hybridoma 3: 223-232 (1984).

36. P. Ashorn and K. Krohn, Characterization and partial purification of human milk fat globule membranes by polyacrylamide gel electrophoresis and immunoblotting using monoclonal antibodies. Int. J. Cancer 35: 179-184 (1985).

37. H. Sekine, T. Ohno and D.W. Kufe, Purification and characterization of a high molecular weight glycoprotein detectable in human milk and breast carcinoma. J. Immunol. 135: 3610-3615 (1985).

38. P.A.W. Edwards, Heterogeneous expression of cell-surface antigens in normal epithelia and their tumors, revealed by monoclonal antibodies. Brit. J. Cancer, 51: 149-160 (1985).

39. M.G. Ormerod, P. Monaghan, D. Easty and G.C. Easty, Asymmetrical distribution of epithelial membrane antigen on the plasma membranes of human breast cell lines in culture. Diagn. Histopathol. 4: 89-93 (1981).

40. M. Abe and D.W. Kufe, Sodium butyrate induction of milk-related antigens in human MCF-7 breast carcinoma cells. Cancer Res. 44: 4574-4577 (1984).

41. N. Berry, D.B. Jones, J. Smallwood, I. Taylor, N. Kirkham, and J. Taylor-Papadimitriou, The prognostic value of the monoclonal antibodies HMFG1 and HMFG2 in breast cancer. Brit. J. Cancer 51: 179-186 (1985).

42. J. Burchell, D. Wang and J. Taylor-Papadimitriou, Detection of the tumour-associated antigens recognized by the monoclonal antibodies HMFG-1 and 2 in serum from patients with breast cancer. Int. J. Cancer 34: 763-768 (1984).

43. T. Feizi, Demonstration by monoclonal antibodies that carbohydrate structures of glycoproteins and glycolipids are onco-developmental antigens. Nature (London) 314: 53-57 (1985).

A MULTIPARAMETRIC STUDY BY MONOCLONAL ANTIBODIES IN BREAST CANCER

M.I. Colnaghi, S. Ménard, M.G. Da Dalt, R. Agresti,
G. Cattoretti, S. Andreola, G. Di Fronzo, M. Del Vecchio,
L. Verderio, N. Cascinelli and F. Rilke

Istituto Nazionale Tumori, Via Venezian 1, Milan, Italy

INTRODUCTION

Although the relative 5-year survival rate of breast cancer patients has improved over the past few years, the age-adjusted mortality rate has remained stationary because the age-adjusted incidence rate has increased. A local recurrence or the development of distant metastases after therapy is part of the natural course of the disease. Reliable factors capable of predicting which patients will develop metastatic cancer, and when, are not available yet. Clinical, pathological and biochemical studies contribute to the identification of a number of parameters which can help us predict early recurrences of the disease after radical surgery in women with operable disease. In fact, prognosis seems to be correlated, to a certain extent, with some of them, evaluated separately or in combination. The prognostic factors most commonly taken into consideration include the clinical stage, nodal status and hormone receptor levels (1,2). However, even well-established parameters are not entirely dependable.

For example, in clinically cured $T_1T_2N^-MO$ patients a relapse usually occurs in 25% of cases. As far as hormone receptors levels are concerned some studies report a significantly longer relapse-free interval in patients with estrogen-receptor-positive tumors in comparison to those with estrogen-receptor-negative ones (3,5), other studies show no differences at all (6,7), and still others only give evidence of some differences during the early months of follow-up (8,9). Contradictory results also came from studies on the relationship between progesterone-receptor (PgR) status and the relapse-free interval (9,10).

There are several factors which, other than their bearing on prognosis, are also important for a better understanding of the natural history of a tumor. For example, the nodal status and hormone receptor levels have a certain biological significance. The first seems to reflect the age of the disease from inception to the time of diagnosis (11), the second helps us deduce valuable information on the disease long after their first measurement in the primary tumor. In fact, the hormone receptor levels can inform us of the growth characteristics of the tumor and for this reason ER and PgR assays have now widely replaced clinical parameters for selective hormone therapy in patients with advanced breast cancer. Furthermore, they can supply us with information on the first possible sites of metastases: a patient with an ER positive tumor is more likely to develop bone metastases, whereas those with ER negative tumors tend to develop visceral metastases (12,13).

Breast cancers do differ, as far as their biological behaviour is concerned, and fundamental biological questions such as whether the disease in patients without relapse is different from the disease in patients which develop metastases and die, or whether early breast cancers are chronologically early or biologically indolent, still have no answer. It is therefore unlikely that a single therapy should be appropriate for tumors with different natures. Only a better knowledge of the behaviour of the individual tumor would allow improvement in therapy and may have a great impact on the ability to cure the disease.

Today there is still a great need to discover new reliable factors that can provide us with a better insight of the biology of tumors and help us identify different subgroups of patients which will undergo different courses of the disease and therefore require different kinds of treatment.

In this multiparametric study we evaluated the expression of antigenic determinants identified by some of the MoAbs we produced, on breast tumors in relation to different parameters known to have a certain predicting or biological significance, with the aim of finding new factors with high prognostic values and obtaining further biological information on breast carcinoma.

MATERIAL AND METHODS

Monoclonal antibodies

Monoclonal antibodies reacting with breast carcinomas, were obtained by fusing the murine myeloma P3 with spleen cells from mice immunized with cell membrane preparations from the human breast cancer cell line MCF-7 or from surgical specimens of epithelial tumors (14-18).

Tissue specimens

The prospective study was carried out on frozen sections from surgical specimens. Immunologic tests and DNA content evaluation for each single case were carried out on serial sections of the same surgical specimen.

The retrospective study was carried out on histological sections of mammary tumors from 40 specifically selected patients in follow-up from 5 to 12 years.

Immunologic tests

Immunoperoxidase (IPX) and immunofluorescence (I.F.) tests with MoAbs MBr1, MOv2, MBr8, MOv16 were carried out as previously described (14,17,19,20). The ER-ICA test was carried out by indirect IPX staining with the commercially available anti-ER rat MoAb (Abbot, U.S.A.). Epidermal growth factor and transferrin receptor (EGF-R, Trf-R) evaluations were done by indirect IPX staining respectively with the MoAb R1 kindly provided by Dr. M. Waterfield (ICRF London) and the commercially available anti Trf-R MoAb (Becton Dickinson, U.S.A.). The evaluation of p21 and p53 expression was carried out by indirect IPX staining respectively with the commercially available MoAbs v-H-ras Ab1 and Ab2 (Oncogene Science, Inc. U.S.A.) and the MoAb PAB421 kindly provided by Dr. M. Crawford (ICRF London).

In all of the cases a tumor was considered positive when at least 10% of the cells stained positively.

Hormone receptor and DNA content assays

The hormone receptor levels (DCC method) were evaluated as previously described (21). The DNA content was evaluated essentially according to the method described by Vindelov et al. (22).

Statistical methods

Associations between antigen expression and each prognostic factor were investigated by means of the CHI-SQUARE tests in contingency tables. Survival curves were drawn according to the Kaplan-Meier method (1958). By convention, $p < 0.05$ was taken to be significant.

RESULTS AND DISCUSSION

Table 1 summarizes the multiparametric prospective study in progress at the Istituto Nazionale Tumori, Milan. A series including 14 different monoclonal antibodies raised in our laboratory and reacting with breast tumors were chosen to be tested on 191 cases of ductal and lobular infiltrating primary carcinomas of the breast and their reactivity will be correlated with some of the many factors proven or suggested to have some prognostic value.

Table 1. A multiparametric study

14 MoAbs produced at the Istituto Nazionale Tumori, Milan, tested on 191 cases of ductal and lobular primary breast carcinoma

Reactivity investigated in relation to:

Tumor size (86% $<$2.5cm)	Estrogen receptor
Tumor margin (61% infiltrating)	DCC-method (81% pos.)
Lymphnode involvement (59% N^-)	ER-ICA method (78% pos.)
Grade (8%I; 49%II; 43%III)	Progesterone-receptor (71% pos.)
Kinetic index (77% $<$2.8)	EGF-R (38% pos.)
Menopausal status (39% pre)	Trf-R (73% pos.)
p53 expression (16% pos.)	DNA content (39% diploid)
p21 expression (75% pos.)	Disease progression

In this paper we report some preliminary results which refer to 4 MoAbs, namely MBr1, MBr8, MOv2 and MOv16, whose characteristics are listed in Table 2.

Table 2. Description of MoAbs used in the multiparametric study

MoAb	Immunogen	MoAb Isotype	Ag recognized
MBr1	cell membrane preparation from the MCF-7 cell line	IgM	polysaccharide epitope on a glycolipid, glycoproteins, mucins
MBr8	cell membrane preparation from a breast carcinoma surgical specimen	IgM	unknown
MOv2	cell membrane preparation from an ovarian carcinoma surgical specimen	IgM	polysaccharide epitope on a glycolipid, glycoproteins, mucins
MOv16	cell membrane preparation from an ovarian carcinoma surgical specimen	IgG1	glycoprotein

Table 3 summarizes information regarding the expression of CaMBr1 on breast epithelial cells. According to its distribution it seems to be an antigen related to a functional status: it is, in fact, strongly expressed on normal breast epithelium during the second part of the proliferative phase and the first part of the secretory phase of the menstrual cycle, i.e. from the 8th to the 22nd day. During this period, following the resting status, under hormonal stimulus the breast gland shows a progressive increase of cytoplasmic vacuoles and mitoses (23).

Table 3. Expression of CaMBr1 on breast epithelial cells

Antigen associated with the proliferating and secreting activity of the human mammary gland	
High expression on:	Normal breast epithelial cells during the proliferative and secretory phase of the menstrual cycle (from 8th to the 22nd day)
	Breast glands during pregnancy and lactating mammary glands.

MOv2, MBr8 and MOv16 MoAbs react on normal breast epithelial cells, on the breast glands during pregnancy, on lactating mammary glands and on benign tumors; as regards their relationship with the menstrual cycle, CaMOv2 expression is independent, whereas CaMBr8 and CaMOv16 have not yet been analyzed.

Previously reported data (14,17,19,24) regarding the heterogeneous expression of CaMBr1, CaMOv2, CaMBr8 and CaMOv16 on breast carcinomas are summarized in Table 4 which shows that none of the 4 MoAbs were able to react with the totality of the tumors of a given oncotype. They were therefore considered suitable for an analysis regarding their predicting potential.

Table 4. Expression of CaMBr1, CaMBr8, CaMOv2, and CaMOv16 on breast cancer

Oncotype	Percentage of positivity			
	CaMBr1	CaMBr8	CaMOv2	CaMOv16
Ductal	80	70	52	61
Lobular	78	75	65	75
Mixed	86	77	57	50
Others	56	23	44	31

In Figures 1 and 2 is reported the relationship between the reactivity of each single MoAb and the tumor grade, and, among the factors listed in Table 1, only those which resulted significantly correlated according to the statistical analysis.

Tumors expressing CaMBr1 included a statistically significant higher percentage of ER-ICA and Trf-R positive tumors and of tumors from patients in premenopausal status when compared with those which were MBr1 negative. Moreover, almost all the well differentiated carcinomas (grade I) were MBr1 positive (Fig. 1A).

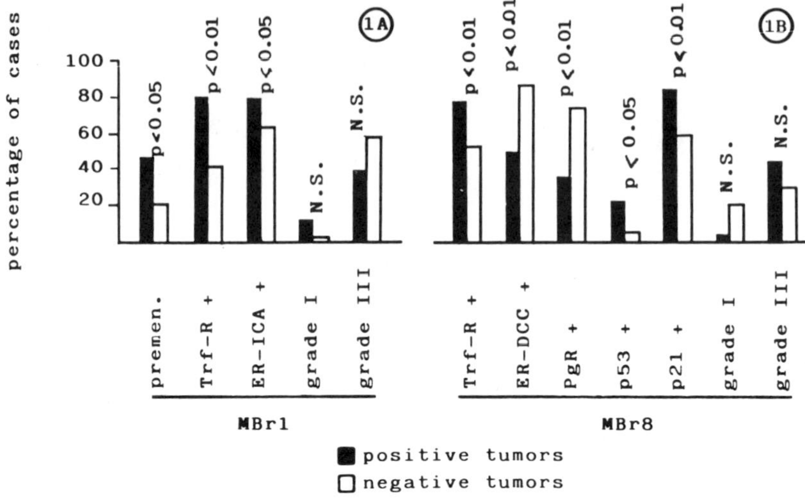

Fig. 1. Relationship of MBr1 and MBr8 reactivities with various parameters. Among tumors MBr1 or MBr8 positive (closed bars) or negative (open bars) the bars represent the percentage of tumors showing the parameter reported below (premen., Trf-R positivity, etc.)

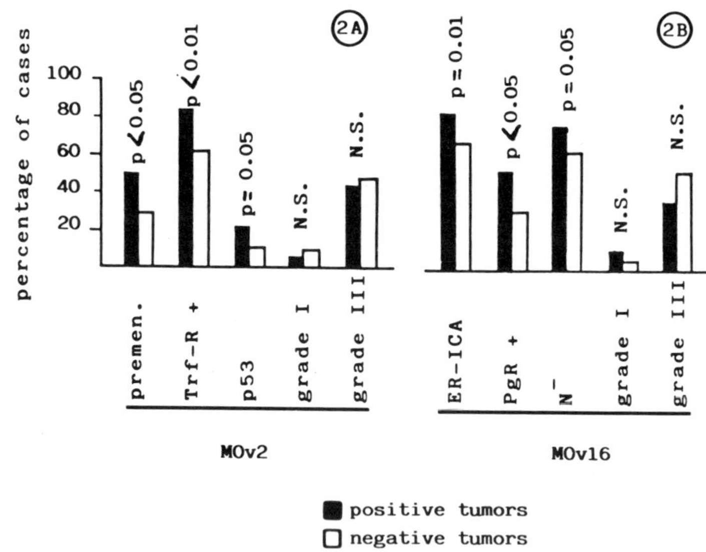

Fig. 2. Relationship of MOv2 and MOv16 reactivities with various parameters. Among tumors MOv2 or MOv16 positive (closed bars) or negative (open bars) the bars represent the percentage of tumors showing the parameter reported below (premen., Trf-R positivity, etc.)

MBr8 reactivity was significantly stronger on Trf-R, p53 and p21 positive tumors, and significantly lower in ER (DCC evaluation) and PgR positive tumors in comparison to the negative ones. As far as grade is concerned, no significant difference was observed, but there seemed to be a tendency towards a lower expression in grade I tumors (Fig. 1B).

CaMOv2 became significantly prominent, in tumors from premenopause patients and in Trf-R and p53 positive tumors (Fig. 2A).

ER (ER-ICA evaluation) and PgR positive tumors, as well as tumors from node negative patients, expressed a significantly higher level of CaMOv16 in comparison to hormone negative tumors or tumors from node positive patients. Finally, as in the case of MBr1, CaMOv16 showed a tendency towards higher expression in grade I tumors (Fig. 2B).

Table 5. Retrospective study on 40 breast cancer patients in premenopausal status treated, after relapse, with oophorectomy

Analyzed parameters	20 patients with a 100% survival after 5 years (Median survival time of patients dead after relapse: 7 years)		20 patients with a 0% survival after 5 years (Median survival time of patients dead after relapse: 2.5 years)	
Stage	No.	%	No.	%
I	1/20	5	1/20	5
II	10/20	50	12/20	60
IIIa	5/20	25	3/20	15
IIIb	3/20	15	3/20	15
IV				
X	1/20	5	1/20	5
ER (DCC)				
(+)	9/20	45	8/20	40
(+/-)	3/20	15	4/20	20
(-)	0/20	-	2/20	10
(N.D.)	8/20	40	6/20	30
Nodal status				
(+)	14/20	70	16/20	80
(-)	6/20	30	4/20	20

In brief, the expression of the determinant defined by the MBr1 MoAb seems to be associated with functional changes in the breast gland related to hormonal stimuli, CaMOv16 appears to be related to a pattern of differentiation, whereas CaMOv2 and CaMBr8 tend to be present in less differentiated tumors in which the hormonal regulatory function seems to be bypassed or integrated by other factors such as transferrin or oncogene-related products. Only the results of the follow-up now in progress will clarify the meaning of these results. However, 3 of our reagents (MBr1, MBr8 and MOv2), due to their persistent reactivity on paraffin sections, were analyzed in a retrospective study which revealed a predicting capability for two of them and suggested interesting biological implications. Table 5 summarizes some information on the 40 selected patients in follow-up from 5 to 12 years who entered the retrospective study and on their tumors on which the three reagents were tested. MBr1 gave 43% positivity, MBr8 59% and MOv2 54%. Patients were divided into two groups according to their survival evaluated 5 years after diagnosis (100% versus 0%) and the median survival rate of those dead after relapse (7 years versus 2.5 years). Known prognostic factors such as clinical stage, hormone receptor levels and nodal status did not help to identify the population with a poor prognosis; in fact the percentages referring to the various parameters were almost identical in both groups (Table 5) due to the adopted selective criteria.

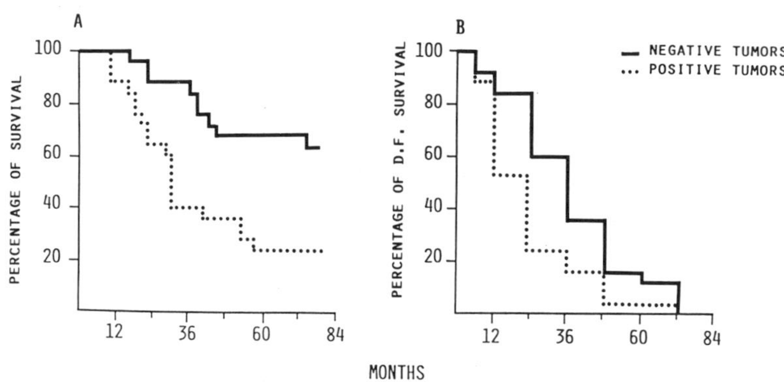

Fig. 3. Relationship of CaMBr1 expression with survival (A) and disease free survival (B).

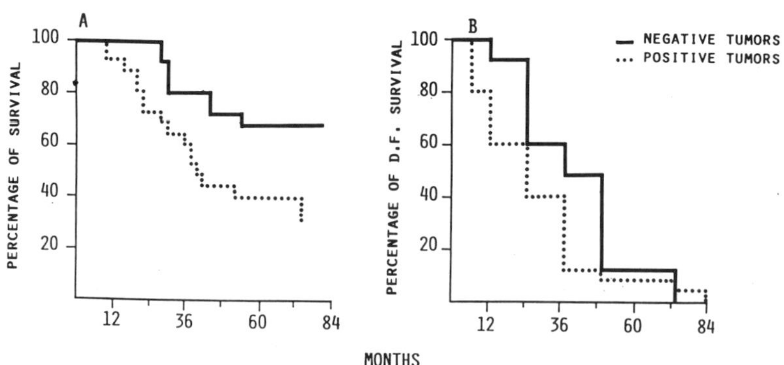

Fig. 4. Relationship of CaMBr8 expression with survival (A) and disease free survival (B).

As reported in Figures 3 and 4, the survival was associated with the expression of CaMBr1 and CaMBr8, whereas no relationship was found with MOv2 (Fig. 5). Despite the small case material the results were statistically significant ($p < 0.006$) in the case of MBr1.

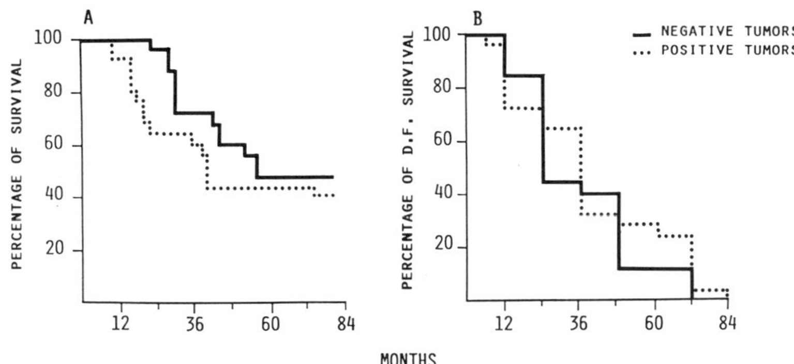

Fig. 5. Relationship of CaMOv2 expression with survival (A) and disease free survival (B).

When MBr1 and MBr8 which gave evidence of a correlation with a poor prognosis were evaluated together, i.e. the survival of 10 patients with MBr1 and MBr8 positive tumors was compared to the survival of 10 patients with MBr1 and MBr8 negative tumors, the difference after 10 years was even stronger: a 20 versus about 80% survival rate (Fig 6).

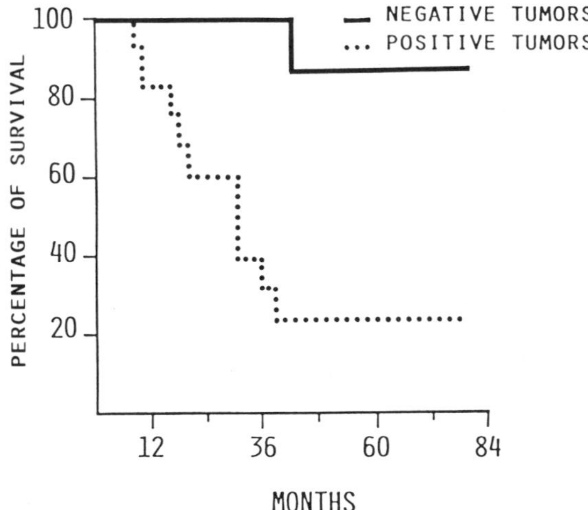

Fig. 6. Relationship of MBr1 + MBr8 expression with survival

It therefore seems that two of the three reagents tested in the retrospective study have a strong predicting capability even in those cases where already validated prognostic factors failed; however these data need to be confirmed by the results of the wider prospective study. With reference to the other reagent, MOv16, which correlates with known prognostic indicators such as node status and hormone levels, unfortunately it could not be tested retrospectively and we must therefore wait for the results of the follow-up of the prospective study to establish its predicting value.

From our study we can also deduce some interesting biological speculations which however still require further clarification. For example, with reference to the MBr1 receptor, which is strongly associated with a poor prognosis and whose expression fluctuates in relation to the menstrual cycle, we found that it may be expressed in different molecular forms according to various functional situations. In fact, CaMBr1 was only found on glycoproteins in the resting glands in postmenopausal status; whereas in tumors, in the breast during pregnancy and in lactating mammary glands it was also associated with glycolipids (data not shown). It has been reported that membrane glycolipids have an important role in the maturation (25) or regulation (26) of cell growth factor receptors. In keeping with this finding we found that CaMBr1 and Trf-R expressions were strongly associated on tumors and now further studies are in progress in order to elucidate the meaning of this association.

A clearer understanding of the MBr1 receptor influence on some important functions of the cell life and of its interference in proliferative processes could help us reach a better understanding of the biology of breast cancer.

REFERENCES

1. B. Salvadori, M. Greco, C. Clemente, R. De Lellis, V. Delledonne, D. Galluzzo, P. Piotti, V. Sacchini, R. Bufalino, E. Marubini, A. Morabito and N. Cascinelli: Prognostic factors in operable breast cancer. Tumori 69: 477 (1983).
2. R. W. Blamey, C.W. Elston, J.L. Haybittle and K. Griffiths, Prognosis in breast cancer: The Nottingham-Tenovus Trial, in: "Commentaries on research in breast disease". R.D. Bulbrook, D.J. Tailor, Eds., Alan R. Liss, New York (1983).
3. M. A. Rich, P. Furmanski and S.C. Brooks: Prognostic value of estrogen receptor determinations in patients with breast cancer. Cancer Res. 38: 4296 (1978).
4. T. Cooke, W.D. George, R. Shields, P. Maynard and K. Griffiths: Oestrogen receptors and prognosis in breast cancer. Lancet i: 995 (1979).

5. H. Westerberg, S.A. Gustafsson, B. Nordenskjold, C. Silfversward and A. Wallgren: Oestrogen receptor level and other factors in early recurrence of breast cancer. Int. J. Cancer 26: 429 (1980).

6. A. Howell, D.M. Barnes, R.N.L. Harland, J. Redford, V.H.C. Bramwell, M.J.S. Wilkinson, R. Swindell, D. Crowther and R.A. Sellwood: Steroid-hormone receptors and survival after first relapse in breast cancer. Lancet i: 588 (1984).

7. B. H. Mason, I.M. Holdaway, P.R. Mullins, L.H. Yee and R.G. Kay: Progesterone and estrogen receptors as prognostic variables in breast cancer. Cancer Res. 43: 2985 (1983).

8. R. Hahnel, T. Woodings and A.B. Vivian: Prognostic value of estrogen receptors in primary breast cancer. Cancer 44: 671 (1979).

9. J. M.T. Howat, D.M. Barnes, M. Harris, and R. Swindell: The association of cytosol oestrogen and progesterone receptors with histological features of breast cancer and early recurrence of disease. Br. J. Cancer 43: 629 (1983).

10. M. F. Pichon, C. Pallud, M. Brunet and E. Milgron: Relationship of presence of progesterone receptors to prognosis in early breast cancer. Cancer Res. 40: 3357 (1980).

11. A. H.G. Paterson, V.P. Zuck, O. Szafran, A.W. Lees and J. Hanson: Influence and significance of certain prognostic factors on survival in breast cancer. Eur. J. Cancer Clin. Oncol. 18: 937 (1982).

12. J. F. Stewart, R.J.B. King, S.A. Sexton, R.R. Millis, R.D. Rubens and J.L. Hayward: Oestrogen receptors, sites of metastatic disease and survival in recurrent breast cancer. Eur. J. Cancer 17: 449 (1981).

13. F. C. Campbell, R.W. Blamey, C.W. Elston, R.I. Nicholson, K. Griffiths and J.L. Haybittle: Oestrogen-receptor status and sites of metastasis in breast cancer. Br. J. Cancer 44: 456 (1981).

14. S. Ménard, E. Tagliabue, S. Canevari, G. Fossati and M.I. Colnaghi: Generation of monoclonal antibodies reacting with normal and cancer cells of human breast. Cancer Res. 43: 1295 (1983).

15. S. Canevari, G. Fossati, A. Balsari, S. Sonnino and M.I. Colnaghi: Immunochemical analysis of the determinant recognized by a monoclonal antibody (MBr1) which specifically binds to human mammary epithelial cells. Cancer Res. 43: 1301 (1983).

16. E. G. Bremer, S.B. Levery, S. Sonnino, R. Ghidoni, S. Canevari, R. Kannagi and S.I. Hakomori: Characterization of a glycolipid antigen defined by the monoclonal antibody MBr1 expressed in normal and neoplastic epithelial cells of human mammary gland. J. of Biological Chemistry 23: 14773 (1984).

17. E. Tagliabue, S. Ménard, G. Della Torre, P. Barbanti, R. Mariani-Costantini, G. Porro and M.I. Colnaghi: Generation of monoclonal antibodies reacting with human epithelial ovarian cancer. Cancer Res. 45: 379 (1985).

18. S. Miotti, S. Aguanno, S. Canevari, A. Diotti, R. Orlandi, S. Sonnino and M.I. Colnaghi: Biochemical analysis of human ovarian cancer-associated antigens defined by murine monoclonal antibodies. Cancer Res. 45: 826 (1985).
19. R. Mariani-Costantini, M.I. Colnaghi, F. Leoni, S. Ménard, S. Cerasoli and F. Rilke: Immunohistochemical reactivities of a monoclonal antibody prepared against human breast carcinoma. Virchows Archiv. A. Pathol. Anat. 402: 389 (1984).
20. R. Mariani-Costantini, P. Barbanti, M.I. Colnaghi, S. Ménard, C. Clemente and F. Rilke: Reactivity of a monoclonal antibody with tissues and tumors from the human breast: Immunohistochemical localization of a new antigen and clinico-pathologic correlations. Am. J. Pathol. 115: 47 (1984).
21. G. Di Fronzo, C. Clemente, V. Cappelletti, P. Miodini, D. Coradini, E. Ronchi, S. Andreola and F. Rilke: Relationship between ER-ICA and conventional steroid receptor assays in human breast cancer. Breast cancer research and treatment, in press (1986).
22. L. L. Vindeløv, Ib.J. Christensen and Nis.I. Nissen: A detergent-Trypsin method for the preparation of nuclei for Flow cytometric DNA analysis. Cytometry 3 (5): 323 (1983).
23. T .A. Longacre and S.A. Bartow: A correlative morphologic study of human breast and endometrium in the menstrual cycle. The American J. of Surgical Pathol. 10(6): 382 (1986).
24. E. Tagliabue, G. Porro, P. Barbanti, G. Della Torre, S. Ménard, F. Rilke, M.I. Colnaghi: Improvement of tumor cell detection using a pool of monoclonal antibodies. Hybridoma 5: 107 (1986).
25. M. B. Omary and I.S. Trowbridge: Biosynthesis of the human Transferrin receptor in cultured cells. J. Biol. Chem. 256: 12888 (1981).
26. E. G. Bremer, J.Schlessinger and S. Hakomori: Ganglioside mediated modulation of cell growth. Specific effects of G_{M3} on Thyrosine phosphorylation of the epidermal growth factor receptor. J. Biol. Chem. 261: 2434 (1986).

MOLECULAR AND IMMUNOLOGICAL ANALYSIS OF MUCIN MOLECULES PRODUCED BY NORMAL AND MALIGNANT HUMAN MAMMARY EPITHELIAL CELLS

Sandra Gendler, Joy Burchell, Andrew B. Griffiths
and Joyce Taylor-Papadimitriou

Imperial Cancer Research Fund
P O Box 123, Lincoln's Inn Fields
London WC2A 3PX, U.K.

INTRODUCTION

The mammary gland is a complex tissue containing several lineages, including the luminal or secretory epithelial cells and the basal or myoepithelial cells which line the ducts and alveoli. These two cell types can be distinguished in tissue sections by immunohistochemical staining with monoclonal antibodies to structural components and to functional products characteristic of each cell type. Such studies have focused attention on the luminal or secretory epithelial cell lineage, since the dominant cell in breast cancers expresses both the simple epithelial keratins and the mucin molecules expressed by the luminal epithelial cells in the normal gland[1]. In these particulars the breast cancer cell resembles other adenocarcinomas, such as those from the colon, lung and ovary.

A large number of antibodies have been developed which react with the mucins expressed by normal and malignant mammary epithelial cells[2], and some of these antibodies are being used in the clinic in the diagnosis and treatment of cancer. Few of the epitopes recognized by these antibodies have been identified, and many are characterized only by their spectrum of reactivity with normal tissues and with tumours. Even using these ill-defined reagents, however, it is becoming clear that the mucins are expressed in a complex fashion[3] and that there is a need to find approaches to analyze these molecules at the structural level.

THE MILK OR MAMMARY MUCIN

Mucins are characterised as large glycoproteins, containing 50-60% carbohydrate in which the sugar side chains are O-linked to serines and threonines through the sugar N-acetyl-galactosamine. A component with these characteristics is present in milk and the MFG and has been purified by Shimizu and Yamauchi, and termed PAS-O[4]. Other workers have called this component NPGP[5] or EMA[6]. Using an antibody affinity column we have purified the material carrying the HMFG-1 epitope from human milk. On Western blots the component shows a diffuse band of high molecular weight (>400K) which is reactive with both the HMFG-1 and HMFG-2 antibodies[3]. Using a silver stain for glycoproteins other bands are apparent in the purified preparations, including a glycoprotein of MW 68kd, but these can be selectively removed by size exclusion chromatography to give a pure preparation of the high molecular weight material. The purified component is rich in glycine, serine and proline and shows an amino acid composition similar to the material biochemically purified by Shimizu and Yamauchi[7]. This component we have called the milk or mammary mucin.

Glycoproteins Immunologically Related to the Milk Mucin Expressed by Breast Cancers

When antibodies reactive with the milk mucin are used to detect components produced by breast cancer cells on Western blots, more than one band is generally observed and the mobility of these bands in acrylamide gels is faster than that of the milk mucin. There is also individual variability in the apparent molecular weight of the components between different tumours and cell lines. Figure 1 shows the reactivity of a series of antibodies with gel separated extracts of MCF-7 cells on a Western blot. All the antibodies appear to be recognising the same 2 bands of molecular weight 320kd and 430kd. If other cell lines are used these high molecular weight bands show differing mobilities and certain antibodies, such as HMFG-2 and M8, can detect lower molecular weight components[2]. Recently, a mucin has been identified in urine which carries the epitopes defined by HMFG-1 and HMFG-2 and a number of other tumour associated antigens recognised by monoclonal antibodies[8]. This urinary mucin was originally identified by its lectin binding ability and shows a genetic polymorphism which is inherited in a Mendelian fashion[9]. Immunoblotting analysis using HMFG-1 and HMFG-2 to probe tumour and urine samples from the same individual indicates that the heterogeneity observed among tumours in the high molecular weight components is due to this genetic polymorphism (MS in preparation). However, this does not explain the presence of lower molecular weight bands observed in some tumours which may reflect abortive processing of the mucin. Such abortive processing is indicated by the observation that HMFG-2 reactive components accumulate in the Golgi of certain breast cancer cell lines[2]. A difference in the processing of the mucin in the lactating mammary gland may also explain the apparent higher molecular weight (low mobility in gels) of the component produced *in vivo* by the fully differentiated secretory cell.

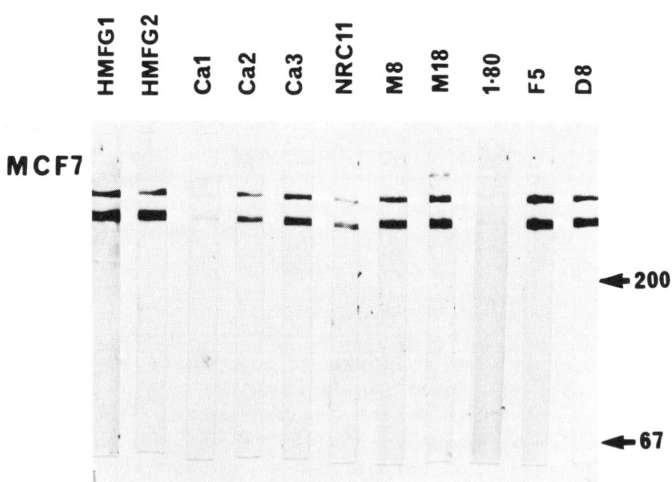

Fig. 1. Immunoblot of MCF-7 whole cell lysates with various monoclonal antibodies. Cell lysate from MCF-7 cells was separated on SDS acrylamide gels, transferred to nitrocellulose paper and incubated with the antibodies indicated in the figure and described in reference 2.

Purification of HMFG-2 Reactive Material from Breast Cancer Cell Lines

Although it is assumed that the components expressed by breast cancer cells which are immunologically related to the milk mucin are coded for by the same gene(s) as that coding for the mucin, this has not been formally proven. In an attempt to obtain material for amino acid analysis, we purified the antigen carrying component from T47D and MCF-7 cells using an HMFG-2 affinity column. Although the material obtained was not in fact sufficient for accurate analysis, an interesting observation was made. Thus while immunoblotting of the purified material with HMFG-2 showed only high molecular weight bands, a periodic acid silver stain demonstrated the presence of a glycoprotein of similar molecular weight (68kd) to that which co-purified with the milk mucin. It is still not clear whether this glycoprotein is a subunit of the mucin or an unrelated artefact. It is however immunologically related to the high MW component since monoclonal antibodies raised against the HMFG-2 purified material show a reactivity with both components[2].

Another approach to obtaining structural information about the core protein of the putative mucins expressed by breast cancer cells is to select for cDNAs coding for the protein from a library made from a breast cancer cell line. We have taken this approach and our strategy has been to use antibodies developed against the core protein of the milk mucin to select clones from a λ gt11 expression library prepared from mRNA of MCF-7 cells.

Stripping of the Milk Mucin and Preparation of Antibodies to the Core Protein

Because the carbohydrate in the milk mucin is attached by O-linkage to serines and threonines and forms more than 50% of the content of the molecule, it is not possible to remove it with enzymes or mild chemical procedures. Deglycosylation was accomplished however by treating the mucin with hydrogen fluoride for 3 hours at room temperature (carried out by D. Lamport, Michigan State University). A partially stripped preparation was also obtained by treating the purified material with HF for 1 hour at 4°C. That the mucin was totally stripped of carbohydrate by the three hour treatment was confirmed by the lack of reactivity of the product with lectins including Helix pomatia aglutinin (HPA), a lectin that specifically binds to the linkage sugar N-acetylgalactosamine. The partially stripped material showed an increased reactivity with HPA and decreased reactivity with peanut aglutinin indicating that the peripheral oligosaccharides had been removed. The iodination of stripped material followed by gel electrophoresis and autoradiography showed that while the partially stripped material was of high molecular weight, the totally stripped material contained a major band around 68kd and a minor one at 72kd. Amino acid analysis of this material showed it to be the same as that of the unstripped mucin[7].

The two preparations of partially and totally stripped mucin were used to prepare polyclonal and monoclonal antibodies. Monoclonal antibodies were selected by their reaction with the stripped material and two which were unreactive with the unstripped mucin but strongly reactive with both the totally and partially stripped material were chosen for use in screening plaques from a λgt11 cDNA expression library constructed from MCF-7 cells[10].

Selection and Characterisation of Partial cDNA Clones Coding for the Core Protein of the Mammary Mucin Gene

Using first the polyclonal antiserum to the stripped milk mucin followed by screens with the monoclonal antibodies which were selected as described above, seven cross-reactive clones were selected from the library, the largest being 1.8kb[11]. This cDNA recloned into pUC8 has been termed pMUC10 and used in Southern blots of restriction enzyme digests of DNA from different individuals. The results show that there appears to be one gene which exhibits extensive restriction fragment length polymorphisms (figure 2). Northern blots (carried out under conditions of high stringency) of RNA from breast cancer cell lines, normal breast tissue and cultured cells from milk show that hybridizing messages around 4.7kb and 6.4kb are expressed in all these breast epithelial cells. Figure 3 shows a Northern blot of breast cancer cell lines probed with pMUC10. No mucin-related message was detectable in fibroblasts or the non-epithelial breast cancer cell line Hs578T. The polymorphism and tissue specific expression of the gene are in agreement with the observations made at the glycoprotein level, and support the idea that we have indeed isolated a cDNA corresponding to part of the gene coding for the mammary mucin as expressed in MCF-7 cells. The fact that the antibodies used to select the cDNA were raised against the core protein of the milk mucin also indicates that the core proteins of the molecules expressed by normal and malignant breast epithelial cells are immunologically related.

Reaction of antibodies to the core protein with breast tissues and tumours

One of the antibodies (SM-3) which was developed against the core protein and used in the above cloning studies has been found to react with sections of breast cancers in an immunohistochemical staining technique, and initial studies with normal breast tissues and benign tumours indicate that the reaction with breast cancers is highly specific. Results obtained so far show a negative or weak focal reaction with normal resting, pregnant and lactating breast and most benign tumours. Of the latter the papillomas showed the most reactivity, which was still weak and heterogenous compared to the strong reaction shown by this antibody on 20 out of 22 breast carcinomas.

The determinant recognised by the antibody is destroyed by formalin fixation, although it is resistant to fixation in methacarn; the results illustrated in Figure 4 were therefore obtained using methacarn fixed, paraffin embedded tissues. For comparison the reaction of the antibody HMFG-2 was also examined on the same tissues using identical fixation procedures. This antibody is widely used in cancer diagnosis and had previously been thought to be preferentially expressed by breast cancers as compared to normal breast tissue and benign breast tumours. However, the studies leading to this conclusion had been done using formalin fixed tissues and tumours. A reexamination of the reaction of HMFG-2 with methacarn fixed material showed that in most benign tumours, around 60% of normal lobules in the resting breast and all of the epithelial structures in the pregnant and lactating breast gave a positive reaction with this antibody. Similarly, the range of normal tissues giving a positive reaction with HMFG-2 was also increased using methacarn fixed material. A reaction with antibody SM-3, however, was only detectable (and then as a weak focal stain) in salivary gland and sebaceous gland and in the distal kidney tubules. Figure 4 illustrates some of the staining patterns seen with the antibody SM-3 as compared with the antibody HMFG-2.

The lack of reaction of the SM-3 antibody directed to the core protein of the mammary mucin with most normal tissues, together with its consistent

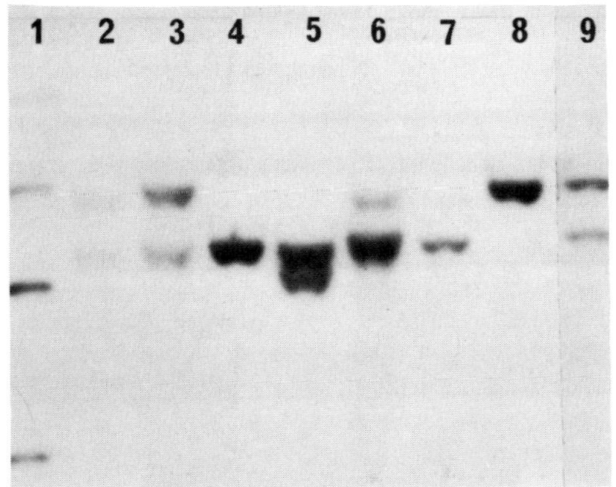

Fig. 2. Polymorphic human DNA fragments detected by hybridization with pMUC10 probe. Genomic DNA samples prepared from the white blood cells from 4 individuals (tracks 2-5) and from 4 cell lines (track 6 = ZR-75-1, 7 = BT20, 8 = fibroblasts, 9 = MCF-7) were digested to completion with EcoRI, fractionated by electrophoresis through 0.6% agarose and transferred to Biodyne nylon membrane. The filter was hybridized to the pMUC10 DNA insert which was labelled with [α-^{32}P]dCTP by the method of random priming. Track 1 is DNA of 1353, 1078, 872, 603bps.

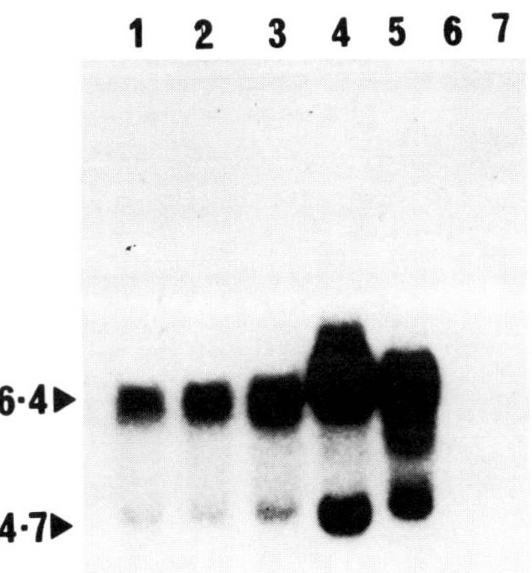

Fig. 3. Northern blot hybridization analysis of mammary breast mucin mRNA. 10μg of total RNA from MCF-7 cells (tracks 1,2,3, three preparations), T47D cells (track 4), normal mammary epithelial cells from human milk (track 5), fibroblasts (track 6) and the carcinosarcoma cell line Hs578T (track 7) were separated in a 1.3% agarose/glyoxal gel, blotted onto nitrocellulose paper and hybridized to the pMUC10 EcoRI insert labelled with ^{32}PdCTP.

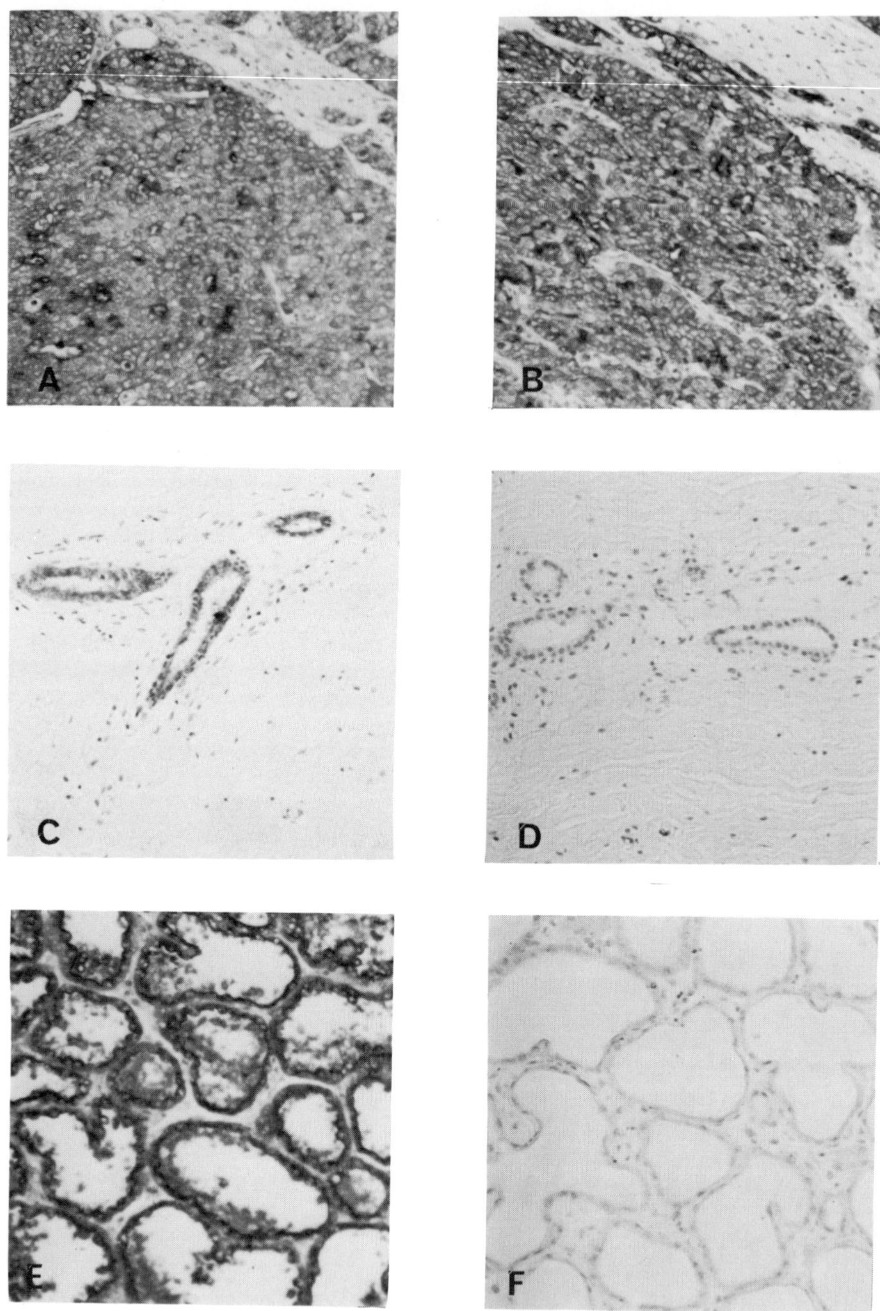

Fig. 4. Indirect immunoperoxidase staining of mammary tissue. Methacarn fixed sections of breast carcinoma (A,B), normal resting (C,D) and lactating breast (E,F) were reacted with the monoclonal antibodies HMFG-2 (A,C,E) and SM-3 (B,D,F) and the binding visualized by incubating with peroxidase conjugated rabbit anti-mouse followed by the substrate.

reaction with breast cancers (>90%) suggest that this antibody could be an extremely important tool in the diagnosis and therapy of breast cancer. Moreover, since SM-3 is directed to the milk mucin core protein and reacts with breast cancers but not with normal breast tissues the reactive epitope must be masked in normal tissue, but not in cancer tissue. This suggests that the mucin molecule is underglycosylated in most breast cancers.

COMMENTS

Many of the tumour associated determinants defined by monoclonal antibodies have been found to be carried on epithelial mucins. Much of the work relating to these molecules and the characterisation of epitopes on them has been concerned with the carbohydrate component. A different spectrum of carbohydrate epitopes appear to be present on mucins expressed by different epithelial tissues and the carcinomas derived from them, and it has also been suggested that tissues and carcinomas may be classifiable by the detailed structure of the oligosaccharide component of the mucin they express. In contrast to the work emphasizing the carbohydrate component, we have begun to study the core protein of the mammary mucin and to develop antibodies to this portion of the molecule. Our results suggest that the core protein of the mammary mucin is coded for by one polymorphic gene, indicating that the core protein for other tissue mucins is either identical to that of the milk mucin or coded for by genes which do not cross-hybridize. Cloning of genes from libraries prepared from epithelial tissues other than breast should resolve this question.

A dramatic observation with far reaching implications coming from these studies is that epitopes on the core protein normally masked in non-malignant breast tissues are exposed in a high proportion of breast cancers. It will be of interest to see whether underglycosylation of mucins is a general feature of carcinomas, and whether this reflects a general defect in glycosylation of proteins in these cells.

REFERENCES

1. J. Taylor-Papadimitriou, E.B. Lane and S.E. Chang, Cell lineages and interactions in neoplastic expression in the human breast, in: "Understanding Breast Cancer: Clinical and Laboratory Concepts", M. Rich, J.C. Hager and P. Furmanski, eds., Marcel Dekker Inc., New York, p. 215 (1983).
2. A. B. Griffiths, J. Burchell, J. Taylor-Papadimitriou, S. Gendler, A. Lewis, K. Blight and R. Tilly, Immunological analysis of mucin molecules expressed by normal and malignant mammary epithelial cells, Int. J. Cancer (submitted).
3. J. Burchell, H. Durbin and J. Taylor-Papadimitriou, Complexity of expression of antigenic determinants recognised by monoclonal antibodies HMFG-1 and HMFG-2, in normal and malignant human mammary epithelial cells, J. Immunol. 131:508 (1983).
4. M. Shimizu and K. Yamauchi, Isolation and characterisation of mucin-like glycoproteins in human milk fat globule membranes. J. Biochem. 91:515 (1982).
5. R. L. Ceriani, J. A. Peterson, J. Y. Lee, R. Moncada and E. W. Blank, Characterisation of cell surface antigens of human mammary epithelial cells with monoclonal antibodies prepared against human milk fat globule, Som. Cell Genet. 9:415 (1983).
6. M. G. Ormerod, K. Steele, J. M. Westwood and M. Mazzin, Epithelial Membrane Antigen: partial purification assay and properties, Br. J. Cancer 48:533 (1983).
7. J. Burchell, S. Gendler, J. Taylor-Papadimitriou, A. Girling, A. Lewis, R. Millis and D. Lamport, Monoclonal antibodies to the

core protein of the mucin found in human milk show improved tumour specificity, Cancer Res. (submitted).

8. D. Swallow, B. Griffiths, M. Bramwell, G. Wiseman and J. Burchell, Detection of the urinary "PUM" polymorphism by the tumour-binding monoclonal antibodies Ca1, Ca2, Ca3, HMFG-1 and HMFG-2, Disease Markers (in press).
9. S. Karlsson, D. M. Swallow, B. Griffiths, G. Corney and D.A. Hopkinson, A genetic polymorphism of a human urinary mucin, Ann. Hum. Genet. 47:263 (1983).
10. P. Walter, S. Green, G., Greene, A. Krust, J.-M. Bornert, J.-M. Heltsch, A. Staub, E. Jensen, G. Scrace, M. Waterfield and P. Chambon, Cloning of the human estrogen receptor cDNA. Proc. Natl. Acad. Sci. USA. 82:7889 (1985).
11. S. J. Gendler, J. M Burchell, T. Duhig, D. Lamport, R. White, M. Parker and J. Taylor-Papadimitriou, Cloning the cDNA coding for differentiation and tumour-associated mucin glycoproteins expressed by human mammary epithelium, Proc. Natl. Acad. Sci. USA. (submitted).

SINGLE CELL HETEROGENEITY IN BREAST CANCER

Jerry A. Peterson

John Muir Cancer & Aging Research Institute
2055 N. Broadway
Walnut Creek, CA 94596 USA

INTRODUCTION

Although single cell heterogeneity in breast and other tumors has become a well-established observation, neither the underlying reasons for it nor its biological significance are yet clearly understood. However, it exemplifies the dynamic nature of a tumor cell population; it may play an important role in the effectiveness of breast cancer therapy, especially with the new possibilities for monoclonal antibody (MoAb) therapy; and it also could be used in improving diagnosis and prognostic evaluation. The type of single cell heterogeneity addressed in this paper is quantitative heterogeneity, especially that which has been revealed with monoclonal antibodies to surface antigens, but it must be emphasized that quantitative single cell heterogeneity has also been observed for other cell components, such as enzymes (1), secretory products (2), and hormone receptors (3).

Since the production of the first monoclonal antibodies to breast epithelial cells in 1980 (4), the most antigenic component on the surface of these cells has been found to be a high molecular weight mucin-like glycoprotein complex (5). Most monoclonal antibodies produced to date that have some specificity to breast (tumor and/or normal), that have been made either against breast epithelial cell membranes [usually the human milk fat globule membrane (4,5,6)] or breast tumor cells (7-13), have been found to identify epitopes on this mucin-like complex. Our present studies in single cell heterogeneity presented here have been carried out with the monoclonal antibody Mc5 which identifies this mucin (5). This MoAb, identifies an epitope that is present on almost all breast carcinomas, both as cultured breast epithelial cells and in histological sections.

MATERIALS AND METHODS

Breast cell lines (BT-20, MCF-7, T47D, SKBR-3) were cultured in Dulbecco's modified medium plus 10% fetal bovine serum and penicillin/streptomycin as described previously (14). Primary cultures of breast epithelial cells were prepared as described previously (15). For determination of rate of phenotypic variability (RPV), single cell suspensions were seeded on glass coverslips in culture dishes, allowed to form colonies (approximately 5 days), fixed with acetone, stained by immunoperoxidase techniques with Mc5, the colonies scored for quantitative variants, and the RPV determined as described previously (14). For effect of hormone treatments on RPV, the cell suspensions were seeded in the above medium but containing "stripped serum" and the appropriate steroid concentrations, fixed and scored as above. The "stripped serum" was fetal bovine serum treated with activated charcoal to reduce the endogenous steroid concentrations (16). The single cell antigen concentration was determined with a photometer (Microscope Spectrum Analyzer, Farrand Optical Co., Valhalla, N.Y.) attached to a standard microscope, where relative fluorescent intensity was read at 535 nm for fluorescein (15) and relative immuno-peroxidase staining read as percentage transmittance at 540 nm and expressed as absorbance (14). In the histological sections the readings were taken through a circular area of 2μm in the cytoplasm of each cell. One hundred percent transmittance was set on unstained tumor cells, or if none were present, on adjacent unstained connective tissue. Histopathological paraffin-embedded sections were obtained from the Pathology Department of John Muir Memorial Hospital, Walnut Creek, CA from primary breast tumors diagnosed as infiltrating ductal carcinomas in the years 1976, 77, 78. All patients had estrogen receptor determinations and to date follow-up and/or cause of death to be the result of the breast cancer. Glucose 6-phosphate dehydrogenase and 6-phosphogluconate dehydrogenase were detected on a single cell basis using histochemical staining procedures (17), and quantitative variants scored in clonal colonies for determination of RPV as described elsewhere (2).

RESULTS AND DISCUSSION

Quantitative assessment of single cell heterogeneity

The monoclonal antibody, Mc5, which was prepared using delipidated human milk fat globule membranes as the immunogen, binds to breast epithelial cells from both normal breast and breast carcinomas (5). The large mucin-like glycoprotein identified by Mc5 has been designated NPGP (non-penetrating glycoprotein) because it does not enter a 7% polyacrylamide gel upon electrophoresis due to its large molecular weight (> 400,000 daltons) (5). Using a microphotometer attached to a microscope the single cell NPGP content detected by immunoperoxidase techniques in normal and cancerous breast epithelial cells in culture was measured, revealing a 10-fold or greater range in the single cell distribution for both normal and tumor cells (Figure 1). Therefore, single cell heterogeneity in breast epithelial surface antigens is a normal property that is also exhibited in breast carcinomas. An unusual aspect of the staining of breast carcinoma cells with Mc5 is that in some tumors the staining was cytoplasmic as well as on the cell surface. In contrast, for normal breast tissue, NPGP was detected only on the apical surface of the epithelial cells facing the lumen and in some secreted material in the lumina of the ducts and alveoli.

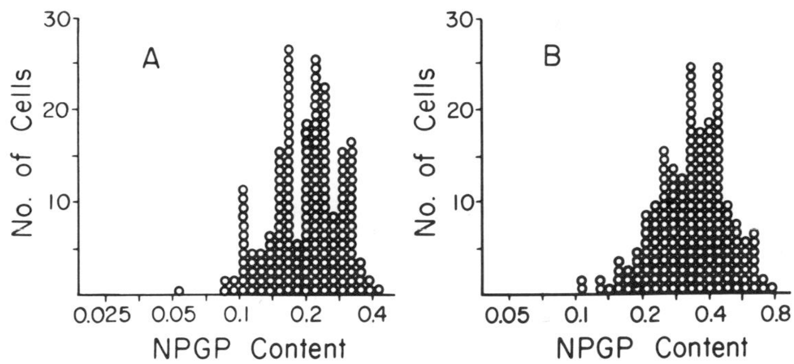

Figure 1. Single cell distribution in specific surface antigens (NPGP) in normal breast epithelial cells cultured from a reduction mammoplastie (A) and a breast carcinoma cell line, SKBR-3 (B). The cultured cells were stained, using immunoperoxidase techniques, with Mc5 that identifies the large molecular weight mucin-like glycoprotein (NPGP). Relative NPGP content in single cells was determined with a microscope photometer.

In order to assess the significance of single cell heterogeneity of surface antigen expression in breast cancer we have devised two quantitative methods for measuring and comparing breast cell heterogeneity. Both methods rely on assessing the single cell NPGP content in cells stained by either immunoperoxidase or immunofluorescence techniques. In the first method where degree of heterogeneity is expressed as the coefficient of variation (C.O.V.), breast cells can be evaluated as a monolayer cultures or in histological sections. Routinely, fifty to a hundred cells chosen at random are measured with a microscope photometer for single cell NPGP content and the coefficient of variation (standard deviation divided by the mean absorbance = C.O.V.) is calculated. The C.O.V. is an expression of the range of single cell variation in the breast tumor cell population at a fixed moment in time. The second method relies on the ability to obtain cultures of breast epithelial cells and to clone them. Single cells are cloned on the surface of a culture vessel and allowed to form small colonies. The colonies are fixed and stained by immunoperoxidase or immunofluorescence techniques and the colonies scored for the presence or absence of visually discernible quantitative variants (14,15). From the proportion of colonies that have no variants we determine the rate of phenotypic variability (RPV) which is an expression of the rate per cell per generation that quantitative variants arises in a colony (2). Both C.O.V. and RPV are quantitative assessments of cell heterogeneity; however, C.O.V. reflects the range of cell heterogeneity at a moment in time, while RPV is a measure of the rate of single cell diversification (18,19).

Using RPV to compare cultured normal and malignant breast epithelial cells (14,15), we have determined that breast epithelial cells cultured from breast carcinomas have about a

10-fold higher RPV than cells cultured from normal breast (Table 1). Cells cultured from normal appearing areas of a breast, peripheral to a breast carcinoma, have intermediate values (Table 1). With regard to the comparison of level of NPGP expression and heterogeneity among normal patients or among breast cancer patients, there is considerable variation in both the means and in the C.O.V.s with both groups (Table 2). Although the breast carcinomas and also the normal cells peripheral to a carcinoma tend to have higher C.O.V.'s than normal epithelial cells from reduction mammoplasties (Table 2).

Table 1. Comparison of rates of phenotypic variability (RPV) in expression of a breast cell surface antigen (NPGP) in clonal colonies of epithelial cells cultured from normal and cancerous tissues

Cell source	RPV ($X\ 10^{-2}$) Mean	(Range)
Normal breast (7)[a]	<0.119 ± 0.021	(<0.047 - 0.159)
Tissue peripheral to breast carcinoma (5)	0.310 ± 0.055	(0.192 - 0.368)
Breast Carcinomas (7)	1.21 ± 0.46	(0.175 - 3.4)

[a]Numbers in parenthesis are number of tissue samples (patients) in each group.

<u>Comparison of antigen content, RPV, and C.O.V. in different breast carcinoma cell lines</u>

In order to assess the heritability of NPGP content and single cell heterogeneity (C.O.V. and RPV), we have compared three different breast carcinoma cell lines BT-20, MCF-7, and T47D. We have done this since in our initial studies, we observed that although breast carcinoma cells had a higher RPV then normal breast epithelial cells there was considerable variation among different tumors (15) and cell lines (14). It is of interest to determine if this observation has any prognostic significance and/or if there are genetic differences among patients. As shown in Figure 2, the three breast carcinoma cell lines had different mean NPGP contents where BT-20 < MCF-7 < T47D. It was also observed that BT-20 was more heterogeneous, having a higher C.O.V., T47D was the least heterogeneous (lowest C.O.V.) and MCF-7 had an intermediate value (Table 3). In order to evaluate if both C.O.V. and RPV were consistent in measuring quantitative heterogeneity, we

Table 2. Quantitation of a cell surface antigen (NPGP) in normal, peripheral, and neoplastic breast epithelial cells.

	Cell Source	NPGP content/cell (relative fluorescence)[a]	C.O.V.[b]
Normal			
51E	(33%)[c]	55.8 ± 5.9[d] (25)[e]	53
48E	(40%)	37.4 ± 2.8 (42)	49
123E	(94%)	139.1 ± 8.6 (50)	44
112E	(100%)	66.7 ± 3.1 (50)	33
191E	(73%)	116.5 ± 5.1 (50)	31
337E	(51%)	118.2 ± 10.7 (50)	64
344LE	(93%)	210.6 + 18.4 (50)	62
Means		106.3 ± 7.8	48 ± 5
Peripheral to carcinoma			
90P	(79%)	22.1 ± 1.6 (50)	51
173P	(23%)	83.3 ± 8.0 (50)	68
336P	(17%)	113.8 ± 15.2 (50)	94
346P	(36%)	163.6 + 20.4 (50)	88
Means		95.6 ± 11.3	75 ± 10
Carcinoma			
336T	(7%)	143.7 ± 20.2 (43)	92
346T	(36%)	132.2 ± 11.1 (50)	59
343T	(26%)	263.7 ± 26.8 (51)	72
PH140[f]	(36%)	71.8 + 5.4 (50)	53
Means		152.7 ± 15.9	69 ± 9

[a] The relative NPGP content is estimated in individual cells stained with the monoclonal antibody Mc5, by immunofluorescence techniques, using a microscope spectrum analyzer (wave length, 535 mm). Only cells deemed positive by eye were measured.

[b] C.O.V. = Coefficient of variation

[c] Numbers in parentheses indicate percentage positive cells.

[d] Mean ± Standard error of mean.

[e] Numbers in parentheses indicate number of single cells measured.

[f] PH140 is from a metastasis of breast carcinoma to skin.

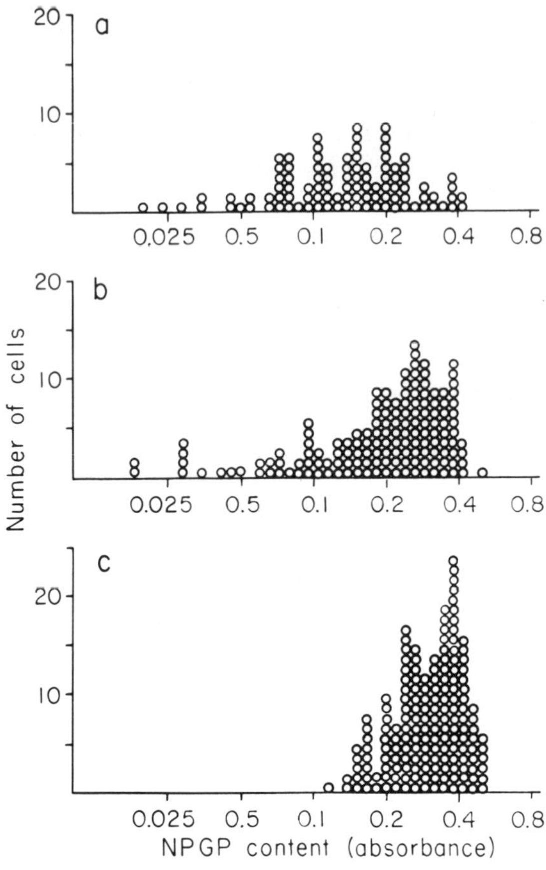

Figure 2. Single cell distribution in specific surface antigen (NPGP) content in three breast carcinoma cell lines, BT-20 (A), MCF-7 (B) and T47D (C). The cultured cells were stained with the monoclonal antibody, Mc5, using immunoperoxidase techniques. NPGP content per cell was determined with a microscope photometer.

compared them in these three cell lines and as seen in Table 3 there is a direct correlation between RPV and C.O.V. Also, it was observed that there was an indirect correlation between the mean NPGP content and cell heterogeneity, expressed either as C.O.V. or RPV (Table 3). The significance of this latter indirect correlation is not yet clear, although a similar indirect correlation is observed when NPGP content and its heterogeneity (C.O.V.) was assessed in histological sections of breast carcinomas (see below). Since these three cell lines have been cultured extensively and still maintained their characteristic antigen contents and RPV's, we can conclude that antigen content and the rate of single cell diversification (RPV) are heritable properties in these cell lines. The question still remains as to whether this represents genetic differences among the patients from which the cells were derived or differences among unique characteristics of the tumor cell populations.

Table 3. Comparison of single cell heterogeneity as measured by coefficient of variation (C.O.V.) and rate of phenotypic variability (RPV), and antigen content in three breast carcinoma cell lines, BT-20, MCF-7, and T47D, stained by immunoperoxidase technique with the monoclonal antibody Mc5 that identifies the large mucin-like surface glycoprotein, NPGP.

Cell Line	NPGP Content	C.O.V.	RPV ($X10^{-2}$)
BT-20 (5)[a]	0.112 ± 0.01[b]	54 ± 3	5.0 ± 0.29
MCF-7 (8)	0.212 ± 0.018	47 ± 6	3.53 ± 0.5
T47D (6)	0.360 ± 0.014	24 ± 3	0.93 ± 0.14

[a] Number in parentheses indicate number of independent assays

[b] Means ± standard error of mean

Single cell heterogeneity and prognosis

In order to evaluate the possible importance of single cell heterogeneity in prognosis in breast cancer, we have undertaken a retrospective study of a group of breast cancer patients with infiltrating ductal carcinoma diagnosed in the years 1976, 1977 and 1978. Paraffin-embedded sections of the breast tumors from initial surgery were stained by immunoperoxidase techniques with the MoAb, Mc5. As mentioned earlier, an unusual but often occurring aspect of the staining pattern of these mucin-like molecules in breast carcinomas is that in some tumors there is considerable cytoplasmic staining, while normal breast epithelial cells stain only on the surface. In order to assess in a quantitative manner the degree of single cell heterogeneity, for each stained tumor section we measure the intensity of cytoplasmic staining in single cells using a microscope photometer. For each patient, cytoplasmic staining intensity of 50 tumor cells selected at random was measured per slide and the mean absorbance calculated. From the mean and standard deviation, the C.O.V. was determined (see Materials and Methods). As can be seen in Figure 3, there was considerable variability from patient to patient in both the mean intensity of cytoplasmic staining and in the degree of cell heterogeneity (C.O.V.). There was also a tendency for the more heterogeneous tumor cell populations to be among the tumors that have the lower mean intensity of staining (Figure 3), recalling the results with the cell lines. There was no correlation between the degree of differentiation of the tumors and either the cytoplasmic staining intensity or the cell heterogeneity (C.O.V.) (Figure 3). In order to attempt to sub-divide the patients with regard to the degree of cell heterogeneity in cytoplasmic staining we divided Figure 3 into four quandrants. All of the patients fell into three of them, group A, B and C which represented tumors with: low mean intensity, high heterogeneity (group A); low mean intensity, low heterogeneity (group B); and high mean intensity, low heterogeneity (group C), respectively. The dividing lines making up the quadrants were at the average C.O.V. and average intensity of the studied patients, respectively. By analyzing the percentage of patients in the three groups that were alive after 8 years it was found that the best survival was for patients in group B where 74% (17/23) were alive at 8 years. A lower percentage survival was seen in the other groups; for group A it was 29% (3/8) and for group C it was 26% (4/11). Group A was significantly different from group B ($p < 0.05$) and group C significantly different from group B ($p < 0.01$) as analyzed by the chi-squared test on a 2 x 2 Contingency Table. These preliminary results suggest that detailed analysis of single cell heterogeneity in histological sections can have prognostic significance, and leads to a new approach to prognosis taking into consideration the single cell heterogeneity of the breast tumor cell population.

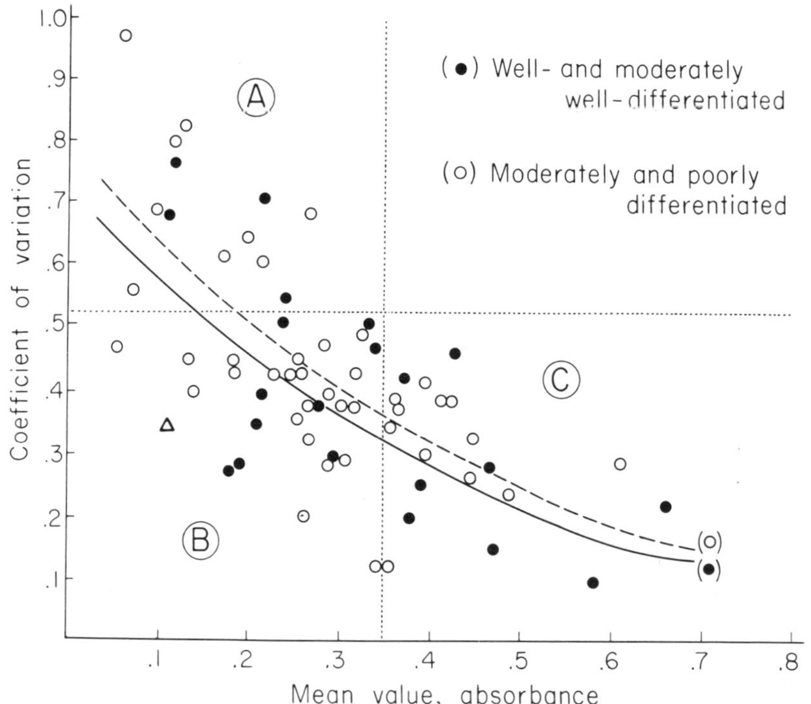

Figure 3. Relationship between mean intensity of cytoplasmic staining with Mc5 and heterogeneity (C.O.V.) in single tumor cells of histological sections of infiltrating ductal carcinomas. (●) Well- and moderately well- differentiated tumors grouped together. (○) Moderately and poorly-differentiated tumors grouped together. Solid line = curve obtained by regression analysis for more differentiated tumors (R_2 = 0.47). Dashed line = curve obtained by regression analysis for less differentiated tumors (R_2 = 0.23). (△) Value for lactating breast. Vertical and horizontal dotted lines are at average mean values and average C.O.V., respectively.

Single cell heterogeneity and monoclonal antibody therapy

With the development of monoclonal antibodies that have tissue and tumor specificity, the prospects for using them in therapy of breast cancer has become evident. An obvious problem in obtaining the effective killing of all tumor cells in the body would be the expected heterogeneity of breast tumor cell populations and the presence of antigen negative cells.

A strategy for overcoming the heterogeneous nature of most epitopes identified with monoclonal antibodies is the cocktail approach, whereby a collection of monoclonal antibodies to different epitopes of the same molecule or of different molecules would be used in combination. The rationale behind this approach is that even though each monoclonal antibody identifies epitopes that are not present on some tumor cells, most cells should have at least one of the several epitopes identified by the "cocktail". An alternative approach to overcoming the problem presented by tumor cell heterogeneity is to use radiolabelled antibodies, whereby the tumor tissue or metastasis would be destroyed even though the antibody does not bind to each cell by the fact that the radioisotope will irradiate and kill cells within the immediate area around which the antibody binds. A third approach could be to use various means to manipulate either the antigen content thereby increasing the number of cells within the tumor that have an effective antigen level, or to use various drugs or hormones to manipulate the rate of cell diversification (e.g., RPV) whereby theoretically slowing down the rate of generation of phenotypic variants (phenotypic drift).

With regard to antigen density and effectiveness of monoclonal antibody therapy, it would be expected that the greater the density of the antigen target the more likely effective killing with the monoclonal antibody would be obtained. Selecting MoAbs to high prevelence antigens and also finding factors that increase antigen target concentration could be approaches to improving therapeutic effectiveness.

With regard to the selection of epitopes that are more prevalent in a tumor we have found as a result of our production of a collection of antibodies against the large mucin-like glycoprotein (NPGP), that some epitopes are more prevalent than others. This suggests a cell heterogeneity in the synthesis, completion, and complexity of this molecule(s). An example is the comparison of binding to breast cells of a rat monoclonal antibody and the mouse monoclonal antibody Mc5, both of which identify this mucin-like complex. MCF-7 cells stained simultaneously by immunofluorescence techniques with these two antibodies demonstrates that they recognize different epitopes and that some cells will have both epitopes while other cells will have either one or the other. The monoclonal antibody, Mc5, stained almost all of the MCF-7 cells while the rat monoclonal antibody stained only a small percentage (2-5%). This double staining was possible by using two different secondary antibodies, a goat-anti-mouse antibody labelled with fluoroscein and a goat-anti-rat antibody labelled with rhodamine.

Another approach to improving monoclonal antibody therapy would be to select target antigens that exhibit less cell heterogeneity or a reduced rate of cell diversification. Even for the same antigen, different patients may present different degrees of cell heterogeneity which may reflect different genetic make-ups. This latter possibility is suggested by the comparison presented above for the three breast cell lines. Preliminary evidence suggesting that different components of the same tumor cell population can have different RPVs is found in the comparison of RPV for surface antigens and for two enzymes detected by histochemistry. For example, BT-20 cells have similarily high RPVs with regard to NPGP content and also two enzymes, glucose 6-phosphate dehydrogenase and 6-phosphogluconate dehydrogenase (Table 4). On the other hand, MCF-7 cells have a high RPV for NPGP content, but have a lower RPV for the two enzymes (Table 4). In contrast, T47D cells have a low RPV with regard to NPGP content but higher RPV for the enzymes (Table 4).

Table 4. Comparison of rates of phenotypic variability (RPV) for surface antigens and constitutive enzymes in different human breast carcinoma cell lines.

	Rate of Phenotypic Variability (X 10^{-2})		
Cell Line	NPGP[a]	G-6-PD[b]	6-Ph-D[c]
BT-20	5.0	4.0	5.4
MCF-7	4.6	1.2	1.9
T47D	0.92	5.2	3.2

[a] NPGP = Nonpenetrating glycoprotein
[b] G-6-PD = Glucose 6-phosphate dehydrogenase
[c] 6-Ph-D = 6-phosphogluconate dehydrogenase

In order to explore the possibility of manipulating cell heterogeneity, we have examined various steroid hormones and their effect on RPV. As shown in Figure 4, estrogens reduced the RPV by at least 2-fold with physiological concentrations of the hormone compared to control medium. The fetal bovine serum used in the experiments was treated with charcoal to remove the endogenous steroid hormones (16). Very low concentrations of 17ß-estradiol reduced the RPV significantly; however, unnaturally high concentrations again increase the rate of phenotypic variability (Figure 4). A biphasic effect of steroid hormones is often observed (20). In contrast, the antiestrogen, tamoxifen, increases the RPV and the effect is dose dependent, while progesterone has no effect on the RPV with MCF-7 cells (Figure 4). The differential effects of these three sex hormones appears to be specific to the action of the hormones on this cell line, since MCF-7 cells are known to have high levels of estrogen receptors, but they have very low levels of progesterone receptors (21). In order to further examine the significance of the presence of specific receptors on the effect of steroid hormones on RPV we treated T47D cells with progesterone and examined the effect on RPV. T47D cells, in contrast to MCF-7 cells, have high levels of progesterone receptors (21). As shown in Figure 5, progesterone increased

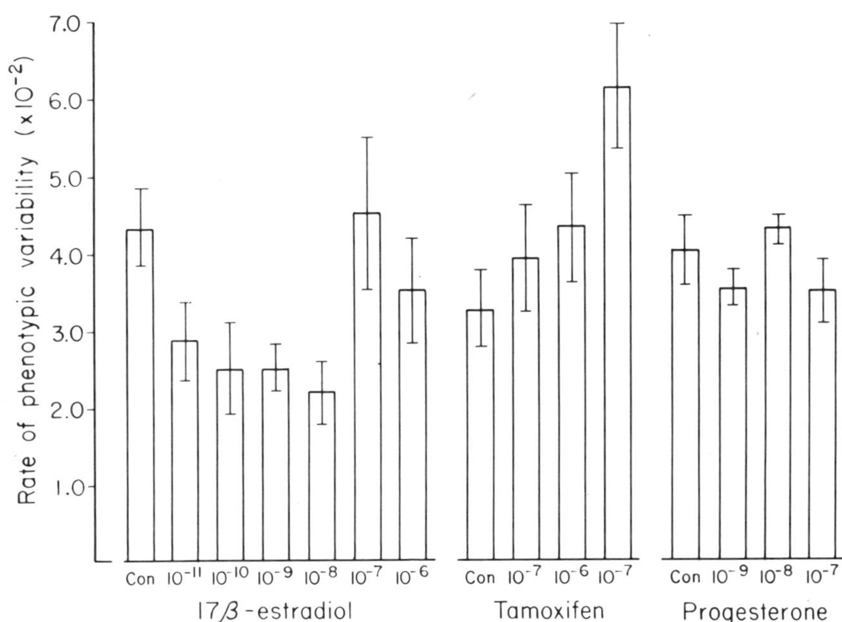

Figure 4. The effect of 17β-estradiol, tamoxifen, and progesterone on the rate of phenotypic variability (RPV) in the breast carcinoma cell line MCF-7. Molar concentrations of hormones are indicated along abscissas. Con = control media containing "stripped" fetal bovine serum with no added hormones (see Materials and Methods).

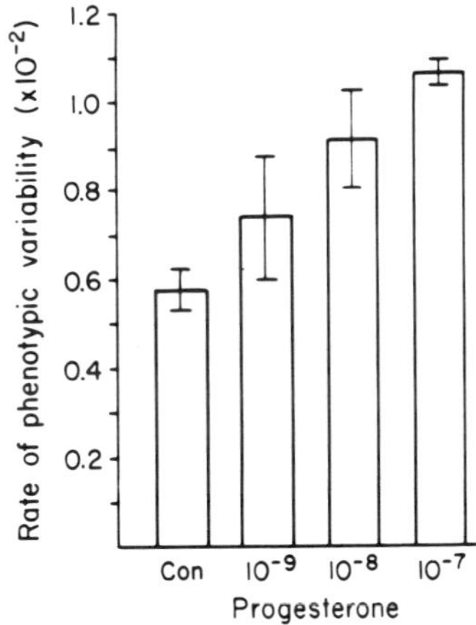

Figure 5. The effect of progesterone in the rate of phenotypic variability (RPV) in the breast carcinoma cell line T47D. Molar concentrations of progesterone are indicated along abscissas. Con = control media without added hormones (see Materials and Methods).

the RPV and the effect was dose dependent. This ability of steroid hormones to alter the RPV suggests that the rate of generation of phenotypic variants can be manipulated and that by combining specific hormones and other treatments with therapuetic drugs, it may be possible to improve the effectiveness of the treatment.

ACKNOWLEDGEMENT

This work is supported by NIH Grant No. CA39931.

REFERENCES

1. J.A. Peterson, The widespread nature of phenotypic variability in the form of a geometric progression, J. Theorectical Biol. 102:41-53 (1983).

2. J.A. Peterson, Analysis of the discontinuous variation in albumin synthesis at the cell per cell level, Somatic Cell Genetics 5:641-651 (1979).

3. F. Kodama, G.L. Green and S.E. Salmon, Relation of estrogen receptor expression to clonal growth and antiestrogen effects on human breast cancer cells. Cancer Res. 45:2720-2724 (1985).

4. J. Taylor-Papadimitriou, J.A. Peterson, J. Arklie, J. Burchell, R.L. Ceriani and W.F. Bodmer, Monoclonal antibodies to epithelial-specific components of the human milk fat globule membrane: Production and reacton with cells in culture, Int. J. Cancer 28:17-21 (1981).

5. R.L. Ceriani, J.A. Peterson, J.Y. Lee, R. Moncada and E.W. Blank, Characterization of cell surface antigens of human mammary epithelial cells with monoclonal antibodies prepared against human milk fat globule, Somat. Cell Genetics 9:415-427 (1983).

6. J. Hilkens, F. Buijs, J. Hilgers, P. Hageman, J. Calafat, A. Sonnenberg and M. Van der Valk, Monoclonal antibodies against human milk fat globule membranes detecting differentiation antigens of the mammary gland and its tumors, Int. J. Cancer 34:197-206 (1984).

7. L. Papsidero, G. Croghan, M. O'Connell, L. Valenzuela, T. Nemoto and T. Chu, Monoclonal antibodies (F36/22 and M7/105) to human breast carcinoma, Cancer Res. 43:1741-1747 (1983).

8. D. Kufe, G. Inghirami, M. Abe, D. Hayes, H. Justi-Wheeler and J. Schlom, Differential reactivity of a novel monoclonal antibody (Df3) with human malignant versus benign breast tumors, Hybridoma 3:223-232 (1984).

9. A. Frankel, D. Ring, F. Tringale and S. Ma-Hsieh, Tissue distribution of breast cancer-associated antigens defined by monoclonal antibodies, J. Biol. Response Mod. 4:273-286 (1985).

10. D. Colcher, P. Hand, M. Nuti and J. Schlom, A spectrum of monoclonal antibodies reactive with human mammary tumor cells, Proc. Natl. Acad. Sci. USA 78:3199-3203 (1981).

11. C. Foster, P. Edwards, E. Dinsdale and A. Neville, Monoclonal antibodies to the human mammary gland, Virchows Arch 394:279-293 (1982).

12. I. Ellis, R. Robins, C. Elston, R. Blamey, B. Ferry and R. Baldwin, A monoclonal antibody, NCRC 11, raised to human breast carcinoma, Histopathology 8:501-516 (1984).

13. F. Ashall, M. Bramwell and H. Harris, A new marker for human cancer cells. 1. The Ca antigen and the Cal antibody, Lancet 2:1-11 (1982).

14. J.A. Peterson, R.L. Ceriani, E.W. Blank and L. Osvaldo, Comparison of rates of phenotypic variability in surface antigen expression in normal and cancerous breast epithelial cells, Cancer Res. 43:4291-4296 (1983).

15. R.L. Ceriani, J.A. Peterson and E.W. Blank, Variability in surface antigen expression of human breast epithelial cells cultured from normal breast, normal tissue peripheral to breast carcinomas, and breast carcinomas, Cancer Res. 44:3033-3039 (1984).

16. E.R. Stanley, R.E. Palmer and V. Shun, Development of methods for the quantitative in vitro analysis of androgen-dependent and autonomons Shionugi carcinoma 115 cells, Cell 10:35-44 (1977).

17. J. Chayen, L. Bitensky and R.G. Butcher, "Practical Histochemistry", John Wiley and Sons, NY pp. 204-209 (1973).

18. J.A. Peterson, W.L. Chaovapong and A.A. Dehgnan, Quantitative phenotypic variation of single normal and malignant cells from liver and breast occurs along a geometric series, Somatic Cell and Molecular Genetics 10:331-334 (1984).

19. J.A. Peterson, Analysis of variability in albumin content of sister hepatoma cells and a model for geometric phenotypic variability ("Quantitative Shift Model"), Somatic Cell and Molecular Genetics 10:345-357 (1984).

20. S.P. Tam, T.K. Archer and R.G. Deeley, Biphasic effects of estrogen on apolipoprotin synthesis in human hepatoma cells: Mechanism of antagonisms by testosterone, Proc. Natl. Acad. Sci. USA 83:3111-3115 (1986).

21. K.B. Horwitz, D.T. Zava, A.K. Thilagar, E.V. Jensen and W.L. McGuire, Steroid receptor analyses of nine human breast cancer cell lines, Cancer Res. 38:2434-2437 (1978).

MONOCLONAL ANTIBODY STUDIES OF DRUG RESISTANCE

William L. McGuire, Suzanne A. W. Fuqua, and Lynn G. Dressler

Department of Medicine/Oncology, University of Texas Health Science Center at San Antonio
7703 Floyd Curl Drive, San Antonio, Texas 78284

INTRODUCTION

A major problem in the control of metastatic disease is the outgrowth of cells which display simultaneous resistance to a number of therapeutic drugs.[1] This multidrug resistance (MDR) involves resistance to some of the most commonly used anticancer drugs. Several mammalian cell lines are available which model this human pleiotropic cross-resistance to chemotherapeutic agents.[2-7] These drug-resistant cell lines afford an in vitro system to study molecular mechanisms of resistance. Studies in such model systems indicate that reduced cellular accumulation of the affected drugs is a major factor, so that membrane alterations may be involved in drug resistance. In the well-characterized colchicine-resistant Chinese hamster ovary (CHO) system selected by Bech-Hansen et al.,[3] it is clear that multidrug resistance has a genetic basis. The degree of both drug resistance and reduced membrane permeability is correlated with the elevated expression of a plasma membrane glycoprotein with a molecular weight of 170,000 daltons, termed P-glycoprotein or P170.[8-13] Recently, a 600-base pair (bp) complementary DNA (cDNA) encoding part of the P-glycoprotein was obtained from a λgt11 expression vector library of a multidrug resistant CHO cell line.[12] Using this cDNA as a probe in Southern blot analyses, it was shown that P-glycoprotein gene sequences are conserved among hamster, mouse, and human DNA.

Using the novel approach of in-gel DNA renaturation,[14] Roninson et al. provided direct evidence that gene amplification underlies the process of drug resistance in CHO cells.[15] These authors showed that the degree of drug resistance correlates with the number of copies of the amplified domain.

Utilizing a probe from one of the commonly amplified segments, they cloned a continuous domain of about 120 kilobases (kb) from the hamster genome that is amplified in CHO MDR.[16] Within the domain a gene was identified which encodes a messenger RNA (mRNA) transcript of 5 kb, whose level of expression correlates with the degree of drug resistance in CHO cells. The presence of common amplified sequences in resistant human KB carcinoma cells was also identified using the in-gel DNA renaturation technique.[17] Segments of human DNA sequences homologous to the CHO MDR gene were cloned and designated _mdrl_ and _mdr2_.[18]

It is clear that gene amplification appears with drug selection; human tumor cells _in vivo_ and human tumor cell lines amplify their genes with relative ease.[19] For example, amplified cellular oncogenes have been found in human patients[20] and clinical resistance to methotrexate can be achieved via amplification of the dihydrofolate reductase (DHFR) gene.[21] But in clinical studies in which the increase in DHFR gene copy number has been established, the amplification is only 5-fold.[21,22] In human MDR cell lines it is hypothesized that resistance is initially accompanied by elevated expression of the _mdrl_ gene without major amplification of the genomic sequences.[23] Thus, gene amplification may not be the only mechanism for the development of drug resistance in human tumor cells.

We recently reported the production and characterization of the 265/F4 monoclonal antibody, which reacts with the P170 protein in colchicine-resistant CHO cells.[24] Unlike P170 monoclonal antibodies described by others,[13] this antibody is able to detect the P-glycoprotein in live, unfixed resistant cells.[24] This permitted us to examine the hypothesis that sorting for increased P-glycoprotein expression by fluorescence-activated cell sorting techniques should select cells with increased drug resistance.

We report here the cloning of a cDNA encoding P170 utilizing our monoclonal antibody. We show that the P170 gene is expressed in an adriamycin-resistant subline of the human MDA-231 breast cancer cell line, but not control drug-sensitive human breast cancer cells.

RESULTS

Drug Resistance Enrichment

We confirm that sorting live CHO cells for increased P-glycoprotein increases drug resistance. This was made possible with our 265/F4 monoclonal antibody, which has the ability to recognize the P-glycoprotein on live, intact cells. By flow cytometry, we were able to enrich the percentage of cells expressing P170 from 31% to 63%. Western blots provided further evidence that the sorted, cloned cells were enriched for P170. The P170 enrichment was accompanied by a remarkable increase in drug resistance. The resistant "parent" CHO/C5 was only 117-fold less sensitive to colchicine than the drug-sensitive

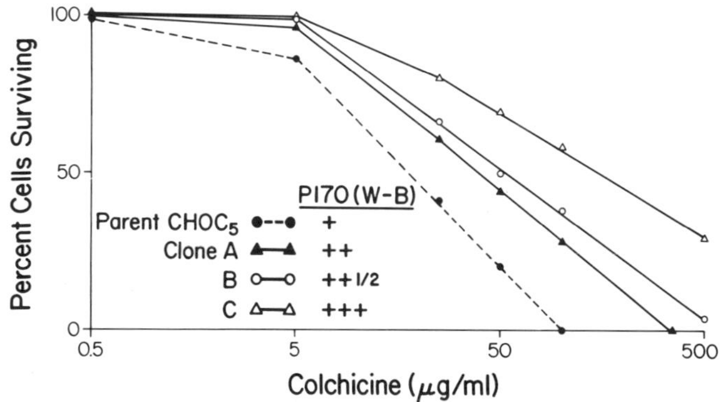

Fig. 1. Drug resistance profile of cell lines enriched for P170. Methodology to be published elsewhere (T. Shenkenberg et al.).

CHO/AB. In the sorted, cloned cells (Clone C, Figure 1), however, 1333-fold increase in drug resistance was observed. The correlation of degree of drug-resistance with the amount of P-glycoprotein has also been suggested by other investigators studying a variety of CHO resistant mutants and revertants.

In vitro data also indicate a correlation between P-glycoprotein and pleiotropic drug resistance in various other mammalian species.[13] In human cells, increased expression of P-glycoprotein with concomitant multidrug resistance has been demonstrated in a leukemic lymphoblast line.[25] Bell et al. recently reported the detection of P-glycoprotein in two patients with ovarian cancer who were clinically resistant to chemotherapy.[26] Thus, it appears that the multidrug resistance phenotype associated with the P-glycoprotein may occur in human tumors. Detection of this membrane glycoprotein in human tumor biopsies might therefore predict for drug-resistance and allow for better treatment strategies.

Isolation of a cDNA which Detects P170 Expression in a Human Breast Cancer Cell Line

We have used a specific monoclonal antibody[24] to isolate a P-glycoprotein cDNA clone from an expression vector library. This clone has the potential to be a powerful tool to study the molecular mechanisms of acquired drug resistance. Though the degree of cross-resistance and the drugs involved in the process of drug resistance vary among different cell lines, suggesting a multicomponent, complex system, there is considerable evidence to link the overproduction of the P-glycoprotein to drug resistance.[8-13] Elevated expression of the P170 protein correlates with the degree of amplification in the CHO system,[12] and the P170 gene is the only one of five genes consistently amplified in independently-derived, drug-resistant hamster cell lines.[27] Others have reported the cloning of a P170 cDNA utilizing a monoclonal antibody which recognizes an epitope that is conserved between mouse and human proteins.[12] The monoclonal antibody used in the present study differs in that it recognizes an epitope on the CHO antigen which is not conserved, at the protein level, in the human antigen.[24] In addition, this monoclonal antibody is able to detect P170 on the surface of intact, live CHO MDR cells. These results suggest that our cDNA clone encodes a P170 sequence at least partially exposed on the exterior of the cell.

We have demonstrated elevated expression of the P-glycoprotein gene in human breast cancer cells selected for resistance to adriamycin. P170 gene probes recognize two mRNA species in hamster and one mRNA in human cell lines.[28] We find that the human P170 mRNA is slightly larger than the corresponding mRNA species in hamster cells. The smaller hamster mRNA may represent a spliced message; a distinct, but related gene; or an artifact of RNA degradation. At least two related genes, the overexpression of one or all, may be associated with the drug-resistant phenotype. Future studies are directed at determining if there is a correlation between the level of expression of the P170 gene(s) and the extent of drug resistance in resistant human breast cancer sublines. A clear parallel was seen between the extent of drug resistance and expression of the mdrl gene in KB carcinoma cells,[23] but there is conflicting evidence in other human cell lines.[28]

Elevated expression of the P170 gene is not solely the result of gene amplification in human cell lines, as in the CHO/P170 system. Increased expression of the P170 sequence in human cells can occur without gene amplification.[23] Amplification of the DHFR gene in patients receiving conventional dosages of methotrexate is only five-fold,[21,22] suggesting that amplification during the course of chemotherapy is not a prerequisite parameter for the development of resistance as activation and expression of specific genes. Expression of P170 gene(s) may be a common mechanism of multidrug resistance in human cell lines. It is not known what transcriptional control mechanisms activate expression of the genes involved in MDR in human tumor cells; it may be that regulatory mutations in P170 gene(s) or other genes are necessary to turn on the MDR phenotype in the clinical setting. The P170 cDNA described here, combined with additional MDR gene probes,[12,18,27,28] will be invaluable in defining these mechanisms.

Only limited studies have been reported examining the expression of P170 in clinical tumor samples.[26] Experiments are in progress to assess parameters of tumor aggressiveness (steroid receptor status, proliferative rate, and ploidy) in relation to specific MDR gene expression in clinically resistant human breast tumors.

ACKNOWLEDGMENT

This work was supported in part by NIH Grant CA 30195.

REFERENCES

1. G. A. Curt, N. J. Clendininn, and B. A. Chabner, Drug resistance in cancer, Cancer Treat. Rep. 68:87 (1984).
2. V. Ling, N. Kartner, T. Sudo, L. Siminovich, and J. R. Riordan, Multidrug-resistance phenotype in Chinese hamster ovary cells, Cancer Treat. Rep. 67:869 (1983).
3. N. T. Bech-Hansen, J. E. Till, and V. Ling, Pleiotropic phenotype of colchicine-resistant CHO cells: cross-resistance and collateral sensitivity, J. Cell Physiol. 88:23 (1976).
4. J. L. Biedler, T. Chang, M. B. Meyers, R. H. F. Peterson, and B. A. Spengles, Drug resistance in Chinese hamster lung and mouse tumor cells, Cancer Treat. Rep. 67:859 (1983).
5. J. L. Biedler and H. Riehm, Cellular resistance to actinomycin D in Chinese hamster cell in vitro: cross-resistance; radioautographic; and cytogenetic studies, Cancer Res. 30:1174 (1970).

6. D. Kessel and H. B. Boxmann, On the characteristics of actinomycin D resistance in L5178Y cells, Cancer Res. 30:2695 (1970).
7. V. Ling, Genetic aspects of drug resistance in somatic cells, in: "Fundamentals in Cancer Chemotherapy--Antibiotics Chemotherapy," R. Schabel, ed., S. Karger, Basel (1978).
8. D. Garman and M. S. Center, Alterations in cell surface membranes in Chinese hamster lung cells resistant to adriamycin, Biochem. Biophys. Res. Commun. 105:157 (1982).
9. R. L. Juliano and V. Ling, A surface glycoprotein modulating drug permeability in Chinese hamster ovary cell mutants, Biochim. Biophys. Act 455:152 (1976).
10. V. Ling, Drug resistance and membrane alterations in mutants of mammalian cells, Can. J. Genet. Cytol. 17:503 (1975).
11. V. Ling and L. H. Thompson, Reduced permeability in CHO cells as a mechanism of resistance to colchicine, J. Cell Physiol. 83:103 (1974).
12. J. R. Riordan, K. Deuchars, N. Kartner, N. Alon, J. Trent, and V. Ling, Amplification of P-glycoprotein genes in multidrug-resistant mammalian cell lines, Nature 316:817 (1985).
13. N. Kartner, D. Evernden-Porelle, G. Bradley, and V. Ling, Detection of P-glycoprotein in multidrug-resistant cell lines by monoclonal antibodies, Nature 315:820 (1985).
14. I. B. Roninson, Detection and mapping of homologous, repeated and amplified DNA sequences by DNA renaturation in agarose gels, Nucleic Acids Res. 11:5413 (1983).
15. I. B. Roninson, H. T. Abelson, D. E. Housman, N. Howell, and Varshavsky, A, Amplification of specific DNA sequences correlates with multidrug resistance in Chinese hamster cells, Nature 309:626 (1984).
16. P. Gros, J. Croop, I. Roninson, A. Varshavsky, and D. E. Housman, Isolation and characterization of DNA sequences amplified in multidrug-resistant hamster cells, Proc. Natl. Acad. Sci. USA 83:337 (1986).
17. A. T. Fojo, J. Whang-Peng, M. M. Gottesman, and I. Pastan, Amplification of DNA sequences in human multidrug-resistant KB carcinoma cells, Proc. Natl. Acad. Sci. USA 82:7661 (1985).
18. I. B. Roninson, J. E. Chin, K. G. Choi, P. Gros, D. E. Housman, A. Fojo, D. W. Shen, M. M. Gottesman, and I. Pastan, Isolation of human mdr DNA sequences amplified in multidrug-resistant KB carcinoma cells, Proc. Natl. Acad. Sci. USA 83:4538 (1986).
19. M. Fox, Gene amplification and drug resistance, Nature 307:212 (1984).
20. K. Alitalo and M. Schwab, Oncogene amplification in tumor cells, Adv. Cancer Res. 47:43 (1985).
21. R. C. Horns, W. J. Dower, and R. T. Schimke, Gene amplification in a leukemia patient treated with methotrexate, J. Clin Oncol. 2:1 (1984).
22. M. D. Cardman, J. H. Schornagel, R. S. Rivest, S. Srimat-Kondada, C. S. Portlock, T. Duffy, and J. R. Bertino, Resistance to methotrexate due to gene amplification in a patient with acute leukemia, J. Clin. Oncol. 2:16 (1984).
23. D. W. Shen, A. Fojo, J. E. Chin, I. B. Roninson, N. Richert, I. Pastan, and M. M. Gottesman, Human multidrug-resistant cell lines: Increased mdrl expression can precede gene amplification, Science 232:643 (1986).
24. B. Lathan, D. P. Edwards, L. G. Dressler, D. D. Von Hoff, and W. L. McGuire, Immunological detection of Chinese hamster ovary cells expressing a multidrug resistance phenotype, Cancer Res. 45:5064 (1985).
25. W. T. Beck, T. J. Mueller, and L. R. Tanzer, Altered surface membrane glycoproteins in vinca alkaloid-resistant human leukemia lymphoblasts, Cancer Res. 39:2070 (1979).
26. D. R. Bell, J. H. Gerlack, N. Kartner, R. N. Buick, and V. Ling, Detection of P-glycoprotein in ovarian cancer: a molecular marker associated with multi-drug resistance, J. Clin. Immunol. 3:311 (1985).

27. A. M. Van der Blick, T. Van der Velde-Koerts, V. Ling, and P. Borst, Overexpression and amplification of five genes in a multi-drug-resistant Chinese hamster ovary cell line, Mol. Cell Biol. 6:1671 (1986).
28. K. W. Scotto, J. L. Bielder, and P. W. Melera, Amplification and expression of genes associated with multidrug resistance in mammalian cells, Science 232:751 (1986).

THE USE OF MULTITUMOR/TISSUE (SAUSAGE) BLOCKS FOR IMMUNOHISTOLOGIC SCREENING OF MONOCLONAL ANTIBODIES

Hector Battifora

City of Hope National Medical Center

Duarte, California 91010

ABSTRACT

We have developed a method of embedding 100 or more different tissue samples in a multi-compartmentalized paraffin block averaging 1 cm. in diameter, the multitumor/tissue (sausage) block. These blocks allow the simultaneous immunohistologic testing of numerous tissue samples on a single slide with one drop of antibody. Because all of the tissue samples are treated equally during immunostaining, most sources of variation are removed and comparative and semiquantitative studies are facilitated.

The composition of the sausage blocks vary according to their intended use. Sausage blocks containing a wide spectrum of neoplasms and normal tissues are suitable for screening of hybridoma supernatants during the early phases of monoclonal-antibody production. This permits economical and rapid screening for antibody specificity and sensitivity and simultaneously selects those useful for immunohistochemistry. Tissues fixed with various fixatives as well as unfixed, freeze-dried tissues can be incorporated in the same sausage block. This makes possible the identification and selection of the most appropriate specimen handling method for each antigen/antibody system. Sausage blocks prepared with tumor samples from preselected groups of patients with established clinical behavior may be used to screen for markers of biological significance.

INTRODUCTION

The somatic hybridization method to produce monoclonal antibodies in vitro[1] has resulted in great advances in the clinical applications of immunohistology. Monoclonal antibodies to molecules of possible clinical value can now be produced with relative ease. However, the development of techniques for efficient screening and fast determination of clinical applications of these new antibodies has lagged behind. Most current methods of screening for monoclonal antibodies are based on solid phase assays which allow only a limited identification of specificity. Immunohistologic studies thus become necessary as a secondary screening procedure. These are usually done on slides which contain one or, at best, a few specimen samples, a costly and time consuming system.[2] Placement of multiple tissue samples in a single slide increases the efficiency of immunohistologic evaluation of antibodies.[2]

We have developed a method by which a large number of normal or tumor tissues can be mounted on a paraffin block of conventional size, the multi-tumor/tissue (sausage) block (MTTB). Such blocks facilitate rapid and inexpensive immunohistologic testing of antibodies against a large group of different tissues and/or neoplasms mounted on a single conventional glass slide, and they require a minimal amount of antibody solution. Direct screening of hybridoma supernatants by immunohistology using sections from sausage blocks thus becomes a practical means to ascertain the specificity, and approximate sensitivity of antibodies. In addition, if tissues with a variety of fixatives are incorporated into the sausage block, the choice of optimal fixative can be identified at the same time.

MATERIALS AND METHODS

The method of preparation of the sausage blocks has been previously published[3] and will be only briefly outlined here.

Tissue Samples

Portions of tissues which have been pre-embedded in paraffin, are selected, removed from their paraffin blocks, deparaffinized in xylene, and rehydrated in ethanol to a final concentration of 50%, cut into slender, rod-like pieces which have an average cross-sectional area of 1 mm^2 and are about 10 mm long. Alternatively, prospectively collected, fixed or freeze-dried tissues may be used with appropriate adjustments to the method.

Method of preparation

Combinations of rods obtained from as many as 100 different paraffin blocks are stacked in parallel over a piece of sausage casing or comparable membranous tissue. The tissue rods are tightly wrapped in the casing, the resulting sausage is routinely processed back to paraffin, and is embedded with the tissue rods perpendicular to the face of the block. Multiple compartments can be created during the rolling of the tissue rods into the sausage casing, thus separating the tissue samples by predefined criteria, (fig 1).

Between 750 and 1,000, 5 micron thick slides can be prepared from an average sized MTTB. If care is taken to keep all of the rods in a straight, parallel stack during preparation of the MTTB, the tissue samples are positioned nearly identically in all of the sections. This facilitates comparative studies and identification of the various tissue samples by their relative position in the section.

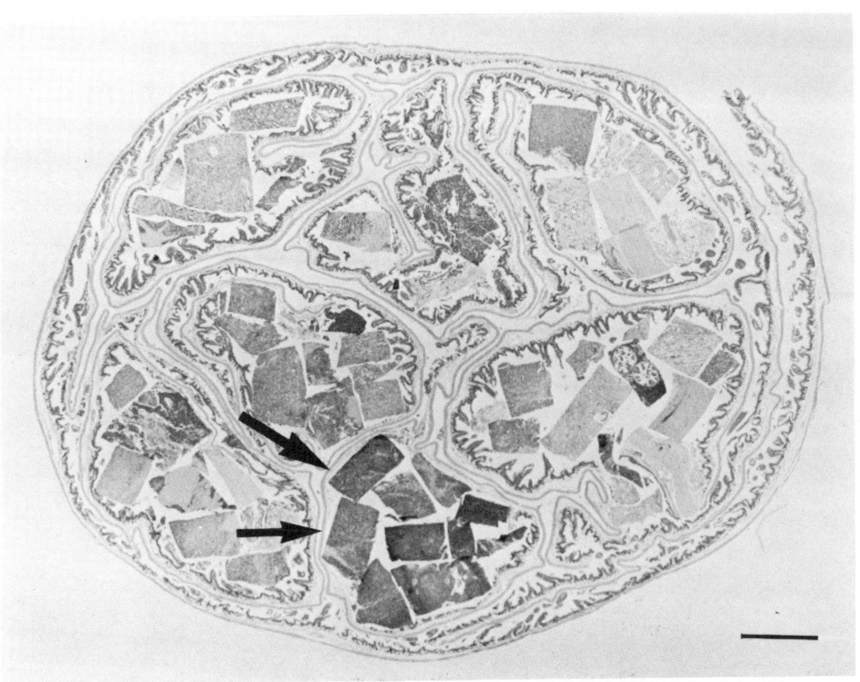

Figure 1. Section of a sausage block containing samples of various types of neoplasms within discrete compartments created during preparation of the block. Stained with antiserum to S100 protein which has stained all samples in the melanoma compartment (arrows). Hematoxylin counterstain, bar = 0.1 cm.

DISCUSSION

One of the best-known advantages of the hybridoma technique is that it enables the production of monoclonal antibodies without the need for identification or prior purification of the antigens. However, because a mixture of many immunogens is used, the number of antibodies generated to irrelevant molecules vastly exceeds the number of those that are generated to molecules of interest. Moreover, rapid decisions have to be made during the early screening of hybridoma cultures so that desired hybridomas are selected and cloned and overgrowth of irrelevant colonies is avoided.[2]

Direct screening of hybridoma supernatants by immunohistologic methods has the advantage over the commonly used RIA and ELISA-based screening, that one can ascertain cell specificity while simultaneously optimizing the search for antibodies which perform well with immunohistochemical methods. However, immunohistologic screening is impractical unless a large number of tissues can be grouped within a small surface area.[4] Thus, one of the most useful applications of sausage blocks is in the detection of tissue-specific antigens or tumor markers during the early stages of hybridoma preparation (figure 2).

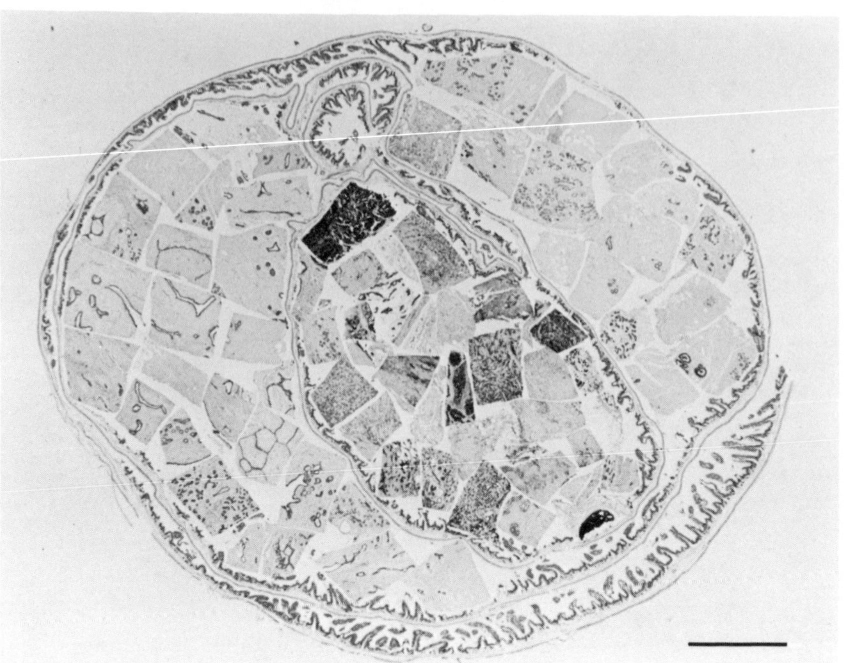

Fig 2. Section of sausage block containing many samples of adenocarcinoma of breast origin in the middle compartment, fibroadenomas in the right compartment and normal breast tissues in the left one. Immunostained with supernatant of monoclonal antibody Mc5 (prepared by Dr. Roberto Ceriani, John Muir Cancer and Aging Research Institute, Walnut Creek, CA). Hematoxylin counterstain, bar = 0.1 cm.

In addition, in the diagnostic immunohistochemistry laboratory, sausage blocks permit rapid and inexpensive evaluation of new reagents for specificity and sensitivity as well as being a practical multipurpose routine control preparation.

There is no evidence that the steps needed to prepare the sausage blocks have deleterious effects on tissue antigenicity. We have investigated the effect of re-processing of paraffin embedded material on antigen preservation with a large number of antibodies which detect antigens of common clinical use. When the sausage sections were compared with sections of the original paraffin blocks, no reduction in the immunoreactivity with any of the antibodies tested was detected.

One possible objection to screening of monoclonal antibodies by immunohistology is that important antigens may be destroyed or masked by the fixation step. Recent methodological advances which permit the preparation of freeze-dried paraffin-embedded blocks using unfixed tissues and with excellent antigen preservation[5] can be readily adapted to the preparation of sausage blocks. Sausage blocks prepared with a comprehensive group of, freeze dried, normal organ samples from several individuals would be particularly useful in the screening of normal tissues to detect unexpected reactivities, an essential step prior to the parenteral administration of monoclonal antibodies. Currently this can only be achieved by examination of numerous individual frozen sections, a tedious and costly procedure.

The small size of the tumor samples in sausage blocks has not been a serious obstacle to their use. Individual tissue samples measure about 1 mm^2, and therefore are not smaller than many endoscopic biopsies. Furthermore, sampling errors can be avoided by careful selection of the tissues to be used in the preparation of the block. Another cause for concern would be possible errors due to heterogeneity of antigen expression, particularly in neoplastic tissues. However, these drawbacks are compensated for, in considerable measure, by the large number of samples included in the block. In our laboratory, many monoclonal antibodies have now been screened by this means, moreover comparative studies using larger, single-slide sections of the same neoplasms used in the preparation of the sausage block have consistently yielded good agreement between the results of the sausage blocks and those of the conventional blocks.

Given the large number of tissues, many with similar histologic appearance, within a sausage block, it is not possible to identify the source of each individual tumor sample. On the other hand, because the tissues may be separated into numerous compartments, it is not difficult for inexperienced observers to identify the various components of the tissue section by referring to a pre-prepared sausage "map". The inability to trace each tumor sample to its patient source is not a serious impediment to the use of the method because it is designed for screening purposes and not for definitive studies. Blocks containing larger but fewer tissue samples, arranged in a way that the individual patient sample can be recognized, with the help of a computer program, are used routinely in our laboratory for comprehensive antibody testing after screening with sausage block slides.

Another advantage of the use of sausage blocks is that they ensure that all the histologic sections are treated equally during processing and immunostaining. This eliminates variations from sample to sample and may permit a more accurate semiquantitave approach to immunohistology. Moreover, because the geographical distribution of the tissue samples varies little from slide to slide, the sections are amenable to computer-aided automatic screening.

Retrospective immunohistologic comparison of defined patient populations, in search for markers of biological significance can be achieved by a system which uses sections from sausage blocks of tumor samples from the groups being compared, within separate compartments. Screening with these sections may help to rapidly and economically identify marker substances of possible prognostic value and worthy of a larger and more detailed study using conventional tissue samples.

REFERENCES

1. Kohler G, Milstein C, Continuous cultures of fused cells secreting antibody of predefined specificity. Nature (Lond) 256:495 (1975)

2. Bastin JM, Kirkley J and McMichael AJ, 1982, Production of monoclonal antibodies: a practical guide, in: "Monoclonal Antibodies in Clinical Medicine", McMichael AJ and Fabre JW, Academic Press, London (1982)

3. Battifora H, The multitumor (sausage) tissue block: Novel method for immunohistochemical antibody testing. Lab Invest 55:244 (1986)

4. Mason DY, Naiem M, Abdulaziz Z, Nash JRG, Gatter KC, and Stein H, 1982, Immunohistological applications of monoclonal antibodies, in: "Monoclonal Antibodies in Clinical Medicine", McMichael AJ and Fabre JW, Academic Press, London (1982)

5. Stein H, Gatter K, Asbahr H, and Mason DY, Use of freeze-dried paraffin-embedded sections for immunohistologic staining with monoclonal antibodies. Lab Invest 52:676 (1986)

ADVANCES TOWARDS CLINICAL RELEVANCE OF BREAST CARCINOMA ASSOCIATED ANTIGENS

Fernando A. Salinas

Advanced Therapeutics Department, Cancer Control Agency of British Columbia, and Department of Pathology, University of British Columbia, Vancouver, B.C. V5Z 4E6, Canada

ABSTRACT

Use of monoclonal antibodies Mc 3 and Mc 8, and the respective human mammary epithelial antigens (HME Ags), has enabled the isolation, characterization and identification of free and bound antigenic moieties extracted from breast carcinoma (BC) patients' sera immune reactants. As a result we have been able to compare and identify reactive similarities encountered with either source of antigens. Both isolated antigens (BCAA), and Mc 3 and Mc 8 monoclonals have been reacted with BC patients' sera grouped according to tumor burden by use of an in vitro model of tumor burden change. Results of this interaction have provided insight into relative concentration of free antigen:antibodies at differing tumor burden load. The effects of circulating immune complexes (CIC) and antibodies on free circulating BCAA levels, and their relationship to tumor burden have resulted in a better understanding of clearance, pathogenetic deposition and ultimate fate of CIC. An evaluation of free circulating BCAA in BC patients' sera demonstrated that despite BCAA not correlating linearly with tumor burden, BCAA represent a useful marker to clinically monitor tumor burden changes.

INTRODUCTION

Our recent studies have been concentrated on the often deranged immune response encountered in cancer patients harboring solid tumors. The diagnostic, prognostic, and therapeutic implications for a better understanding of such an immune response have been overwhelmingly demonstrated in recent reported information concerning biological response modifiers[1]. We have selected breast carcinoma (BC) because of the impact of this disease on the affected population involved. Among the several immune components under study, the humoral reactants have attracted our attention to a greater extent. The novelty of our approach consisted in dealing with the effects of circulating immune complexes (CIC) and antibodies on free circulating antigens and their relationship to tumor burden. To that extent, we have dissected each of the components into its variables to learn more about their relationship. In each case, every effort has been made to maintain the integrity of the in vivo relationship.

Since our earlier reported observations have emphasized primarily the effect of CIC and antibodies on their relationship to tumor burden[2], the present article will concentrate on the antigenic components. These antigens, which have been detected with increased prevalence in fluids from breast carcinoma patients, have been called breast carcinoma associated antigens, denoted hereafter as BCAA. In summary, the isolation techniques used, the preliminary biochemical characterization, the specificity of the moieties detected, and the functional interaction of BCAA and two of the respective monoclonal antibodies raised against human mammary epithelial antigens (HME Ags) with selected breast carcinoma and control sera will be outlined in the following paragraphs. An analysis on the occurrence of free circulating BCAA including details about the detection techniques used will be included, as well as preliminary indications concerning the potential prognostic and tumor-marker roles of BCAA during follow-up of breast carcinoma patients.

Monoclonal Antibodies

The IgG2a monoclonal antibodies (hereafter called Mc 3 and Mc 8) used, kindly supplied by Dr. R.L. Ceriani, John Muir Cancer and Aging Research Institute, Walnut Creek, CA, were prepared against HMEAgs of human milk-fat globule membranes as per details described elsewhere[3]. Mc 3 and Mc 8 biotinylation with biotin-p-nitrophenyl ester (control # 34828, US Biochemical Corp., Cleveland, OH) was performed as described by Kendall et al.[4]

Patient Population under study

One hundred and thirty five BC patients with primary histopathological confirmation of diagnosis were assigned to groups on the basis of objective evaluable tumor burden, as previously described[2,5]. Briefly, Group I included forty-six patients with no evidence of residual tumor at 4 to 6 weeks after surgical excision of all known carcinoma; Group II comprised forty-three patients with limited recurrent disease confined to the chest wall with a tumor mass estimated at < 5 gm; and Group III consisted of forty-six patients known to have advanced regional or distal metastatic disease, with estimated tumor mass at > 5 gm. Serial sample determinations were performed on ten BC patients' sera selected on the basis of known objective clinical episodes of tumor burden changes.

All patients were participants in the breast carcinoma program of the Cancer Control Agency of British Columbia. They were evaluated at 1 to 3 monthly intervals for objective evidence of tumor burden reduction, stabilization, or increase according to criteria reported elsewhere[5,6] in the absence of BCAA results.

In view of reported multiple marker evaluation advantages, and in order to examine how other markers relate to circulating BCAA, patients were monitored for CIC by the fetal liver cell (FLC) or Raji-cell radioimmunoassay (RIA)[7], and anti-XOFA antibodies by isotopic antiglobulin test (IAT)[2,8]. Thirty-five benign breast disease (BBD) patients having biopsy-proven diagnosis of fibrocystic disease or fibroadenoma were similarly evaluated. Seventy normal control sera (NCS) from healthy non-hospitalized volunteers with no known medical illness, were selected for comparison, from the serum bank maintained at the Advanced Therapeutics Department of the Cancer Control Agency of B.C. Also, included from the same source were pretested malignant melanoma, colon and ovarian carcinoma serum samples.

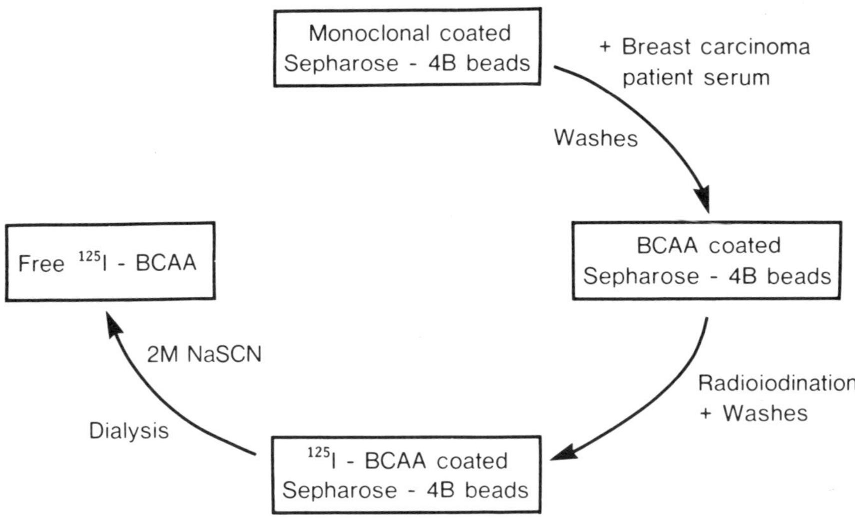

Fig. 1 Schematic representation of BCAA isolation procedure by use of monoclonal antibodies.

TECHNIQUES FOR THE ISOLATION OF BCAA

BCAA have been isolated as free and bound forms from selected breast carcinoma patients' sera in order to achieve further discriminatory capacity. Free circulating BCAA have been isolated by use of monoclonal antibody-coated immunobead procedure. CIC-bound BCAA have been isolated by the polyethylene glycol and the Raji-cell techniques from selected patients' sera with increased (3 to 5-fold over NCS) CIC concentration.

Isolation of BCAA using immunobeads

Both the preparation of monoclonal antibody-coated immunobeads as well as the isolation procedure used were performed as previously described[9]. Briefly, BC patient's serum was incubated with an equal volume of Mc 3 or Mc 8 coated Sepharose-4B immunobeads in PBS, pH 7.2. Immunobeads carrying BCAA recovered from the serum were labeled with ^{125}I, and washed to eliminate unreacted isotope. Bound ^{125}I-BCAA were released from the monoclonal by incubating the immunobeads with sodium thiocyanide or acetate buffer, and dialyzed overnight (Figure 1). A parallel antigen isolation procedure was performed using selected BBD patients' sera.

Results from this isolation technique and the characterization of BCAA from selected BC patients' sera from each tumor burden group was achieved by *in situ* radioiodination of BCAA-coated immunobeads followed by antigen release and subsequent sodium dodecyl sulphate polyacrylamide gel electrophoresis (SDS-PAGE) analysis. BCAA demonstrated increased heterogeneity, while a similar isolation procedure, but using selected BBD sera showed less heterogeneity of breast benign disease antigens (BBDA), as depicted in Figure 2.

Polyethylene Glycol (PEG) Precipitation Method

The test was performed by precipitation of patients' sera containing elevated CIC with 4% polyethylene glycol (PEG-6000, Sigma Chemical Co.,

St. Louis, MO) as described by Digeon et al.[10] and modified by Chia et al.[11] Briefly, precipitates were analyzed by SDS-PAGE as reported earlier[8] for molecular size determination, and characterized by isoelectric focusing. Parallel preparations were evaluated for C3 and IgG by radial immunodiffusion[12]. These results were compared for statistical significance (Student's t test) with normal sera in which the percentages of immunoglobulin and complement components have been previously established. The percentage of these components precipitated by 4% PEG in excess of the normal mean plus two standard deviations was considered to represent immune complexes.

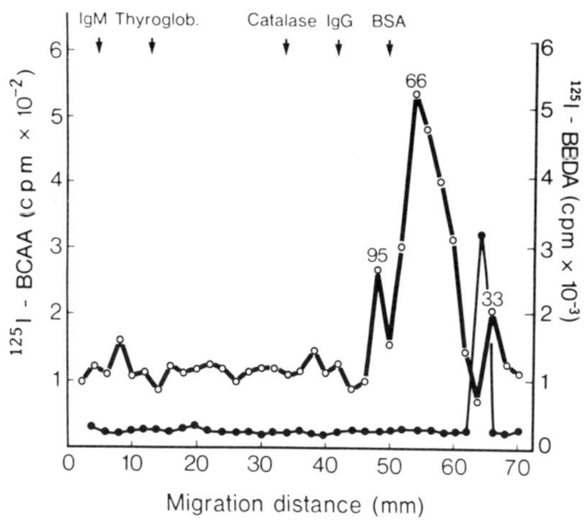

Fig. 2 Representative SDS-PAGE profiles of isolated ^{125}I-BCAA (o——o) and ^{125}I-BBDA (•——•). Standard proteins listed at top were used as reference markers. Estimated Mr (X 10^3) noted on major peaks.

Raji-cell bound CIC Method

This procedure was performed essentially as previously described[13]. The recovery of cell-bound BCAA was accomplished by either: a) incubation of Raji-cell bound radioiodinated CIC with isotonic citrate buffer. After sedimentation, radioactivity associated with both pellet and supernatant was determined, or b) Raji-cells with bound radioiodinated CIC were solubilized with triton in Tris-NaCl-EDTA buffer, and the separation of antigen from antibody was achieved by fractionation on a linear sucrose density gradient 5-35% W/V in dissociation buffer formed in 5 ml cellulose nitrate tubes as described earlier[7] or by SDS-PAGE analysis.

Both separation techniques were demonstrated to retrieve relevant information. The Raji-cell bound CIC method yielded 0.2 to 0.5 mg BCAA/ml serum and 0.4 to 0.9 mg IgG/ml serum. Results of a representative set of

Table 1 Isolation and Characterization of BCAA

CHARACTERISTICS DETERMINED	SELECTED BREAST CARCINOMA PATIENTS Raji-cell Method			PEG Precipitation Method		
TUMOR BURDEN GROUP[a]	I	II	III	I	II	III
ANTIGEN MOIETY						
Total protein yield (mg/ml)	0.2	0.3	0.5	1.2	0.8	0.9
Isoelectric focusing, pI	4.5-5.0	4.5-5.0	4.5-5.0	5.0-5.5	5.4-5.7	5.0-5.3
Mr x 10^3 by SDS-PAGE	34 & 70	31 & 68	34 & 70	34 & 72	34 & 72	34 & 72
ANTIBODY MOIETY						
Total protein yield (mg/ml)	0.4	0.5	0.5	0.8	0.6	0.7
Isoelectric focusing, pI	8.5-8.8	8.5-8.8	8.5-8.8	9.3	9.3	9.3

[a] Grouped by tumor burden as per text.

serum samples from 3 patients are shown in Table 1. Also shown in the same table are results from the PEG precipitation method. This technique demonstrated a higher yield for BCAA (0.8 to 2.0 mg/ml serum) and associated IgG (0.6 to 0.8 mg/ml serum) than the first method described. Raji-cell isolated BCAA demonstrated a common broad isolectric focusing point (pI = 4.5 to 5.0), while associated IgG moieties showed a pI = 8.5 to 8.8. SDS-PAGE determined apparent molecular weights showed heterogeneous moieties approximately at Mr = 34000 and 70000 for BCAA. Similarly determined molecular weights and isolectric focusing points with PEG-extracted BCAA demonstrated minor differences as illustrated in Table 1. The differences observed, although most likely accounted for by the different isolation approaches used, remained to be further investigated.

<u>The specificity of BCAA binding to Mc 3 and Mc 8</u>

The specificity of isolated BCAA from 9 selected BC patients' sera (3 from each tumor burden group) to both Mc 3 and Mc 8 were examined by use of slab gel SDS-PAGE Western blotting procedure, essentially as previously reported[14]. The samples after peroxidase-conjugated goat anti-mouse IgG enzyme-linked immunodetection were measured for band density by a densitometer, model 620 (Bio-Rad Inc., Richmond, CA). The results showed a major single-band reactivity at Mr = 33000 for all BCAA tested. Regardless of tumor burden of patients' sera used for BCAA extraction, a 10-fold stronger band density was observed with Mc 8 than Mc 3. Parallel analysis performed with antigens isolated from 9 selected BBD patients' sera demonstrated minimal reactivity with either monoclonal used (Figure 3).

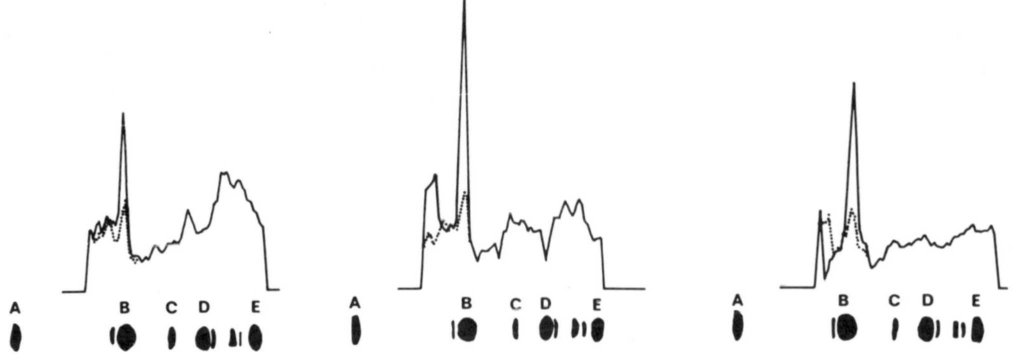

Fig. 3 Immunoblot profiles of Mc 8-detected BCAA isolated from Groups I, II and III (left to right) BC (solid lines) and BBD (broken lines) patients' sera, as determined by densitometer. Protein markers: A, trypsin inhibitor, Mr 21,500; B, carbonic anhydrase, Mr 31,000; C, ovalbumin, Mr 45,000; D, bovine serum albumin, Mr 66,200; and E, Phosphorylase B, Mr 92,500).

Functional Characterization of BCAA, Mc 3 and Mc 8.

The interaction of isolated antigens or monoclonal antibodies with selected BC patients' sera was studied by use of an in vitro model that simulates tumor burden changes[2,15]. By using this model, CIC size changes were examined by titration of either Mc 3 or Mc 8 with selected Group I, II and III BC patients' sera. Conversely, this model was used to simulate defined increases in tumor burden by addition of BCAA to autologous or allogenic patients' sera. The reaction mixture was analyzed for CIC size changes by the SDS-PAGE technique.

The results showed that when serially diluted (50 ul of 1:32 to 1:2048) Mc 3 or Mc 8 were mixed with each of selected Group I, II or III BC patients' sera, changes in patients' sera CIC levels were observed. Maximal CIC changes were achieved with Mc 3 and Mc 8 at 1:128 dilution for Group I, 1:2048 and 1:32 dilution for Group II, and 1:512 and 1:32 for Group III sera, respectively. At optimal Mc 3 and Mc 8 dilution effects, CIC levels were reduced by 32 and 28% for Group I, reduced by 64 and 65% for Group III, but increased by 89 and 41% for Group II patients, respectively (Table 2). However, in a parallel experiment, no CIC change was observed by use of an "indifferent" monoclonal anti-p 97a melanoma associated antigen (Hybritech Inc., La Jolla, CA). Upon addition of ^{125}I-BCAA to BC patients' sera, size analysis of major CIC moieties by SDS-PAGE demonstrated a 1 to 8-fold dissociation of CIC, as compared to unreacted BC serum samples. Autologous combinations resulted in mainly small (7.7S) CIC for Group I and III and intermediate size (9 to 12S) for Group II patients' sera. However, BCAA in allogenic combinations resulted in small CIC for Group I, and intermediate size for Groups II and III. A parallel control determination was performed on BBD sera with two sets of BCAA isolated from BC Groups I, II and III patients. The results showed lack of reactivity as demonstrated by unchanged CIC size moieties in all combinations tested.

Table 2 CIC concentration changes in BC patients serum upon reaction with Mc 3 and Mc 8[a].

BC Group[b]	CIC CONCENTRATION CHANGES[c]				
		Mc 3	Mc 8	Mc 3	Mc 8
	Initial CIC	Final CIC		% Change	
I	96	65	69	32	28
II	74	139	104	89	41
III	176	61	63	65	64

[a] 50 µl of 1:8 diluted patients' serum was reacted with optimally diluted Mc 3 and Mc 8.
[b] Patients' tumor burden grouped as per text.
[c] Average of triplicate determinations of CIC concentration evaluated by Raji-RIA, expressed as µg AHG/ml of serum.

DETECTION OF BCAA IN TUMOR-BURDEN GROUPED BC PATIENTS

One hundred and thirty five BC, twenty each of sarcoma and malignant melanoma, ten each of colon and ovarian carcinoma, thirty-five BBD patients and seventy NCS were evaluated for free circulating BCAA concentration. Reference standard curves made by use of Raji-cell isolated BCAA as well as HME Ags demonstrated minimal quantitative differences when reacted with either Mc 3 or Mc 8, thus the use of BCAA standard reference curves as illustrated in Figure 4 was implemented for the three-step radio-ligand assay. This assay was performed essentially as previously described[9] with minor noted modifications[16]. Test sera (50 ul undiluted) from cancer patients and controls were incubated with packed immunobeads (100 ul). Beads were then reacted with biotin-conjugated Mc 8 or Mc 3 (50 ul). After washing, beads were again incubated with 3 ug of ^{125}I-labeled avidin (control # 28227, US Biochemical Corp.), and their radioactivity determined. The least detectable BCAA concentration was approximately 5 ng/ml serum with a combined intra- and interassay coefficient of variation = 9%. The cut-off value (<20 ng/ml serum) used for classification of results as either normal or elevated was selected on the basis of preliminary results, as analyzed by the Statland et al.[17] technique to minimize the cost of misclassifications.

The results using Mc 8 as detection agent showed significant elevated levels (μ = 105 ng/ml, $p < 0.001$, Mann-Whitney test) of BCAA in one hundred and two of one hundred and thirty-five (76%) BC patients as compared to background levels (<20 ng/ml) in twenty each sarcoma and malignant melanoma patients, and seventy NCS. Slight increases in BCAA levels were observed in ovarian and colon carcinoma, and BBD samples. In 95% of Group II patients elevated BCAA concentration was 3-fold higher than that observed in Group I patients, and 4-fold higher that that of Group III patients tested (Table 3). There was a relationship between tumor burden and their respective mean free-BCAA levels.

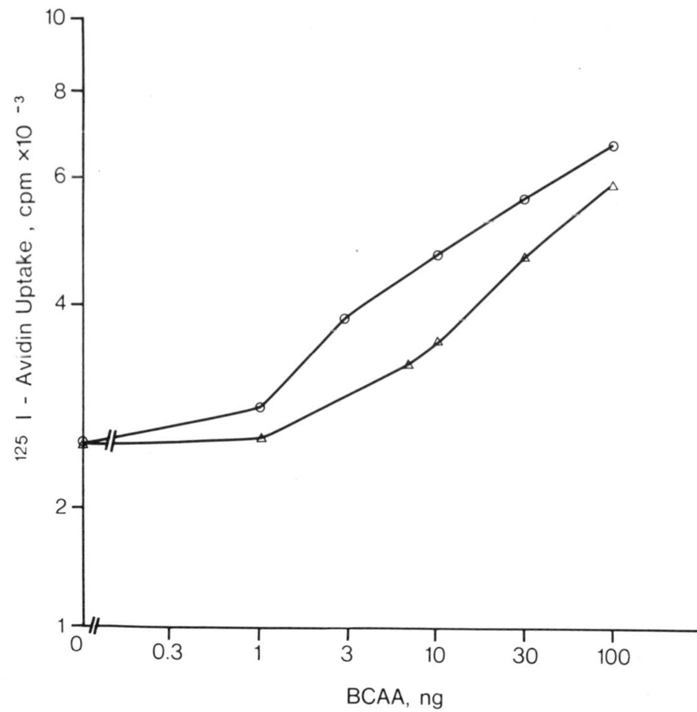

Fig. 4 Typical standard curves for Raji-cell extracted BCAA by a three-step radio-ligand assay. Each point (O = Mc 3, Δ = Mc 8) represents the mean of triplicate determinations.

Table 3. Evaluation of BCAA levels in BC sera by the three-step radioligand immunoassay technique.

Samples tested	BCAA ng/ml (mean ± s.e.)	n elevated[a] / n tested	Percent Elevated	vsNCS[b]
BC Gp. I [c]	70 ± 14	31/46	67	$p \leqq 0.04$
BC Gp. II	197 ± 21	41/43	95	$p \leqq 0.04$
BC Gp. III	50 ± 7	30/46	65	$p \leqq 0.04$
BBD	48 ± 9	20/35	57	$p \leqq 0.04$
M. Melanoma	≦ 20	0/10	0	N/S
Sarcoma	≦ 20	0/10	0	N/S
Ovarian Ca	32 ± 10	3/10	30	N/S
Colon Ca	28 ± 6	3/10	30	N/S
Normal Controls	≦ 20	0/70	0	--

a BCAA elevated values are > 20 ng/ml serum.

b Statistical significance determined by Mann-Whitney test, N/S = not significant.

c Patients' tumor burden grouped as per text.

Adsorption of CIC from sera and testing of residual BCAA

The question of whether the BCAA evaluated was free circulating antigen or bound to CIC or other serum molecules was further investigated. Selected BC patients' sera adsorption with FLC or Raji-cell was performed essentially as described earlier[18]. Both cell types are known to express C3 receptors on the cell surface, thus capable of high affinity immune complex binding[7]. Briefly, 5 X 10 FLC or Raji-cells were used for adsorption and then aliquots of sera prior to and after adsorption were evaluated for BCAA. Cell-adsorption pellets enriched in CIC resulting from these procedures were subsequently treated with isotonic citrate buffer, pH 3.2, in order to release bound BCAA. Resulting BCAA samples were concurrently evaluated by the 3-step radioligand assay. The results demonstrated minimal differences between levels of BCAA before and after adsorption, as illustrated in Table 4. It also demonstrated that target-cell CIC pellets consistently showed minimal BCAA levels.

PREDICTIVE VALUE OF BCAA

Twenty-six patients' sera were retrospectively evaluated for circulating BCAA during intervals at which there were changes in clinical course as reflected by either objective evidence of tumor burden increase or reduction, as compared to twenty-six patients whose tumor burden and BCAA ratio (mean = 1.03) remained unchanged (Table 5). The BCAA ratio for those twenty-six patients whose tumor burden changed, depended on initial and final tumor burden. For six patients with early episodes of increasing tumor burden (Group I to II), there was a concurrent decreased BCAA ratio (mean = 0.25) (Table 6). For eight patients with late episodes of increasing tumor burden (Group II to III) there was concurrent increased BCAA ratio (mean = 8.3) in all. Also those patients who experienced tumor burden regression to Group I showed decreased BCAA levels 4 to 8 weeks later (Table 7), and in four patients presenting tumor burden reduction from Group III to II, there was decreased BCAA ratio (mean = 0.3)

Table 4 BCAA Levels in BC Patients' Sera before and after CIC adsorption

BC Group[a]	Original BCAA ng/ml	BCAA post-adsorption FLC	BCAA post-adsorption Raji-cells	BCAA in CIC pellet FLC	BCAA in CIC pellet Raji-cells
I	214	243	240	< 20	< 20
I	104	104	112	35	< 20
I	86	80	150	< 20	< 20
I	380	290	385	35	24
II	340	320	440	50	42
II	232	250	240	32	35
II	200	210	214	24	35
II	250	268	300	31	30
II	420	336	432	31	28
II	225	214	232	28	< 20

[a] Patients' tumor burden grouped as per text.

TABLE 5 Serum BCAA in BC patients at timed intervals

Tumor Burden	Time[a]	BCAA ng/ml[b] Initial	Final	BCAA Ratio Initial/Final
STABLE				
Group I[c]	7 ± 4	26 ± 8	26 ± 8	1.0 ± 0.2
Group II	6 ± 4	179 ± 72	190 ± 72	0.9 ± 0.1
Group III	8 ± 5	36 ± 30	32 ± 21	1.1 ± 0.2

[a]Interval between serum samples (months) ± S.D.
[b]No statistical differences between initial and final BCAA levels (mean ± S.D.) as calculated by Mann-Whitney test.
[c]Patients' tumor burden groups I, II, & III, n = 14, 5, & 7.

Serial sample determinations were performed on twelve selected BC patients over a 21 to 66-month (median = 28) period. The overall BCAA results demonstrated a tendency to fluctuate with increased values for tumor burden Group II, and lower levels for both Group I and III patients. Using the criterium for evaluation of tumor burden size change (50%), an

TABLE 6 Serum BCAA in BC patients at timed intervals

Tumor Burden[a] PROGRESSION	Time[b]	BCAA ng/ml[c] Initial	Final	BCAA Ratio Initial/Final
I to II	6	< 20	42	0.5
I to II	12	30	110	0.3
I to II	3	27	144	0.2
I to II	4	31	132	0.2
I to II	15	< 20	150	0.1
I to II	6	22	140	0.2
II to III	11	200	60	3.3
II to III	2	110	36	3.1
II to III	9	220	20	11.0
II to III	5	110	36	3.1
II to III	2	660	< 20	33.0
II to III	3	298	52	5.7
II to III	1	236	< 20	11.8
II to III	5	290	120	2.4

[a]Patients' tumor burden grouped as per text.
[b]Interval between serum samples (months).
[c]Statistical differences, initial and final BCAA levels for group changes I to II, $p \leqq 0.004$; II to III, $p \leqq 0.002$; by Mann-Whitney test.

TABLE 7 Serum BCAA in BC patients at timed intervals

Tumor Burden[a] REGRESSION	Time[b]	BCAA ng/ml[c] Initial	Final	BCAA Ratio Initial/Final
II to I	4	200	< 20	10.0
II to I	5	330	< 20	16.5
II to I	2	340	40	8.5
II to I	6	470	54	8.7
II to I	2	69	< 20	3.5
II to I	3	350	40	8.8
II to I	2	232	42	5.5
II to I	4	104	< 20	5.2
III to II	2	37	124	0.3
III to II	1	108	292	0.4
III to II	2	52	340	0.2
III to II	1	35	200	0.2

[a]Patients' tumor burden grouped as per text.
[b]Interval between serum samples (months).
[c]Statistical differences, initial & final BCAA levels for group changes II to I, $p \leqq 0.001$; & III to II, $p \leqq 0.02$, by Mann-Whitney test.

assessment of how BCAA changes related to tumor burden was undertaken. The results showed that in nine of twelve patients, BCAA changes antedated 9 times (3 regressions and 6 progressions) clinical objective evidence of tumor burden changes by 8 to 24 (mean = 16) weeks. Concurrent changes in BCAA levels and tumor burden were observed in three patients, while a 2-month delay was noted in the remaining patient. In all patient follow-ups, an irregular inverse relationship between BCAA and CIC levels was noted. A profile representative of one of these patients, including ongoing clinical and therapeutic interventions, is illustrated in Figure 5.

OVERVIEW AND CONCLUDING REMARKS

The availability of monoclonal antibodies (Mc 3 and Mc 8) and the respective antigen, HME Ags, has enabled the isolation, characterization, and epitope identification of free and bound antigenic moieties extracted from immune reactants occurring in BC patients' sera. This feature has allowed us to compare and identify the qualitative reactive similarities encountered with either antigen source. Whereas, HME Ags consistently demonstrated components at Mr = 95000, 66000 and 33000, patient-extracted antigens (BCAA) more frequently showed moieties at Mr = 33000, and sometimes at Mr = 66000. Whether, this is an expression of monomer-dimer aggregation phenomenon or rather that of precursor moieties, is yet to be investigated. Regardless of the ultimate outcome, HME Ags and BCAA account for a single band reactivity upon Western blot analysis by use of either Mc 3 or Mc 8. Monoclonal antibodies prepared against HME Ags, as well as free and bound BCAA extracted antigens were interacted with BC patients' sera, grouped according to tumor burden, by use of an earlier described _in vitro_ model of tumor burden change[2,15]. Under the defined experimental

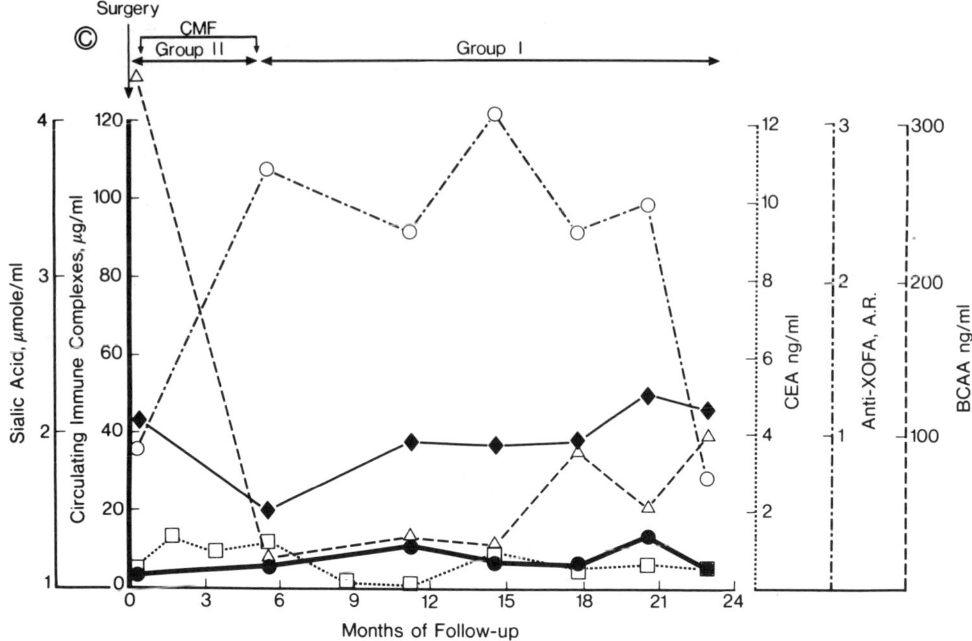

Fig. 5 Representative profile of a BC patient for BCAA (Δ), FLC determined CIC (●), anti-XOFA (o), CEA (□) and sialic acid (◆), including ongoing clinical and therapeutic interventions (CMF = adjuvant chemotherapy).

conditions described, the present evaluation with Mc 3 and Mc 8 (Table 2) and that of BCAA, suggested that Group III patients' CIC were close to or at antigen:antibody equivalence, Group II patients' CIC were in antigen excess, while Group I patients' CIC were in relative antibody excess. By addition of optimal concentration of BCAA to selected BC patients' sera, we assessed how tumor burden changes related to BCAA concentration, size and composition of immune complexes. We have observed that CIC formation and dissociation illustrated a kinetic balance of CIC-size changes as they relate to antigen and antibody concentration. In addition, results of the effects of CIC and antibodies on free circulating BCAA levels, and their relationship to tumor burden may have direct implications on the understanding of clearance, pathogenetic deposition and ultimate fate of CIC.

A modified three-step radioligand immunodetection assay for quantitation of free circulating BCAA in patients' sera has been developed[16]. An overview of assay results demonstrated that although BCAA levels do not correlate linearly with tumor burden, BCAA represent a useful marker to monitor tumor burden. The clear pattern emerging from our studies demonstrated that, associated increased BCAA level to Group II tumor burden, and decreased BCAA level to Groups I and III, was further substantiated by results from our serial sample BCAA determinations. In view of the above results, an extended retrospective survival study to further examine the role of BCAA concentration at diagnosis, as well as during follow-up of BC patients, is currently underway. By use of univariate and multivariate analyses, an evaluation of the role that BCAA and other clinical parameters may have in predicting disease-free interval, and overall survival, is contemplated. Preliminary results of this study suggested BCAA as a prospective adjunct tumor marker for the clinical monitoring of BC patients.

ACKNOWLEDGEMENTS

I thank K.H. Wee and K.L. Lee for their technical assistance, Dr. R.L. Ceriani, John Muir Cancer and Aging Research Institute, Walnut Creek, CA., for kindly supplying HME Ags, Mc 3 and Mc 8. Andy Coldman, Division of Epidemiology, Biometry and Occupational Oncology, CCABC, for assistance in statistical analysis. Terry Nuyten, Bio-Rad Laboratories, Ltd., for assistance in densitomiter determinations, and Linda Wood and Joan Bethune for their secretarial expertise. Figure 2 and Tables 6 and 7 reprinted with permission from Salinas et al (1987), copyright Cancer Research, Inc.

REFERENCES

1. R.K. Oldham, Biological response modifiers program, J. Biol. Resp. Modif. 1:81 (1982).
2. F.A. Salinas, K.H. Wee, and H.K.B. Silver, Clinical relevance of immune complexes, associated antigen and antibody in cancer, in: "Immune Complexes and Human Cancer", pp. 55-109, F.A. Salinas and M.G. Hanna, Jr., eds., Plenum Publ. Co., New York (1985).
3. R.L. Ceriani, J.A. Peterson, J.Y. Lee, R. Moncada, and E.W. Blank, Characterization of cell surface antigens of human mammary epithelial cells with monoclonal antibodies prepared against human milk fat globule, Somatic Cell Genetics 9:415 (1983).
4. C. Kendall, I. Ionescu-Matin, and G.R. Dreesman, Utilization of the biotin/avidin system to amplify the sensitivity of the enzyme-linked immunoadsorbent assay (Elisa), J. Immunol. Method 56:329 (1983).
5. H.K.B. Silver, K.A. Karim, M.J. Gray, and F.A. Salinas, High performance liquid chromatography quantitation of n-acetylneuraminic acid in malignant melanoma and breast carcinoma, J. Chromat. Biomed. Applic. 224:381 (1981).
6. H.K.B. Silver, K.A. Karim, and F.A. Salinas, Significance of sialic acid and carcinoembryonic antigen as monitors of tumor burden among patients with carcinoma of the ovary, Surgery, Gynae & Obst. 153:209 (1981).
7. F.A. Salinas, K.H. Wee, and H.K.B. Silver, Immune complexes and human neoplasia: detection and quantitation of circulating immune complexes by the fetal liver cell assay, Cancer Immunol. Immunother. 12:11 (1981)
8. F.A. Salinas, H.K.B. Silver, K.M. Sheikh, and S.B. Chandor, Natural occurrence of human tumor-associated anti-fetal antibodies during normal pregnancy, Cancer 42:1653 (1978).
9. F.L. Ceriani, M. Sasaki, H. Sussman, W.M. Wara, and E.W. Blank, Circulating human mammary epithelial antigens in breast cancer, Proc. Natl. Acad. Sci. USA 79:5420 (1982).
10. M. Digeon, M. Laver, J. Riza, and J.F. Bach, Detection of circulating immune complexes in human sera by a simplified assay - with polyethylene glycol, J. Immunol. Method 16:165 (1977).
11. D. Chia, E.V. Barnett, J. Yamagata, D. Knutson, C. Restivo, and D. Faust, Quantitation and characterization of soluble immune complexes precipitated from sera by polyethylene glycol, Clin. Exp. Immunol. 37:399 (1979).
12. G. Mancini, A.O. Carbonara, and J.F. Heremans, Immunochemical quantitation of antigens by single radial immunodiffusion, Immunochem. 2:235 (1965).
13. A.N. Theofilopoulos, R.A. Eisenberg, and F.J. Dixon, Isolation of circulating immune complexes using Raji cells: separation of antigens

from immune complexes and production of antiserum, J. Clin. Invest. 61:1570 (1978).

14. S.J. McDougal, S.M. Kennedy, M.Hubbard, S.W. Browning, V.C.W. Tsang, E.F. Winton, and F.C. McDuffie, Antigen detection in immune complexes by a modified staphylococci binding assay and Western blot analysis, Clin. Immunol. Immunopath. 38:184 (1986).
15. F.A. Salinas, K.H. Wee, and H.K.B. Silver, Tumor burden and its relationship to antigen, size and composition of immune complexes, in: "31st Colloquium Prot. Biol. Fluids", pp. 749-752, H. Peeters, ed., Pergamon Press Ltd., Oxford, England (1984).
16. F.A. Salinas, K.H. Wee, and R.L. Ceriani, Significance of breast carcinoma-associated antigens as a monitor of tumor burden: characterization by monoclonal antibodies, Cancer Res. 47:907 (1987).
17. B.E. Statland, P. Winkel, M.D. Burke, and R.S. Golen, Quantitative approaches used in evaluating laboratory measurements and other clinical data, in: "Clinical Diagnosis and Management of Laboratory Methods," pp. 525-534, J.B. Henry, ed., W.B. Saunders Co., Philadelphia (1979).
18. F.A. Salinas, and K.H. Wee, Prognostic and pathogenetic implications of immune complexes in cancer, in: "Advances in Immunity and Cancer Therapy," 2:189, P.K. Ray, ed., Springer-Verlag Inc., New York (1986).

SESSION III

DETECTION AND ASSAY OF THE 52K ESTROGEN-REGULATED PROTEASE IN MAMMARY TUMORS

H. Rochefort*+, V. Cavailles*, G. Freiss*, D. Derocq*, G. Salazar*, T. Maudelonde+, S. Khalaf+, H. Rogier°, F. Paolucci°, B. Pau° and M. Garcia*

*Unité d'Endocrinologie Cellulaire et Moléculaire (U148) INSERM, 60 rue de Navacelles, 34100 Montpellier, +Laboratoire de Biochimie Cellulaire Hormonale, Faculté de Médecine, Montpellier, and °Clin Midy Sanofi, Rue du Pr Joseph Blayac, 34082 Montpellier, France

INTRODUCTION

The importance of estrogens in stimulating the growth of human breast cancer is now well recognized, even though the molecular mechanisms of estrogen action are not fully understood (1). Monoclonal antibodies to estrogen-regulated antigens in breast cancer may therefore be of interest both as prognostic markers for breast cancer management and as a means of understanding how breast cancer growth is controlled. Antibodies to the estrogen and progesterone receptors are now available to help clinicians select optimal breast cancer therapies (2). Monoclonal antibodies raised against estrogen induced proteins may also be useful, since some of these proteins can potentially mediate the stimulatory effect of estrogens on breast cancer cells (3,4). The secreted proteins are particularly interesting in this respect since they may display both autocrine and paracrine functions and modulate the growth and invasion of breast cancer cells. We have focused on one of these proteins of 52,000 daltons (52K) which is induced specifically by estrogens and secreted by the MCF7 and ZR75-1 human breast cancer cell lines (5). We first summarize our knowledge of the structure and function of this protein which provides a basis for understanding its use as a marker. We then review the first clinical studies in benign and malignant mastopathies indicating the potential of this protein as a marker of cell proliferation and possibly of tumor invasion.

STRUCTURE AND FUNCTION OF THE 52K PROTEIN

Estrogens stimulate the production of a 52K protein in the culture medium of MCF7 and ZR75-1 human mammary cancer cells, whereas antiestrogens have no agonist effect on this protein (4). Since this finding, our laboratory has raised monoclonal antibodies against this protein (6), purified it to homogeneity (7) and identified it as the precursor of a cathepsin-D-like lysosomal protease bearing mannose 6-P (phosphate) signals on its N-glycosylated chains (8,9). It can be reinternalized in the same cells which secrete it. Two *in vitro* biological activities of the protein have been detected. It is able to stimulate the growth of MCF7 cells (10), and when activated by the removal of the N-terminal fragment (giving a 51K protein), both the secreted and its processed cellular forms (48K, 34K, and 14K) show an acidic protease activity on various substrates including proteoglycans (8) and basement membrane (Morisset et al., in preparation). In the hormone-dependent MCF7 cells, estrogens markedly increase the amount of secreted 52K protein (5) and also the synthesis of the corresponding cellular proteins (11) which are produced at a basal level, in the absence of estrogens.

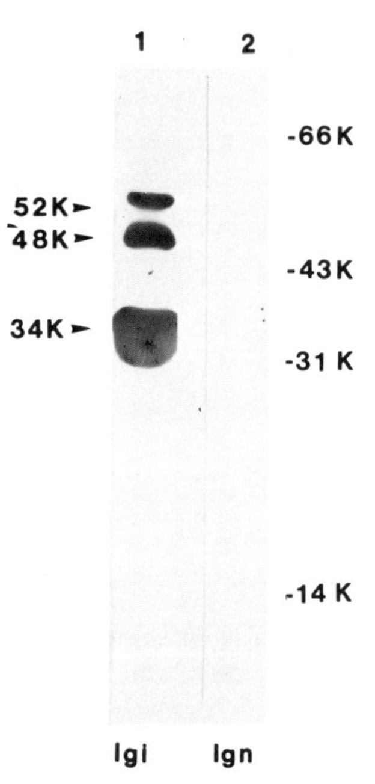

Figure 1. Western immunoblot of the cellular 52K-related proteins. MCF7 cells were lysed in NP40 buffer and the cell lysate was partially purified on Con-A-Sepharose. Aliquots of the eluate containing 200, 200, 500, and 300 ng of the 52, 48, 34, and 17K proteins, respectively, were separated by SDS-PAGE and transferred to nitrocellulose. Nitrocellulose strips were immunodetected with the culture supernatants of either M1G8 hybridomas (Igi) or myelomas (Ign) and revealed by a peroxidase conjugated anti-mouse IgG antibody. Reproduced from ref. 7 by permission of the Editor.

MONOCLONAL ANTIBODIES TO THE 52K PROTEIN

Two series of antibodies have been developed, recognizing two distinct parts of the molecule. The first generation of antibodies (6) recognizes both the secreted (52K) and the processed cellular forms (48K and 34K) (Fig. 1). Seven antibodies have been purified and characterized. They recognize three different domains located on the 34K moiety (C terminal) of the 52K precursor (Fig. 2). All clinical studies reviewed here have been performed with these antibodies. The second generation of antibodies has recently been screened by their ability to recognize only the cellular 52K precursor and not the processed products. Two have been purified and characterized (Freiss et al., in preparation) ; they recognize two different epitopes located on the profragment of the molecule (N-terminal end) and therefore interact exclusively with the 52K proenzyme (Fig. 2). With these antibodies, two double-determinant immunoassays have been developed for specifically measuring in cell extracts and biological fluids, the total 52K related proteins (52K, 48K, 34K) on one hand and exclusively the 52K precursor on the other hand.

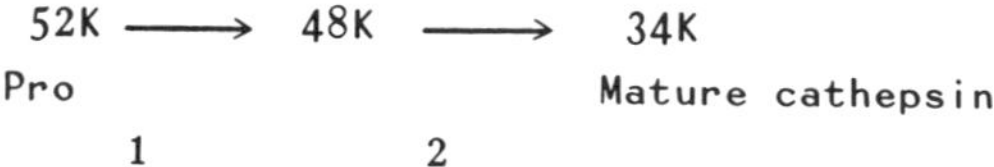

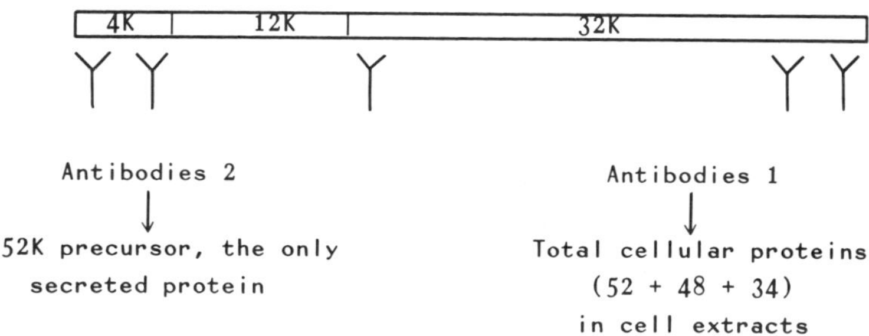

Figure 2. Double-determinant immunoassay of the 52K proteins. The structure of the 52K protein is schematically represented. The two high-mannose N-glycosylated chains of approx. 2,000 daltons each are not represented. Cleavage of the 52K precursor first gives a 48K protein by removal of the profragment and then a 34K protein corresponding to a mature cathepsin-D-like enzyme. Two series of antibodies, 1 and 2, interacting with the 32K and the 4K fragments, respectively, can be used to assay either the total immunoreactive cellular proteins (series 1 antibodies) or exclusively the 52K precursor, which is the only protein to be secreted (series 2 antibodies). Solid phase double-determinant immunoassays have been monitored in both cases (6, Freiss et al., and Rogier et al., in preparation).

IMMUNOPEROXIDASE STAINING OF THE 52K-RELATED CELLULAR PROTEINS IN NON-CANCER TISSUES

Using these monoclonal antibodies, we have examined frozen sections of several human tissues (12) with the peroxidase-anti-peroxidase technique of Sternberger. Negative controls were routinely performed with an excess of antigen, or with irrelevant IgG antibodies showing the staining specificity. Most of the staining was granular in the cytoplasm and corresponded to lysosomes. No plasma membrane staining was detected. Among the different normal tissues studied, the protein appeared to be mostly concentrated in sweat glands and liver, but not in normal uterus or normal resting mammary glands collected by reduction mammoplasties (12). By contrast, immunostaining was observed in 43% of 127 biopsies of benign mastopathies (13). Gynecomastias, fibroadenomas, and fibrous lesions were most often negative. Lobular structures were also mostly negative (adenosis, sclerosing adenosis, atypical lobular hyperplasia). The two groups of mastopathies that were highly stained consisted of cysts over 3 mm in diameter and ductal hyperplasias.

When the different histological types (Table 1) were pooled into proliferative (high-risk) and nonproliferative (low-risk) lesions, according to criteria defined by Dupont and Page (14), we found a significant correlation between proliferation and 52K protein staining. Among the 23% of the lesions that were proliferative, nearly 80% were positive for the 52K protein. The negative cases were all lobular hyperplasia. In the nonproliferative group, only 32% of the tumors were stained. This positivity was due mainly to the presence of cysts. The use of 52K protein staining in predicting high-risk (proliferative) mastopathies therefore appears to be useful, since 91.5% of the 52K-protein-negative lesions were non-proliferative and 60.5% of the 52K-protein-positive (non-cystic) lesions were proliferative.

Table 1. Immunodetection of the 52K protein and breast cancer risk in benign breast disease

Disease	n° cases	52K immunostaining 0	+[a]	++	Risk factor[b]
Gynecomastia	4	4	–	–	x1.0
Fibroadenoma	16	11	4[c]	1[c]	x1.0
Adenosis	23	22	–	1	x1.0
Sclerosing adenosis	6	5	1	–	x1.0
Fibrous mastopathy	39	30	8[c]	1[c]	x1.0
TOTAL 1[d]	88	72(82%)	13(15%)	3(3%)	
Cystic disease					
< 3 mm	13	2	3	8	x1.4 to 4.0
> 3 mm	5	–	2	3	
Ductal hyperplasia	21	–	7	14	x1.8 to 3.0
Solitary papilloma	1	1	–	1	x2.7
Atypical lobular hyperplasia	1	1	–	–	x4.0
TOTAL 2	41	3(7%)	12(30%)	26(63%)	
TOTAL 1 + 2	129	75(58%)	25(19%)	29(22.5%)	

[a] +, 1 to 5% positive epithelial cells ; ++, 5% positive epithelial cells
[b] Relative risk factor according to Azzopardi and Haagensen
[c] Staining in ductal structure
[d] Staining percentages of groups 1 and 2 are significantly different at $P < 0.001$

Reproduced from Ref. 13 with the permission of the Editor.

Table 2. The 52K protein is a marker of mammary cell proliferation.

1. Not detected in resting normal mammary cells, but detected in these cells proliferating in vitro.
2. Higher in proliferative ductal mastopathies (13).
3. More secreted during exponential growth than at confluency in MCF7 and ZR75-1 cells (Derocq D., unpublished)
4. In vitro autocrine mitogenic effect on MCF7 cells (10).

Normal mammary glands are not stained when directly analyzed after surgery (12), but their concentration in 52K-related proteins is markedly increased when they grow in primary culture after collagenase digestion, where 52K immunostaining is generally observed (unpublished results). From the results summarized in Table 2, we conclude that the 52K protein is associated with the proliferation of ductal mammary cells and with cysts, two characteristics that have been shown to increase breast cancer risk (14,15), and that its high cellular concentration is not specific to transformed cells.

IMMUNOHISTOCHEMICAL DISTRIBUTION IN BREAST CARCINOMAS AND ABSENCE OF CORRELATION WITH CYTOSOLIC STEROID RECEPTORS

Among the cancer tissues examined, approximately 64% of the breast carcinomas were stained in tumor cells but not in stroma. Some of the melanomas were also stained. In order to see whether this protein is a marker of hormone responsiveness, we studied 232 primary breast carcinomas collected from April to September 1985, in three French cancer centers (Institut Gustave Roussy, Villejuif ; Centre Antoine Lacassagne, Nice ; Centre Paul Lamarque, Montpellier). The 52K protein was evaluated in frozen sections by immunohistochemistry, and the concentration of estrogen receptors and progesterone receptors were assayed in the cytosol by the classical dextran-coated charcoal method (16).

Altogether, the 52K protein was detected in 64% of the 232 tumor biopsies. In 80% of the 52K-positive tumors, the staining was very heterogeneous and affected only 1 to 30% of the epithelial tumor cells. The staining was generally less homogeneous in breast cancer cells than in proliferative benign mastopathies and in cells bordering the lumen of large cysts. In the four categories of tumors defined according to their positivity for estrogen and progesterone receptors (Table 3a), a similar proportion of tumors was found to be positive for the 52K protein.

Table 3. Absence of correlation between 52K protein and estrogen and progesterone receptors

a. In 232 breast carcinomas(16)			b. Double immunostaining of 35 fine-needle aspirates of breast cancers (17)		
Cytosolic Receptors	52K immunostaining cases n°	%	Groups	cases n°	%
RE-/RP-	37/54	68	RE+/52K+	18	52
RE-/RP+	14/21	67	RE-/52K+	9	26
RE+/RP-	23/31	74	RE+/52K-	4	11
RE+/RP+	75/126	59	RE-/52K-	4	11

a. Accessible estrogen (RE) and progesterone (RP) receptor sites were assayed in tumor cytosol by the dextran-coated charcoal technique. A concentration of 10 fmoles/mg protein is defined as the limit between receptor-positive and receptor-negative patients, both for RE and RP. The amount of cellular 52K protein was evaluated on tissue sections by immunoperoxidase staining. The tumors containing more than 1% stained cells were considered to be 52K-protein-positive tumors.

b. Double-immunostaining of the nuclear RE (Abbott Laboratories, ERICA kit) and of the cytoplasmic 52K protein was performed on breast cancer cell aspirates. The RE was stained in greyish blue by Abbott antibodies (ERICA) and the 52K protein stained red by the D7E3 antibody of series 1. Positivity was defined as more than 3% stained-cells. The validity of this semiquantification is described in (17).

The RE+/RP+ group was not significantly different from the RE-/RP- group or the total population (64%) with respect to 52K-protein immunostaining. Moreover, when the percentage of the 52K-protein-stained cells was plotted against the cytosolic RE and RP concentrations, no statistical correlation, either positive or negative, was observed between the estrogen or progesterone receptor concentration and the amount of 52K positive cells. The absence of correlation between these two types of markers was also shown directly using fine-needle aspirates of breast carcinomas to perform double immunohistochemical staining of the nuclear RE and cytoplasmic 52K protein in the same sample (17). The first results from 35 patients also indicate that the two markers are not correlated. (Table 3b). There were tumor cells with 52K protein and without RE staining, and others with RE and without 52K protein. These data suggest that the amount of 52K protein is not correlated with that of the estrogen receptor in breast cancer cells and that the information given by the evaluation of the 52K protein is different and complementary to that given by the assay of hormone receptors. In order to obtain a better quantification of the concentration of the 52K protein, we then used a solid phase double-determinant immunoassay of the total 52K proteins (13 and H. Rogier et al., in preparation).

IMMUNOASSAY OF THE 52K PROTEIN ACCUMULATED AND SECRETED BY BREAST CANCER CELL LINES

Using two different antibodies recognizing two domains of the 34K cellular product (6), both the precursor (52K) and its cellular products (48K + 34K) are assayed (Fig. 2). The technique was applied both in the culture medium and in the cytosol, to assay the secreted and the total cellular forms, respectively. The concentration of the 52K protein was determined by reference to a standard purified 52K protein assayed by silver staining.

The production and secretion of the 52K protein were compared in several estrogen-receptor-positive (RE+) and negative (RE-) cell lines cultured in 10% fetal calf serum containing estrogens (Fig. 3).

All RE-positive cell lines tested at confluency produced the 52K protein in the presence of estradiol, but its secretion varied markedly according to the cell line. For instance, the secretion by T47D cells was lower that that of MCF7-1 cells, whereas their cytosol concentrations were not very different. The secretion of the protein also varied markedly according to the subline species. For instance, the secretion of 52K protein by the two MCF7 species was quite different. A ZR75-1 line, obtained by courtesy of Dr R.J.B. King, also produced less 52K protein than the one shown here.

Interestingly, this protein was also produced and secreted by the two RE-negative breast cancer cell lines (BT20, MDA-MB231). The secretion of 52K protein by RE-negative cell lines varied according to their degree of confluency and number of passages, and their intracellular concentrations were sometimes higher than in some RE-positive cell lines. The only human mammary cell line producing no measurable 52K protein was the HBL100 line, which was immortalized from normal cells isolated from milk. Other human cancers such as melanoma (M1477) and uterine cervix cancer (Hela) were found to produce and secrete the protein constitutively.

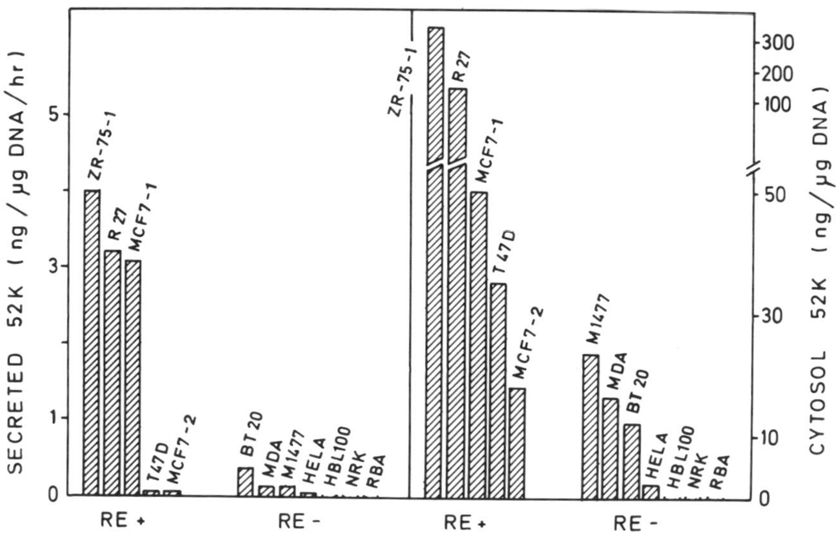

Figure 3. Concentrations of the 52K protein in the culture medium and cytosol of RE-positive and RE-negative epithelial cell lines. The 52K protein was quantified by immunoradiometric assay in the 4-day-conditioned medium and the cytosol of the indicated cell lines. The human cell lines were derived from breast cancers (ZR75-1, R27, MCF7-1, T47D, MCF7-2, BT20, MDA-MB231), melanoma (H1477), cervix carcinoma (Hela) and normal milk mammary cells (HBL-100). The two rat cell lines were from mammary cancer (RBA) and normal kidney (NRK). The cell lines are classified as estrogen receptor positive (RE+) or negative (RE-) according to data in the literature.
Reproduced from (16) by permission of the Editor.

52K PROTEIN CONCENTRATION IN 175 BREAST CANCER CYTOSOLS

We have also completed the first clinical study on 175 cytosols prepared from primary breast cancers in which the 52K protein and the RE and RP sites were assayed (18). The tentative conclusion of this study is summarized in Table 4. The concentration of 52K protein varied markedly according to the patient, as did the proportion of the 52K precursor. The absence of correlation with the estrogen receptor was confirmed. The slight correlation with axillary lymph node invasion indicates that the assay of 52K protein in cytosol may be valuable as a prognostic marker for predicting the degree of invasiveness of breast cancers. This is in full agreement with the proteolytic activity of the protein on basal membrane and proteoglycans.

Table 4

IEMA OF 52K PROTEIN IN CYTOSOL FROM 175 PRIMITIVE BREAST CANCERS

1. A prospective study starting February 1985. Pre- and post-menopausal patients (Centre Paul Lamarque, Montpellier and other Languedoc Hospitals).
2. Concentration of total 52K (secreted + cellular) from 52 to 2,800 U/mg cytosol protein (mean=400).
3. No correlation with RE (r=0.15) and slight correlation with RP (r=0.41).
4. High concentrations of 52K (> 700 U/mg proteins) are correlated with lymph nodes invasion ($p < 0.01$).
5. Variable proportion of the 52K precursor 0% to 42% of the total 52K cellular proteins (52+48+34).
6. Not correlated with Scarff and Bloom grading, tumor size and age of patients.

Cytosol was prepared from nonirradiated breast cancers. The concentration of the 52K protein (total and precursor) was measured by a double-determinant immunoenzymatic assay using our first series of antibodies (see Fig. 2). The concentration of RE was determined by a similar enzymatic assay using Abbott antibodies (kit ER-EIA) and that of RP sites by the classical charcoal assay. Axillary lymph nodes invasion was defined by the pathologist following radical mastectomy. Detailed informations in Ref. 18.

CONCLUSIONS AND PERSPECTIVES

From current studies, it is clear that the 52K protein is not a new marker of hormone dependency but rather a marker associated with tumor proliferation and possibly invasiveness. A retrospective study with the Finsen Institute of Copenhagen on 149 patients clinically followed up for 8 years has recently shown a significant shorter disease-free interval in patients with high total 52K protein concentration (> 400 u/mg protein) than in patients with low concentrations (< 400 u/mg protein) (S. Thorpe et al., in preparation). These preliminary results are further analysed to determine whether or not the 52K protein is an independent prognostic factor. Since the 52K protein concentration is not correlated with the estrogen receptor, its assay in the cytosol of breast cancer may usefully complement that of the sex steroid receptors. Other studies on a larger number of patients, with clinical follow-up for 5 to 10 years, are needed to confirm the usefulness of this marker. The 52K protein can also be detected and semi-quantified in isolated cells collected by fine-needle aspiration before any therapy. By contrast, its assay in the plasma using available antibodies does not seem to be useful since the basal level in normal patients, probably due to liver secretion, is too high. The assay and detection of the 52K precursor alone using the second series of antibodies may provide information supplementary to that obtained with the antibodies recognizing both the precursor and the processed cellular products, since the precursor is the only one to be secreted and to potentially act on neighbouring cells and extracellular matrix. Finally, a better knowledge of the structure of the breast cancer 52K protein compared to that of other cathepsin D proteins may guide us in the development of new antibodies recognizing epitopes more specifically related to the 52K breast cancer protein. In addition to other growth factors (19) and proteases (20) the 52K estrogen-induced protease may have important autocrine and paracrine functions in regulating breast cancer growth and invasion. The first clinical studies support this assumption, since this protease appears to be useful, *via* its different monoclonal antibodies to predict high-risk mastopathies and invasive breast cancers. More generally, the 52K protein illustrates how a rational approach can be used to develop better markers. It also indicates that basic research aimed at understanding the structure and function of proteins possibly involved in mammary carcinogenesis can lead to medical applications.

ACKNOWLEDGEMENTS

We are grateful to the following Anti-Cancer Centers in France (Gustave Roussy, Villejuif; Antoine Lacassagne, Nice; Paul Lamarque, Montpellier) for clinical studies and particularly to Drs Contesso, Delarue, Duplay, Domergue, Simony and Pr Pujol. We are indebted to our colleagues of INSERM U 148 for their studies on the structure and function of the protein (F. Capony, F. Vignon, M. Morisset, I. Touitou) and to M. Egea and E. Barrié for their skillful preparation of the manuscript. This work was supported by the "Institut National de la Santé et de la Recherche Médicale", the "Association pour la Recherche sur le Cancer", the "Fédération Nationale des Centres de Lutte contre le Cancer", Clin-Midy/ Sanofi Laboratories (Collaborative contract n°83052-A), and the Faculty of Medicine of Montpellier.

REFERENCES

1. M.E. Lippman, G. Bolan and K. Huff, The effects of estrogens and antiestrogens on hormone-responsive human breast cancer in long-term tissue culture, *Cancer Res.* 36:4595 (1976).
2. G.L. Greene, N.B. Sobel, W.L. King and E.V. Jensen, Immunochemical studies of estrogen receptors, *J. Steroid Biochem.* 20:51 (1984).
3. H. Rochefort, D. Chalbos, F. Capony, M. Garcia, F. Veith, F. Vignon and B. Westley, Effect of estrogen in breast cancer cells in culture : Released proteins and control of cell proliferation, *in*: "Hormones and Cancer", E. Gurpide, R. Calandra, C. Levy and R.J. Soto, eds, Alan Liss Inc., New York, Vol. 142, pp. 37, (1984).
4. D.J. Adams, D.P. Edwards and W.L. McGuire, Estrogen regulation of specific proteins as a mode of hormone action in human breast cancer, *in*: "Biomembranes", Vol. 11, pp 389, (1983).
5. B. Westley and H. Rochefort, A secreted glycoprotein induced by estrogen in human breast cancer cell lines, *Cell* 20:352 (1980).
6. M. Garcia, F. Capony, D. Derocq, D. Simon, B. Pau and H. Rochefort, Monoclonal antibodies to the estrogen-regulated Mr 52,000 glycoprotein : Characterization and immunodetection in MCF7 cells, *Cancer Res.* 45:709 (1985).
7. F. Capony, M. Garcia, C. Rougeot, J. Capdevielle, P. Ferrara and H. Rochefort, Purification and first characterization of the secreted and cellular 52-kDa proteins regulated by estrogens in human breast cancer cells, *Eur. J. Biochem.* 161:505 (1986).
8. F. Capony, M. Morisset, A. Barrett, J.P. Capony, P. Broquet, F. Vignon, M. Chambon, P. Louisot and H. Rochefort, Phosphorylation, glycosylation and proteolytic activity of the 52K estrogen-induced protein secreted by MCF7 cells, *J. Cell. Biol.* in press (1987).
9. M. Morisset, F. Capony and H. Rochefort, The 52-kDa estrogen-induced protein secreted by MCF7 cells is a lysosomal acidic protease, *Biochem. Biophys. Res. Commun.* 138:102 (1986).

10. F. Vignon, F. Capony, M. Chambon, G. Freiss, M. Garcia and H. Rochefort, Autocrine growth stimulation of the MCF7 breast cancer cells by the estrogen-regulated 52K protein, Endocrinology 118:1537 (1986).
11. M. Morisset, F. Capony and H. Rochefort, Processing and estrogen regulation of the 52-kDa protein inside MCF7 breast cancer cells, Endocrinology 119:2773 (1986).
12. M. Garcia, G. Salazar-Retana, G. Richer, J. Domergue, F. Capony, H. Pujol, F. Laffargue, B. Pau and H. Rochefort, Immunohistochemical detection of the estrogen-regulated Mr 52,000 protein in primary breast cancers but not in normal breast and uterus, J. Clin. Endocrin. Met. 59:564 (1984).
13. M. Garcia, G. Salazar-Retana, A. Pages, G. Richer, J. Domergue, A.M. Pages, G. Cavalié, J.M. Martin, J.L. Lamarque, B. Pau, H. Pujol and H. Rochefort, Distribution of the Mr 52,000 estrogen-regulated protein in benign breast diseases and other tissues by immunohistochemistry, Cancer Res. 46:3734 (1986).
14. W.D Dupont and D.L. Page, Risk factors for breast cancer in women with proliferative breast disease, N. Engl. J. Med. 312:146 (1985).
15. C.D. Haagensen, C. Bodian and D.E.Jr. Haagensen, "Breast Carcinoma Risk and Detection", W.B. Saunders Co, Philadelphia (1981).
16. M. Garcia, G. Contesso, H. Duplay, V. Cavaillès, D. Derocq, J.C. Delarue, B. Krebs, H. Sancho-Garnier, G. Richer, J. Domergue, M. Namer and H. Rochefort, Immunohistochemical distribution of the 52K protein in mammary tumors : A marker associated to cell proliferation rather than to hormone responsiveness, J. Steroid. Biochem., in press (1987).
17. V. Cavaillès, M. Garcia, G. Salazar, J. Domergue, J. Simoni, H. Pujol and H. Rochefort, Submitted for publication.
18. T. Maudelonde, G. Cavalié, S. Khalaf, D. Francès and H. Rochefort, In preparation.
19. R.B. Dickson, K.K. Huff, E.M. Spencer and M.E. Lippman, Induction of epidermal growth factor-related polypeptides by 17ß-estradiol in MCF-7 human breast cancer cells, Endocrinology 118:138 (1986).
20. L.A. Liotta, Tumor invastion and Metastases. Role of the extracellular matrix : Rhoads memorial award lecture. Cancer Res. 46:1 (1986).

DIVERSITY OF ANTIGENIC EXPRESSION ON NORMAL AND MALIGNANT HUMAN MAMMARY CELLS RECOGNIZED BY A NEW PANEL OF MONOCLONAL ANTIBODIES

E. Gerö[1234], Ph. Hageman[1], J. Hilkens[1], J. Sugar[2] and J. Hilgers[14].

[1] The Netherlands Cancer Institute, Antoni van Leeuwenhoekhuis, Division of Tumor Biology, Plesmanlaan 121, 1066 CX Amsterdam, The Netherlands
[2] National Cancer Institute, Oncopathological Research Institute, Budapest, Hungary
[3] Present address: Centocor Inc., 244 Great Valley Parkway, Malvern PA 19355, USA
[4] To whom requests for reprints and available antibody samples have to be addressed

SUMMARY

Mouse monoclonal antibodies were generated to membrane preparations of human primary breast carcinomas. The reactivity patterns were studied on frozen sections of malignant and benign mammary tumors and normal breast tissues by immunoperoxidase staining and on cultured mammary tumor cell lines by immunofluorescence reactions. The diversity of reactivities indicated distinct, unique specificities of the monoclonals.

In the normal mammary epithelium a broad range of binding patterns was found. Several antibodies exclusively stained the luminal epithelium, others reacted with both luminal and myoepithelial cells, and one antibody (130E5) was preferentially reactive with myoepithelium. Four antibodies represent unique markers for epithelial cells: 126E7 is specific for the apical membrane of luminal cells, 125B5 and 126H3 stain the cytoplasm and the lateral-basal membranes of epithelia, whereas 126G5 binds to the cytoplasm of luminal epithelium.

The monoclonals showed a range of positive reactions from 30 to 100 percent in about 30-35 breast cancer cases tested. Seven monoclonals proved to be strongly reactive in a high percentage of malignant cases. All of them had a significant binding also to normal or benign epithelium. However, distribution in malignant cells often lacked the polarized pattern found to be characteristic in normal epithelium.

On in vitro cell lines most antibodies reacted with cell surface determinants; two reacted exclusively with the cytoskeletal network in immunofluorescence test. Several antibodies showed heterogeneous reactivity, revealing a phenotypic diversity among cells in normal mammary epithelium, in primary breast carcinomas and tumor cell lines.

INTRODUCTION

A great variety of antigenic determinants can be found on the cell surface, in the cytoskeleton, in the cytosol or in extracellular products of tumor cells, and their complex composition is characteristic of the histocompatibility phenotype, the tissue origin, the differentiation and functional state of the cell. The cell type and differentiation antigens display a complex distribution in non-neoplastic tissues (Foster et al., 1982b). Malignant cells may express determinants in an elevated concentration compared to normal cells (Ashall et al., 1982, Koprowski et al., 1979, Loop et al., 1981) or to the cells of the corresponding normal tissue (Teramoto et al., 1982, Stramignoni et al., 1983). However, no particular determinant has proved to be able to reliably distinguish between all kinds of normal and malignant cells. A tumor-associated antigenic determinant can be present on a variety of normal cells as well (Atkinson et al., 1982). On the other hand, no individual determinant has been found to be useful for reliable histogenetical identification of a tumor, as both differentiation and tumor-associated antigens can be expressed on a variety of tumors of different organs (Foster et al., 1982, McGee et al., 1982). An antibody raised by White et al. (1985) against the MCF-7 human mammary carcinoma cell line shows organ specificity for breast tumors, with the exception of one cross-reacting colon carcinoma, but as yet only a limited number of tumors from other sites has been tested.

Monoclonal antibodies (MoAbs) are an unique means for recognizing individual determinants (Kohler and Milstein, 1975). A range of MoAbs with known tissue, cell-type and functional specificity helps to identify the tissue or cell type origin of a tumor and to characterize its differentiation stage and cellular composition (Neville, 1982). Monoclonals as differentiation and behavioral markers can be effectively used for distinguishing between the component cell types of an organ, like the mammary gland (Taylor-Papadimitriou et al., 1983, Foster et al., 1982b, Edwards et al., 1982, Hand et al., 1983).

Various antigenic sources have been used for generating MoAbs to normal and neoplastic breast epithelium. The milk fat globule membrane, representing the luminal cell surface of lactating epithelium, has been extensively used for producing polyclonal (Heyderman et al., 1979, Sloane and Ormerod, 1981, Imai and Tokes, 1981) and monoclonal antibodies (Arklie et al., 1981, Taylor-Papadimitriou et al., 1981, Foster et al., 1982, Hilkens et al., 1981, 1984 and Ceriani et al., 1983). Monoclonal antibodies raised to cultured human mammary tumor cells (Papsidero et al., 1983, Thompson et al., 1983, Soule et al., 1983) recognize determinants on various normal and neoplastic tissues. Metastatic mammary tumors cells were applied as immunogen for MoAbs (Colcher et al., 1981), from which one was claimed to detect a determinant associated with carcinomas (Schlom et al., 1980, Stramignoni et al., 1983), but which also reacts with normal breast tissue.

We report a range of MoAbs to primary breast carcinomas with different distribution patterns of binding to the normal and malignant breast epithelium, demonstrating a broad diversity of antigenic determinants which are simultaneously expressed by tumor cells. Some of the antibodies proved to provide new differentiation marker of normal mammary epithelium.

MATERIALS AND METHODS

Primary mammary tumors from two different surgical cancer cases were used for membrane preparations no. 1 and no. 2. The tumor tissue was cut into pieces in ice-cold PBS, homogenized in 0.25 M sucrose solution containing protease inhibitors (0.005% phenyl-methyl-sulphonylfluoride, 50 µg/ℓ soybean trypsin inhibitor and 1 unit/ℓ aprotinin. After a centrifugation of 10,000 g for 20 minutes, the membranes were pelleted by 100,000 g for 60 minutes, resuspended in a cold sucrose solution and were kept frozen until use. The protein content was determined by the Lowry method.

Immunization

BALB/c mice were immunized by intraperitoneal inoculations of membrane enriched preparations containing 200 µg protein in 50 µℓ PBS. Membrane preparation no. 1 was injected 6, 3 and 2 days before fusion 126 (hyperimmunization protocol according Hilkens et al., 1981). For fusions 125 and 130 membrane preparation no. 2 was applied. Fusion 125 was preceeded by three injections 6, 3 and 2 days before the fusion day. In the case of fusion 130, the animals were immunized three times once a week and boosted on week 7, 5-3 days before fusion.

Generation of monoclonal antibodies

Spleen cells from mice immunized with membrane enriched preparations were fused with SP2/0-Ag14 mouse myeloma cells according to the protocol of Oi and Herzenberg (1980). Briefly, 10^8 spleen cells and $2x10^7$ myeloma cells were mixed, pelleted and resuspended in 0.5 ml of 50% solution of polyethylene glycol-1500 in serum free Dulbecco's modified Eagle's medium (DMEM). After one minute, 40 ml serum free DMEM was gradually added. The cells were pelleted at 800 rpm for 6 minutes, resuspended in 40 ml DMEM containing hypoxanthine-aminopterin-thymidine (HAT) and 15% horse serum and distributed in four 96-well tissue culture plates (Falcon). The above selective medium was applied during the first three weeks, and it was first reversed to hypoxanthine and thymidine containing medium followed by DMEM with 15% horse serum. The supernatants were tested for antibody production in an ELISA assay against the immunizing antigen and against ghosts of human red blood cells. The cells from cultures reacting with mammary tumor membrane but not with blood cell membrane were transferred to 1 ml culture and/or cloned by limiting dilution in the presence of $2x10^6$ normal mouse spleen cells/ml as feeder cells. The 1 ml cultures were further tested on frozen sections of human mammary carcinomas by an indirect immunoperoxidase test. Hybridomas showing reactivity with the tumor and/or the normal mammary gland were subcloned. Clones strongly reacting with connective tissue were discarded. The cloned cultures were first screened by ELISA assay and 8-12 positive wells containing one clone were tested on frozen sections. The hybridomas were usually 3, in certain cases 2 or 5 times subcloned. The hybridoma lines were considered stable and monoclonal when at least in two subsequent clonings all the investigated subclones showed an antibody production with identical histological pattern. The stable hybridomas were grown in large amounts and BALB/c mice were i.p. inoculated for ascites production.

Nomenclature

Monoclonal antibodies are designated with a number (125, 126 and 130) corresponding to the serial number of fusion done in the Division of Tumor Biology at The Netherlands Cancer Institute and with a character and number (e.g. E7) referring to the place of primary clone in the microculture plate.

ELISA assay

The membrane enriched preparations in a concentration of 0.2 mg protein/50 µℓ PBS was dried overnight at 37° C into the wells of Falcon microtiter plates. After one washing with PBS, the wells were incubated at 37° C for 60 minutes with 200 µℓ 0.5% gelatin solution in TEN buffer. 50 µℓ solution of monoclonal antibody was added for 30 minutes at 37° C followed by three washes with PBS containing 0.5% Tween-20. 50 µℓ goat anti-mouse Ig peroxidase conjugate (TAGO) in a dilution of 1:2500 was added for 30 minutes at 37° C followed by repeated rinsing. The color reaction as developed with 100 µℓ substrate solution containing 20 mg o-phenylendiamine-dihydrochloride in 10 ml 0.1 M pH 6 phosphate buffer and 5 µℓ 30% H_2O_2. After a 5-10 minute incubation at room temperature in the dark the reaction was stopped with 50 µℓ 2 M H_2O_2 and the intensity was measured at 492 nm in a flow multiscan photospectrometer.

Tissues

The tissues were obtained from the Department of Pathology of the Netherlands Cancer Institute, Amsterdam and from the Oncopathological Research Institute, Budapest. About 30 surgically removed neoplastic and 12 non-neoplastic tumors as well as 6 infiltrated axillary lymph nodes were evaluated in this study. To examine the normal breast epithelium, tissues from four sources were evaluated: a) malignant tumors containing preexisting ducts and acini with preserved structure; b) tissue samples from the area behind the nipple and far from the tumor derived from surgically removed breast of cancer patients; c) benign lesions with preserved normal ducts, and d) a limited number of breast tissues from plastic surgery cases. The tissues were freshly frozen in liquid nitrogen and kept at -70° C. The cryostat sections were allowed to attach to the slides at 37° C, then fixed for 5 minutes in acetone and kept at -70° C until use.

Immmunoperoxidase test

The sections were covered with a solution of monoclonal antibody containing 10% normal goat serum. Undiluted spent medium of hybridoma cultures was applied for 60-120 minutes at 4° C and 1 unit/ml Trasylol was added to avoid the digestion of tissue material. Ascites fluids were generally diluted to 1:100 in PBS, although some of them reacted also in a dilution of 1:10,000 and the reaction was done at room temperature for 30 minutes. After rinsing in three changes of PBS, peroxidase conjugated goat anti-mouse immunoglobulin (TAGO, affinity chromatography purified) in a dilution of 1:20 in PBS with 10% goat serum was added at room temperature for 30 minutes. Following a rinse in three changes of PBS, the color reaction was developed within 10 minutes with a freshly prepared substrate solution of 2 mg 3-amino-9 ethylcarbazole solubilized in 0.5 ml dimethylformamide and diluted in 9.5 ml 0.05 M acetate buffer pH 4.9 and 1 µℓ H_2O_2 was added. The sections were slightly counterstained with haematoxilin (10 sec) and mounted with aquamount.

Human mammary tumor cell lines

The following breast carcinoma cell lines, maintained in DMEM supplemented with 10% FCS and insulin, were applied: MCF-7 (obtained from F. Prop, University of Amsterdam), BT20, Hs578T (from J. Taylor-Papadimitriou, IRFC, London), CAMA 1 (from U. Koldovsky, Dusseldorf), T47D (from American Type Culture Collection, Rockville, MD), SKBR-3 (obtained from Naval Bioscience Laboratory, Oakland, CA). The MPL13 cell line was established from pleural effusion fluid of a breast cancer patient by J. Hilkens (The Netherlands Cancer Institute, Amsterdam).

Immunofluorescence assay on cell lines

For membrane immunofluorescence studies the subconfluent monolayers were washed once with PBS, then detached with 0.2% EDTA in PBS for 5 minutes and washed twice with PBS. The cells were resuspended in 100 µl solution of monoclonal antibodies (undiluted spent medium or ascites fluid in a dilution of 1:100 in PBS), and incubated for 30 minutes on ice. After one washing in PBS, 100 µl FITC labeled goat anti-mouse immunoglobulin (DAKO) was added in a dilution of 1:20 for 30 minutes at 0° C in dark. Following washing the positive cells were counted under a fluorescent microscope. Immunofluorescence staining of fixed cells (IF) was done either after harvesting the cells as in MIF studies, followed by drying onto microscopic slides and fixing for 5 minutes with acetone, or by visualizing the cell structure on growing cells. In the latter case the cells were grown overnight on microscopic slides and fixed with acetone. The slides, after subsequent incubations with the monoclonal antibody and the FITC conjugate for 30 minutes at room temperature, were covered with aquamount and checked under a fluorescence microscope.

Immunoglobulin class and subclass determination

The class and sub-class as well as the light chain type of antibodies was determined from the culture medium of hybridomas by the double diffusion method of Ouchterlony using 1% agar gel in PBS. Specific anti-mouse antisera were obtained from Nordic, Tilburg, The Netherlands.

RESULTS

Generation and selection of hybridomas

In the three fusions 260 hybridomas producing antibodies against the membrane enriched human mammary tumor preparations were obtained. 64 clones, having no reactivity against red blood cells in ELISA assays were selected and further screened on frozen sections of neoplastic breast tissues for their reactivity against breast epithelial cells. During the subsequent clonings, in the case of about 40 monoclonals a significant reactivity against tissues of mesenchymal origin was observed. These hybridomas were discarded. Altogether 17 independent hybridoma lines producing antibodies reactive with neoplastic or with normal mammary epithelium or with both were chosen, 3-5 times cloned and stabilized. Four monoclonals are IgM and thirteen IgG's of various subclasses (Table I). The light chains of all antibodies were of kappa type.

Reactivity against membrane enriched preparations

The monoclonals were tested for their reactivity to the immunizing antigens and against delipidated human milk and milk fat globule membrane by ELISA assay. The highest dilution of ascites fluids showing reactivity and the strength of reaction referring to the antibody reactivity and to the antigen concentration in the preparations were evaluated (Table 1). All of the antibodies reacted with membrane preparation 1, but monoclonal antibodies generated to preparation 1 had considerably weaker and in one case no reaction with preparation 2. Two antibodies generated against preparation 2 reacted weaker with preparation 1 than with 2.

These findings demonstrate that the two immunogens represent different compositions of antigenic determinants. The concentration of certain antigens in the two preparations showed non-coordinated differences, suggesting that these determinants are independent of each other. Only 126E7 had a significant reaction with HMFG membrane. Three other MoAbs reacted weakly and the others did not recognize antigens present in human milk.

Immunohistochemical reactivity on breast tissue

Two antibodies, 125B4 and 126E7, also reacted with formalin fixed tissues. The antigenic determinants recognized by the other antibodies did not resist the formalin fixation and embedding procedure, but the tissue distribution could be tested on frozen material fixed with acetone only. For a better comparison all the antibodies were examined on frozen sections in this study.

The immunoperoxidase reactions were considered to be positive when any significant color reaction was found in the cells. In evaluating the strength of reaction, the percentage of stained cells and the intratissue and intracellular localization of staining were recorded.

Staining incidence in neoplastic and non-neoplastic tumors

The reactivity of monoclonals on human mammary tumor material is summarized in Table II. In primary malignant tumors 7 antibodies had very strong reactions: 125B5, 125H3, 126E7 and 126H12 stained all tumors tested and 125B4, 126G5 and 130B9 reacted with a high (87-95) percentage of the cases. 125E1 and 126A8 were positive in 70-80 percent of malignant tumors, but the reaction was often weak or focal. 126B6, 130E5 and 126E8 had a strong, often heterogeneous reaction in about 40-50 percent of the specimens tested. The remaining 5 antibodies reacted weakly and often only focally, making the evaluation uncertain. Monoclonal antibodies that had the same incidence of positive reactions often stained different specimens.

The tumor cells in lymph node metastases were recognized by all antibodies that were positive on the primary tumors, however, the reactions were often weaker and more homogeneous than in primary tumors. Antibodies 126G5 and 126E7 had a remarkably strong staining, recognizing all the tumor cells.

TABLE 1 REACTIVITY OF MONOCLONAL ANTIBODIES IN ELISA*

No.	Antibody	Isotype	Immunogen No. of membrane preparation	Reactivity against Membrane prep. 1	Membrane prep. 2	HMFG	Skim milk
1	126E7	IgM	1	4++	2+	4+	2+
2	125B5	IgG2b	2	5+	5++	-	-
3	125H3	IgG2b	2	4+	4++	-	-
4	125B4	IgM	2	3+	3+	2+	-
5	126G5	IgG3	1	4++	-	-	-
6	126H12	IgG3	1	5++	4+	-	-
7	130B9	IgM	2	4+	3++	3+	-
8	125E1	IgM	2	2+	2+	-	-
9	126A8	IgG1	1	3+	3±	-	-
10	130E5	IgG	2	3++	3±	-	-
11	126E8	IgG3	1	4++	2+	2+	2+
12	126B6	IgG1	1	5++	2±	-	-
13	125E6	IgG	2	2±	2±	-	-
14	125D9	IgG	2	2+	2+	-	-
15	130C4	IgG	2	2+	2+	-	NT
16	130A3	IgG	2	2±	2±	-	-
17	130F2	IgG	2	2±	2±	-	-

* Numbers: Ig of the highest ascites dilution showing reactivity (e.g.: 4 denotes dilution of $1:10^4$)

Strength of reaction: - negative; ± 2 times; + 3 times; ++ 5-7 times higher than background

NT not tested

TABEL II REACTIONS ON MAMMARY TUMORS

No.	Antibody	Primary malignant lesions: Incidence positive/total	%	Characteristics*: strength in positive cases	binding pattern	Metastases: strength in all cases	Benign lesions: Incidence positive/total	%	Characteristics*: strength in positive	binding pattern
1	126E7	34/34	100	++	am,c,h	++	11/11	100	++	am
2	125B5	31/31	100	++	m,c	+	11/12	92	++	c,blm
3	126H3	32/32	100	++	m,c	+	11/12	92	++	c,blm
4	125B4	30/32	94	++,w+,-	c,m,vh	++	11/12	92	-,++	c,m,vh
5	126G5	29/33	87	++	c,nm	++	8/ 8	100	-,++	c,vh
6	126H12	31/31	100	++	m,am,c	+	12/12	100	++	m
7	130B9	27/28	95	++	c,m	+	12/12	100	++	
8	125E1	25/33	80	w+,+	e,c	+	7/12	58	+	am
9	126A8	20/30	66	w+,+	m,c,am	-,w+	11/12	92	++	
10	130E5	14/25	56	+	m,c,h	-,++	7/11	63	-,++	vh,b
11	126E8	14/31	40	-,w+,++	c,h	-,w+	4/ 9	44	w+	
12	126B6	17/33	50	+	c,m	-,w+	2/12	16	-,w+	
13	125E6	16/31	50	w+	c	w+	3/10	30	w+	
14	125D9	16/30	54	w+	c	w+	2/12	17	-,w+	
15	130C4	10/30	33	w+	c	-,w+	1/10	10	-,w+	
16	130A3	15/29	44	w+	c	-,w+	5/12	42	-,w+	
17	130F2	7/26	38	w+	c	-,w+	1/11	9	-,w+	

* ++ very strong; + strong; w weak reaction; - no reaction
m cell membrane; am apical membrane; nm nuclear membrane; e extracellular matrix; c cytoplasm; a apical side; l lateral side; b basal side; h heterogeneous; vh very heterogeneous

TABEL III REACTIVITY OF MONOCLONAL ANTIBODIES IN NORMAL MAMMARY GLAND*

No.	Antibody	Secretion product	Luminal epithelium	Myoepithelium	Basement membrane	Characteristics of staining	Other reactivities
1	126E7	++	++	-	-	apical m	-
2	125B5	+	++	w+	-	lateral-basal m; c	-
3	126H3	+	++	w+	-	lateral-basal m; c	-
4	125B4	+	++/-	++/-	-	c; circumferential m	blood vessels; capillaries ++
5	126G5	+	+/-	-	-	c; apical side	-
6	126H12	++	++	+	?	c; apical m	blood vessels w+
7	130B9	+	++	++	?	c; circumferential m	blood vessels w+
8	125E1	+	+	-	-	apical m	blood vessels +
9	126A8	+	++	++	-	c; apical m	blood vessels ++
10	130E5	-	-/w+	++	-	c	blood vessel wall +
11	126E8	++	--	-	-	-	-
12	126B6	+	+/-	-	-	c; circumferential m	connective tissue; fibrillar elements
13	125E6	+	w+	-	-	c	-
14	125D9	+	w+	-	-	c	-
15	130C4	-	+/-	-	-	c	lymphocytes
16	130A3	+	w+	-	?	c	-
17	130F2	+	w+	-	-	c	-

* ++ very strong; + strong; w weak reaction; c cytoplasmic staining; m membrane

In benign mammary tumors the incidence of positivity was similar to that found in carcinomas. The only exception was 126A8 reacting in higher percentage and stronger in benign lesions than in carcinomas. However, the binding pattern of some antibodies showed individual and characteristic shifts from benign cases through the better differentiated carcinomas to the infiltrating cells, as it will be described in more detail in the paragraph "Staining patterns".

Reactivity in normal mammary glands

To describe the localization of antibody binding sites in the breast epithelium, we distinguished the luminal epithelium lining the glandular lumen and the basal or myoepithelium bordered by the basement membrane (Figure 1). The luminal epithelium consists of cuboidal cells being radially polarized to the lumen and the cell membrane at the lumen is termed as apical membrane. The myoepithelium is formed by one often not continuous thin layer of elongated cells which are longitudinally polarized along the course of the duct and often have long protrusions. In addition, another cell layer was frequently distinguishable between the luminal and myoepithelial cells. This continuous cell layer consisted of cuboidal cells with longitudinal orientation.

The reactivities and staining patterns are summarized in Table III and Figure 1. Eleven antibodies had strong reactivity with the component cells of the mammary gland. Monoclonal antibodies 126E7, 125E1, 126G5 and 126B6 stained the luminal epithelium only and showed no binding to the myoepithelium. 125B5, 123H3, 126A8, 126H12, 130B9 and 125B4 stained both types of epithelia. 130E5 was predominantly reactive with the myoepithelium. One antibody, 126E8, had no reaction in the normal epithelium, but it strongly stained the occasionally occurring secreted material in the lumen. The intracellular localization of reactivity showed individual patterns at the different antibodies, as it is described in "Staining patterns".

Staining patterns

126E7 stained the apical cell membrane of normal luminal epithelium cells and the secreted material in the lumen. It reacted with all benign and malignant tumors tested. The staining pattern varied according to the degree of differentiation. In benign lesions the staining was predominantly confined to the luminal membranes (Fig. 2 and 3). The well differentiated papillary carcinomas showed a strong luminal membrane staining accompanied by a slight reaction in the apically situated part of the cytoplasm. In invasive carcinomas a strong cytoplasmic reaction was observed being often irregularly polarized within the cells, and the inter- and intracellular lumina were especially strongly stained. Single invading cells showed increased concentration of 126E7 determinants (Fig. 7). In tumor cell groups, however, many cells often remained unstained. Pre-existing normal glands in or near to the malignant tumors often contained only minute amounts of antigen, especially if they exhibited no secretory activity.

125B5 and 125H3 have a staining pattern similar to each other, showing a strong binding to all cells of epithelial origin and to no other components in the breast tissue. In the normal gland they strongly and uniformly stained the luminal cells. The determinants were localized, contrasted with those of 126E7, on the adjacent cell membranes being in contact with one another and with the myoepithelium, whereas the apical membrane showed decreased expression of determinants (Fig. 4). The reaction was always accompanied by a strong, uniformly distributed staining in the cytoplasm. The predominant affinity to the

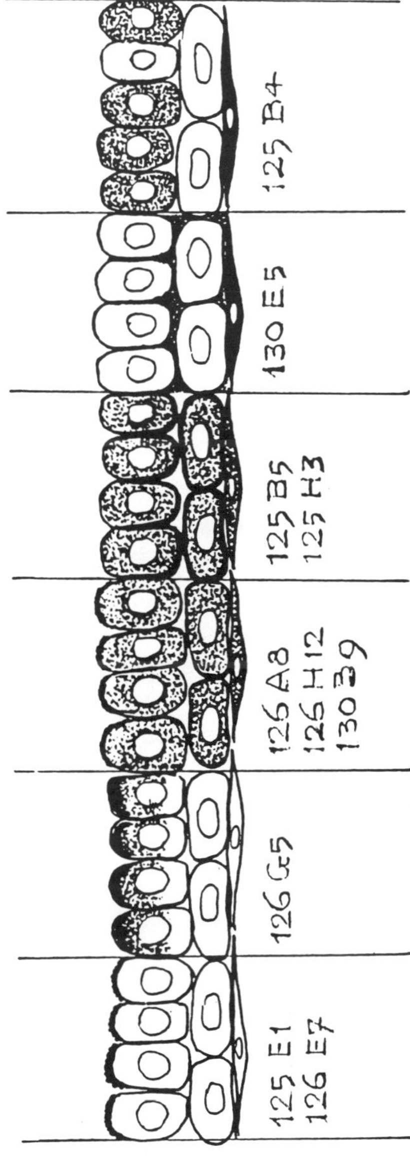

Figure 1. Reaction pattern of monoclonal antibodies on cells of normal mammary duct.

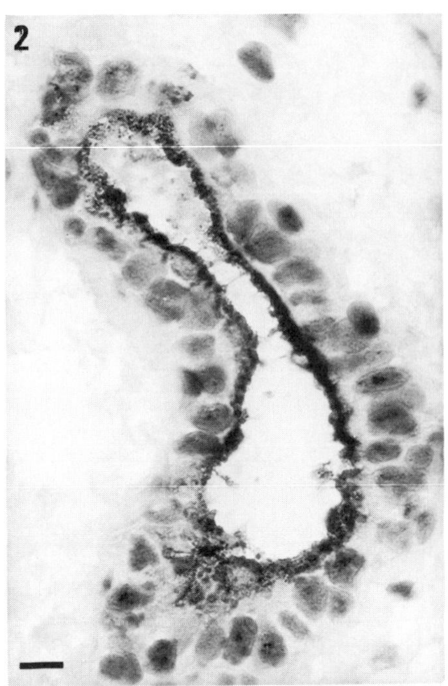

Figure 2. 126E7: reacts with apical membranes of luminal cells of duct in fibroadenoma of the breast. Bar: 10 μ.

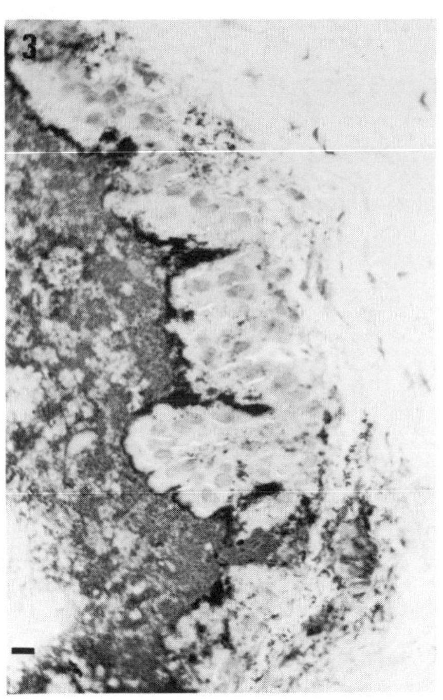

Figure 3. 126E7: stains mainly apical membranes of apocrine metaplasia of the breast. Bar: 10 μ.

laterally and basally situated membranes was conserved in the benign lesions (Fig. 5) and in more differentiated carcinomas, where the orientation of epithelial cells was preserved (Fig. 6). In infiltrating cells and poorly differentiated tumors a circumferential membrane staining was observed. All the tumor cases tested were positive. Using a higher (1:1000 - 1:10,000) dilution of ascites fluid an elevated concentration of determinants on tumor cells compared to the normal glands could be established. 123H3 showed some more heterogeneity in strength of reaction within a tumor and between normal and cancer cells than 125B5.

126G5 represents a specific marker for luminal epithelium, showing no binding to myoepithelium and to any other component of the breast tissues. The antibody recognized cytoplasmic determinants, which were more polarized to the luminal side of the normal cells, whereas the basal side of the cells often remained negative. This staining pattern characterized several benign lesions, such as fibroadenomas (Fig. 8). Pre-existing glands in carcinoma tissues were often considerably weaker in their staining than the malignant cells, or in some cases, a very heterogeneous pattern with strongly stained and completely negative luminal cells adjacent to each other was found (Fig. 9). The same heterogeneous pattern characterized the reactivity in dysplasias. In carcinomas 126G5 had a strong, diffuse binding in the cytoplasm and the nuclear membrane was strongly visible. The adjacent cell membranes were less pronouncedly stained than with 125B5. The carcinoma cells were mainly uniformly stained (Fig. 10), but some heterogenous patterns and a few negative cases were also found. The antibody had a remarkably strong reaction in metastasizing carcinoma cells.

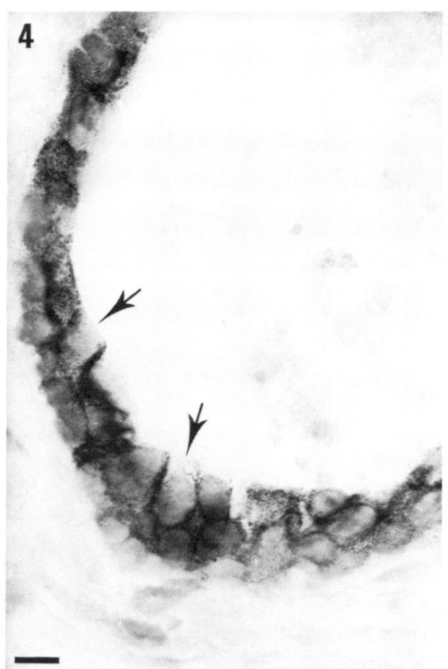

Figure 4. 125B5: reaction on baso-lateral membranes in normal mammary duct. The apical membrane of the luminal cells is negative (arrow). Bar: 10 µ.

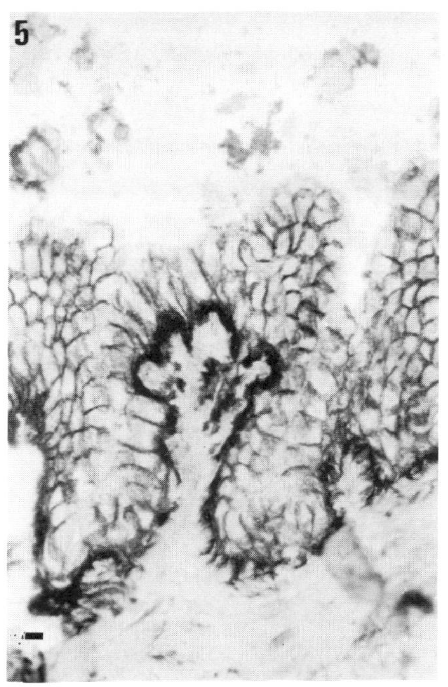

Figure 5. 125B5: strong staining of lateral and basal membranes in an apocrine metaplasia of the breast; the apical membrane of of the cells is negative. Bar: 10 µ.

125B4 stained the circumferential membranes and the cytoplasm. In normal glands it had a very heterogeneous pattern, staining the myoepithelium around the ducts but not around the acini (Fig. 11). In the luminal epithelium often strongly stained and completely negative cells were found near to each other without any reactivity of intermediate strength (Fig. 12). In addition, in some cases completely unreactive or homogeneously stained luminal epithelium was obtained. If more layers of ductal epithelium could be distinguished, the basally situated one proved to be always negative. In the dysplasias the cells showed a heterogeneous pattern. In 94% of malignant tumors 125B4 was reactive, staining mostly all the malignant cells. In some tumors the reactivity was restricted to cells resembling cells of myoepithelial origin. 125B4 had a very pronounced reactivity in blood and lymph vessels and in capillaries.

126H12 and 130B9 stained strongly and uniformly the whole mammary epithelium and reacted with all benign and malignant tumors tested. Both antibodies reacted in the cytoplasm and with the cell membranes. 126H12 had a tendency for apical staining. Both antibodies had, however, a slight reaction with connective tissue and blood vessels.

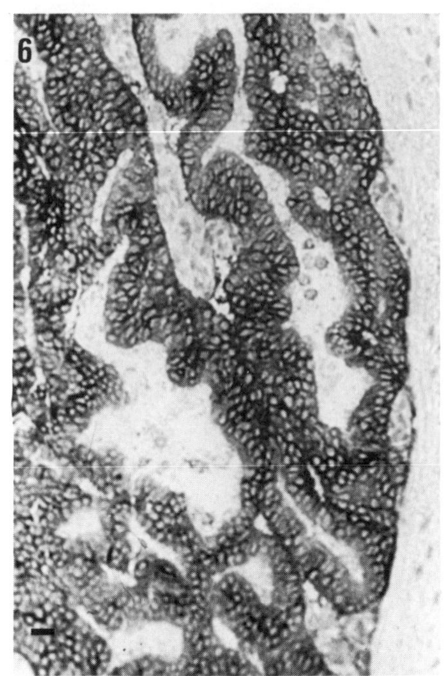

Figure 6. 125B5: stains cells of invasive carcinoma of the breast. Note the absence of apical staining (arrow). Bar: 10 μ.

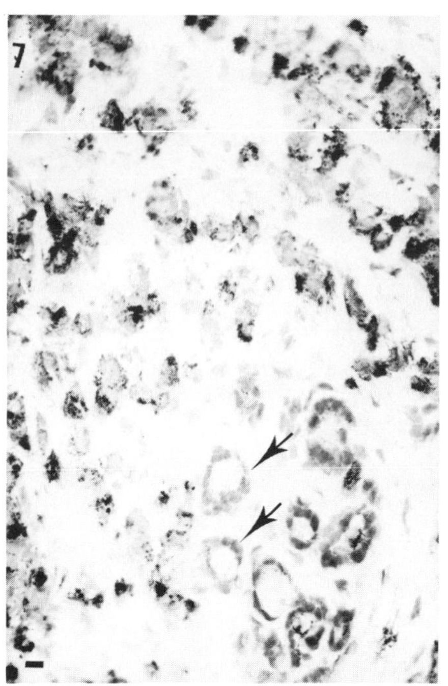

Figure 7. 126E7: reacts strongly with invading cells of a lobular mammary carcinoma. In preexisting normal ducts the reaction is weak or absent (arrow). Bar: 10 μ.

125E1 stained the secreted material in the normal glands and a focal reactivity along the luminal membranes also often appeared. In about the half of the tumor cases 125E1 had a moderately strong, sometimes granulated staining in the cytoplasm. If the tumor cells produced an extracellular matrix, it was predominantly visualized by this antibody. The determinants often appeared in layers in the connective tissue, surrounding the tumor groups and the preserved lobuli, but they were absent from other areas of connective tissue. 125E1 stained the blood vessel walls but not the capillaries.

126A8 reacted strongly with the luminal epithelium and weaker with the myoepithelium. The reaction was localized in the cytoplasm and to the apical membrane. A preferential reactivity for various benign lesions compared to malignant cases was found. In carcinomas the preexisting ducts were often stronger stained than the malignant cells. 126A8 reacted with blood vessels and capillaries.

130E5 is a specific marker for myoepithelial cells exhibiting a consistent, strong reaction in the basal layer along the course of ducts and acini (Fig. 13). The luminal cells stained very weakly and the other tissue components did not react. In benign lesions and in the more well-differentiated carcinomas a pronounced basal polarization of reactivity was detected. In malignant cases a moderately strong, sometimes heterogeneous cytoplasmic binding was observed.

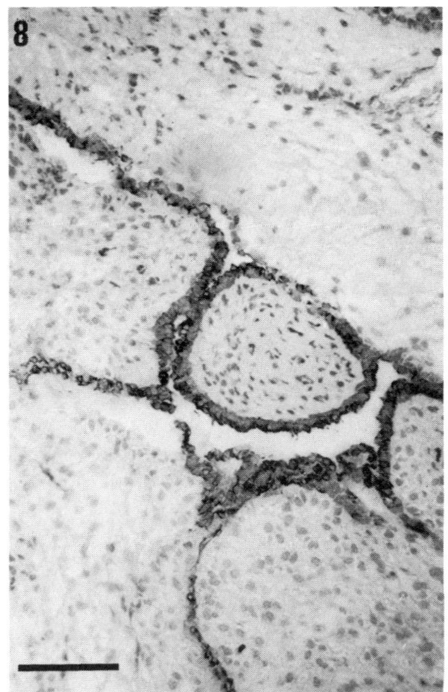

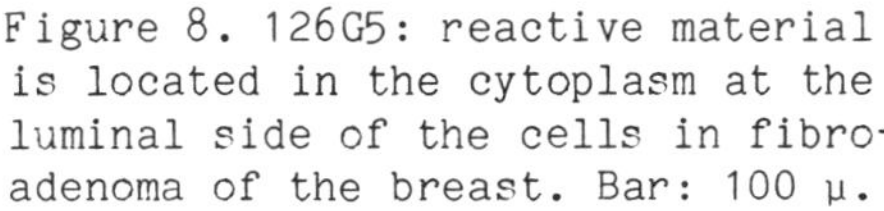
Figure 8. 126G5: reactive material is located in the cytoplasm at the luminal side of the cells in fibroadenoma of the breast. Bar: 100 µ.

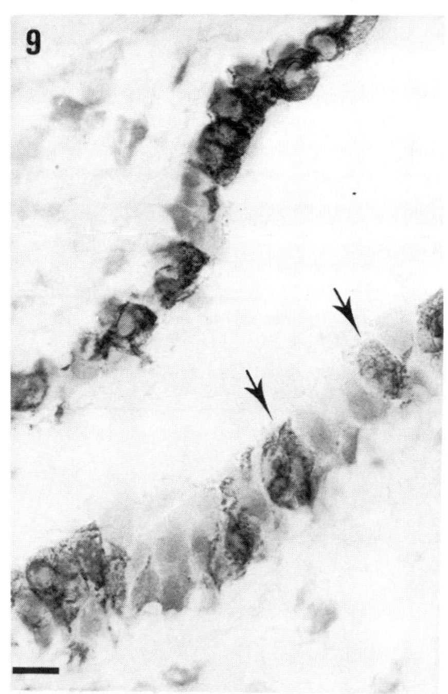

Figure 9. 126G5: heterogeneous staining, strongly positive cells (arrow) border completely negative epithelial cells in a normal mammary duct. Bar: 10 µ.

126E8 strongly stained the secreted material wheras epithelium or other tissue components of the normal breast were negative. However, 40 percent of the cancer cases were positive. Often only some tumor cells were stained, and large areas of the tumor remained negative.

126B6 was often negative in both normal and cancer cells. In the normal gland, if it reacted, only the luminal cells showed affinity to 126B6. In cancer cases the circumferential membrane and the cytoplasm were stained. 126B6 had a characteristic, strong staining in the sclerosing elements of the connective tissue.

126E6, 125D9, 130A3, 130F2 and 130C4 had weak and often only focal staining in the tumor. 130C4 reacted with lymphocytes and macrophages as well.

Reactivity on in vitro cell lines

The cell surface determinants were detected by membrane immunofluorescence test on living cells and the intracellular expression of determinants was visualized after fixing the cells with acetone (Table IV). Monoclonals showing a high incidence of staining in primary mammary tumors proved to be strongly reactive also on cultured mammary tumor cells. Antibodies 125B5, 125H3, 126E7, 126H12 and 130B9 had a strong reaction in all cell lines of carcinoma origin, while the line Hs578T, derived from a carcinosarcoma (Hackett et al., 1977) was negative or weakly stained. All of the above mentioned antibodies

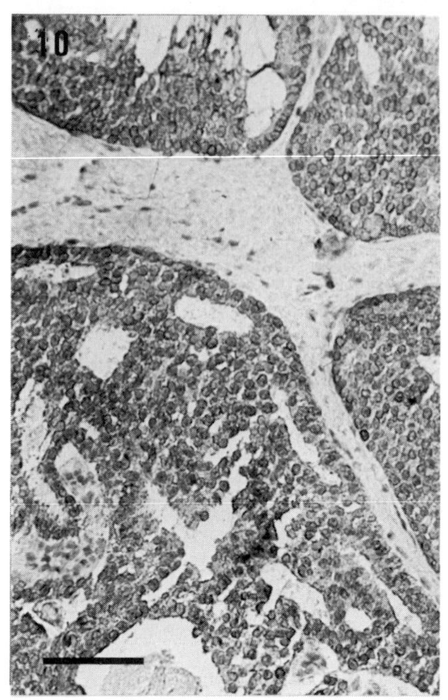

Figure 10. 126G5: homogeneous staining of epithelial cells in breast carcinoma. Bar: 10 μ.

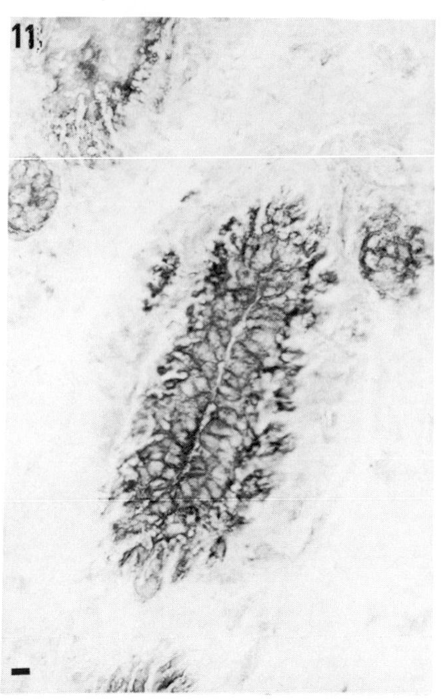

Figure 11. 125B4: strong reaction in myoepithelium. In this duct all epithelial cells are also positive. Bar: 10 μ.

recognized determinants on the cell surface exhibiting a smooth confluent layer (125B5 and 125H3) or roughly distributed granules (126H12) on the cell membrane.

Two antibodies (126G5 and 125B4) visualized an intracytoplasmic filamental structure in acetone fixed cells. 126G5 was characterized by an extremely strong binding to the cytoskeletal network and by a complete lack of cell surface staining (Fig. 14). In five cell lines all the cells were uniformly stained, whereas in Cama and Hs578T lines a heterogeneity could be revealed by 126G5. In the cell line Hs578T the majority of cells were of elongated shape and completely negative for 126G5 determinants. A very small proportion of cells with more round shape and finger-like protrusions, often with two nuclei well distinguishable, were strongly positive. The binding of 125B4 was also predominantly localized in the cytoskeletal structure, but the cell surface was not always completely negative. The reaction in cell line Hs578T was similar to that observed in the case of 126G5.

The myoepithelial cell marker, 130E5, exhibited a cytoplasmic staining in 6 cell lines, including the Hs578T line and often a fine network structure could also be distinguished. The antibody did not recognize cell surface determinants.

Evaluating the results with regard to the cell lines it could be stated that the cultured mammary tumor cells expressed a variety of determinants that are also present in primary tumor cells. The determinants showed a remarkable heterogeneity in their expression among cell subpopulations of certain tumor lines. The phenotypic diversity of the cells of Cama cell line was well demonstrated by the monoclo- nal antibodies that distinguished cell subpopulations within the culture

TABEL IV REACTIVITY OF MONOCLONAL ANTIBODIES ON IN VITRO MAMMARY TUMOR CELL LINES

No.	Antibody	MPL13	T47D*	MCF7*	SKBR3*	BT20	CAMA*	Hs578T*	MPL13**	T47D**	MCF7**	Incidence positive***/total IF	MIF
1	126E7	++	++	++	++	++	70++/30+	+	++	++	++	7/7	3/3
2	125B5	+	++	+	+	+	60++	-/1+	70+	+	++	6/6	3/3
3	126H3	+	++	+	+	+	50++	-	80+	+	+	6/6	3/3
4	125B4	+^{n}	++^{n}++^{n}	-/1++^{n}	+/10++^{n}	+/5++^{n}	80++^{n}	-/++^{n}	90-/10++^{n}	75-/25+	-	5/7	0/3
5	126G5	+++^{n}	+++^{n}	+++^{n}	+++^{n}	+++^{n}	±/1+++^{n}	-/1+++^{n}	95-/5+++^{n}	95-/5+++^{n}	95-/5+++^{n}	5/7	0/3
6	126H12	80±/20++	++	++	+	++	++	+	+	++	+	7/7	3/3
7	130B9	+	+	+	+	++	70++/30+	+	50+	++	+	7/7	3/3
8	125E1	+	+	+	+	-	40+	+	95-/5++^{n}	±	-	6/7	0/3
9	126A8	±	+	+	-	+	80-/20+	±	-	++	90-/10+	3/7	1/3
10	130E5	-/1+	+	+	+	++	80++/20+	++	-	-	-	6/7	0/3
11	126E8	-	-	-	-	-	+	-	-	-	-	1/7	0/3
12	126B6	-	-	-	+	-	-	-	95-/5+	90-/1-+	-	1/7	0/3
13	125E6	-	±	+	+	±	60+	-	-	-	-	3/7	0/3
14	125D9	±	±	±	+	-	+	±	-	-	70-/30+	2/7	0/3
15	130C4	-	±	±	±	-	+	-	-	+	90-/10++	1/7	1/3
16	130A3	±	+	±	+	+	+	+	-	90-/10+	±	5/7	0/3
17	130F2	-	+	-	+	-	+	±	-	90-/10+	-	3/7	0/3

* Detected by immunofluorescence (IF) on acetone fixed cells
** Detected by membrane immunofluorescence (MIF) on living cells
+++ very strong; ++ strong; + positive; ± weakly positive; negative reaction; n network structure is stained; numbers: percentage of cells; 1: 0.1-1%; no numbers: 100% of cells;
*** The reaction is considered to be positive if at least 30% of the cells showed a reaction of + strength

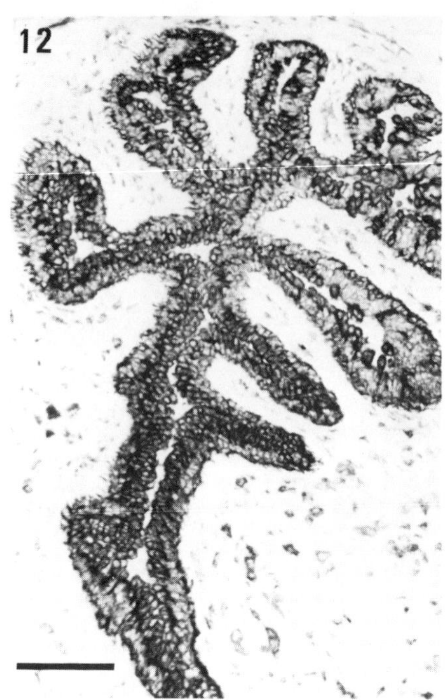

Figure 12. 125B4: heterogeneous staining in duct in a case of lobular carcinoma of the breast. Bar: 100 μ.

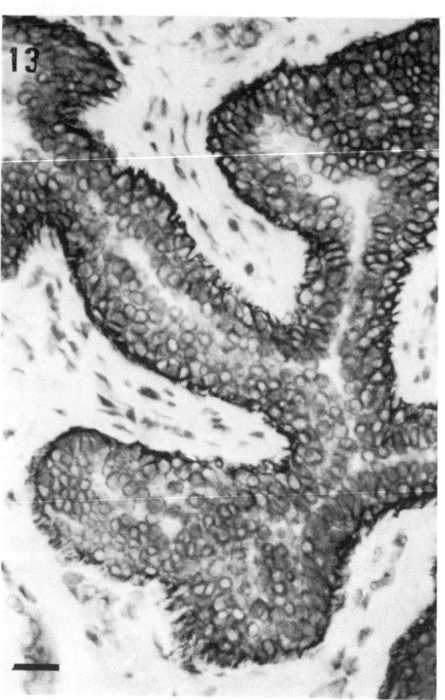

Figure 13. 130E5: positive reaction of myoepithelial cells in normal duct in case of lobular carcinoma of the breast. Bar: 10 μ.

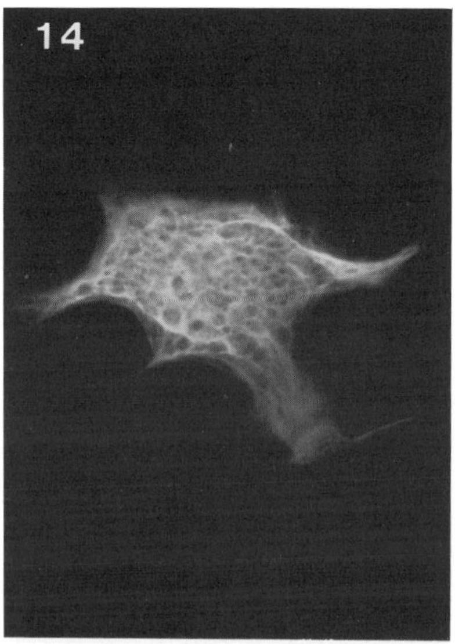

Figure 14. 126G5: Cytoskeletal staining of a mammary epithelial cell in tissue culture. Immunofluorescence.

DISCUSSION

MoAbs were raised to crude plasma membrane preparations of human primary breast carcinoma. The reactivity against the immunizing antigen in ELISA assay demonstrated that some determinants appeared independently of each other in the two membrane preparations. A non-coordinated distribution of determinants was observed in the primary cancer and benign tissues: different ranges of positive cases were found and the localization of staining showed individual patterns with the various antibodies. These findings indicate distinct specificities of the monoclonals. Several tumors and in vitro cell lines were positive for all antibodies demonstrating a broad range of antigenic determinants that simultaneously can be expressed by a tumor cell.

The MoAbs reacted with the plasma membrane or with distinct parts of it, with the cytoplasm, or with the extracellular matrix. Various combinations of the former reactivities were also observed. The binding pattern of this set of antibodies exhibited considerably greater diversity than those generated to milk fat globule membrane. The latter ones are mainly directed to carbohydrate determinants, which appear to be very immunogenic. These structures are strongly expressed on the apical membranes of the lactating breast epithelium (Gooi et al., 1983) and they are also present in the resting mammary gland and in various normal and malignant cells of epithelial origin. The various anti-HMFG antibodies, in spite of the differences in the chemical composition and tissue distribution of the determinants, resemble each other, staining only or predominantly the apical cell surface of the glandular epithelium (Sloane and Ormerod, 1981, Arklie et al., 1981, Foster et al., 1982 a&b, Burchell et al., 1983, Hilkens et al., 1984).

From our panel only one antibody, 126E7, is directed to an HMFG-related, formalin resistant antigenic determinant. The importance of this antibody in detection of neoplastic breast cells is given by the strong reactivity to all mammary tumor cases tested. In ELISA assay 126E7 reacted with HMFG membrane preparation. The histological binding pattern was characterized by a tendency for apical staining in normal and neoplastic breast epithelium. According to preliminary results not reported here, the staining of 126E7 showed significant similarities in extramammary normal and tumor tissues to several other antibodies. Among these are the polyvalent antiserum that recognizes the determinant on "epithelial membrane antigen" (Sloane and Ormerod, 1981), the MoAb 115D8, generated against HMFG, which reacts with the antigen designated MAM-6 (Hilkens et al., 1984), and the antibody MBr1, raised against the mammary cancer cell line MCF7 (Mariani-Costantini et al., 1984).

Two antibodies, 125B5 and 125H3, revealed determinants that are predominantly expressed in the cytoplasm and on lateral and basal membranes of the luminal epithelium. The opposite staining pattern of 126E7 versus 125B5 and 125H12 demonstrates, that in the normal mammary gland the apical and adjacent cell membranes of the luminal epithelial cells express distinct sets of determinants. In malignant tisues this polarization of staining often proved to be lost.

The fourth epithelial marker, 126G5, is specific for luminal cells. As this antibody had no reactivity to any non-epithelial tissues and it stained exclusively the cytoskeletal network of the cells, the antigenic determinant is supposed to be associated with intermediate-sized filaments. In preliminary studies (not shown here) the antibody reacted with a variety of simple epithelia in different normal tissues but it was negative in the epidermis. In this respect the reactivity of 126G5 resembles that of the MoAb LE61 raised to cytoskeleton extracts of a non-primate derived epithelial cell line (Lane, 1982).

125B4 also reacted with cytoskeletal fibrillar components. The staining pattern in normal and malignant tissue sections was often heterogeneous and different from that of 126G5. The MoAb 130E5 was predominantly reactive in the myoepithelium. The above mentioned antibodies and some others showed cell-type specificity within the breast epithelium. These antibodies, as differentiation markers for the mammary (and extra mammary) epithelium, offer means for studying the development and differentiation of epithelial tissues.

Several MoAbs showed a polarized staining in the normal mammary gland, having a restricted binding to the apically (126E7, 126H12, 126G5), laterally-basally (125B5, 125H3) or basally (130E5) oriented determinants. The intracellular distribution pattern of these determinants proved to be a marker for the differentiation stage of tumors. In benign lesions, where the epithelial cells are organized in glandular structures, or in fibroadenomas, the polarized staining pattern was preserved. In carcinomas where the tissue organization is partly or completely disintegrated, a loss of orientation properties of cells was revealed by the antibodies. The determinants exhibited a more extended distribution; the cell surface antigens appeared also in the cytoplasm and along the circumference of the membranes. The 126G5 determinants were more homogeneously distributed within the cytoplasm in malignancies and also in dysplasia than in normal cells.

A remarkable quantitative difference was also observed between normal and malignant cells in the expression of several determinants: generally the 126E7, 126G5, 125E1, 125B4 antigens appeared in higher concentration in cancer than normal cells. However, some of the tested tumors did not express all of these determinants.

The MoAb 126E8 showed a reactivity in 40 percent of primary breast cancer cases and benign lesions, but it was scored to be negative within the normal mammary epithelium. In a preliminary screening on various extramammary epithelia no or very restricted reactivity was observed. Similar properties were reported for the MoAb B72.3 (Nuti et al., 1982) generated to metastatic mammary tumor cells (Colcher et al., 1981). The specificity of the two antibodies is, however, different. Both of them exhibited a heterogeneous staining pattern, but the reactivity of 126E8 was often restricted to a few cells only. The 126E8 determinant was sensitive to formalin fixation. 126E8 reacted with the secreted material of mammary gland and also with gastrointestinal mucin components.

The 130E5 antigen, the marker for normal myoepithelium, was expressed by the majority of cells in the 60 percent of carcinoma specimens, in spite of the fact that these mainly invasive ductal tumors were not of myoepithelial origin. These tumors were also positive with antibodies, that are markers for luminal epithelium. This finding reveals that special caution is required when conclusions are drawn about the cell-type origin of a tumor on the basis of the expression of a single determinant. The origin of 130E5-positive tumors may be a more primitive cell, which has the ability to develop both luminal and myoepithelial characteristics.

In the normal mammary gland and also in reactive glands a layer of epithelial cells was often recognizable, located between the cell layer lining the glandular lumen and the myoepithelium. Considering their position, these cells are supposed to have neither secretory nor contractive function. Therefore, they may represent a lower grade of the differentiation lineage of breast epithelia. This layer of cells reacted neither with luminal nor with myoepithelial cell markers. Malignant cells, although representing a low grade of differentiation and exerting intense metabolic and proliferative activity, displayed considerably higher concentrations of certain antigens than this cell layer. This finding indicates that the expression of certain antigens depends on the functional state of the cells.

Numerous data indicate, that monoclonal antibodies may reveal phenotypic, possibly functional heterogeneity between morphologically identical cellular subsets of normal mammary tissues (Foster et al., 1982b, Edward et al., 1983) or of tumor cells (Miller, F.R., 1982, Nuti et al., 1982, Hand et al., 1983). Several antibodies reported here revealed intratumor heterogeneity, as most of the determinants were unevenly distributed among the cells of a primary tumor and of tumor cell lines. Some antibodies such as 125B4 or 126G5 often had a heterogeneous staining in normal luminal epithelium.

The present study demonstrates that MoAbs with distinct specificities against various determinants of breast carcinoma cells could be raised against plasma membrane preparations of primary tumors. Some of the monoclonals represent epithelial markers; several of them can be applied as cell-type markers within the human mammary gland. Antibodies, recognizing determinants present in elevated concentration and/or altered distribution in malignant compared to normal cells, offer means for detecting tumor cells and for studying the differentiation and functional characteristics of neoplasias.

REFERENCES

Arklie J., Taylor-Papadimitriou J., Bodmer W., Egan M., Millis R. Differentiation antigens expressed by epithelial cells in the lactating breast are also detectable in cancers. Int. J. Cancer 28: 23-29 (1981)

Atkinson B.F., Ernst C.S., Herlyn M., Steplewski Z., Sears H., Koprowski H. Gastrointestinal cancer associated antigen in immunoperoxidase assay. Cancer Res. 42: 4820-4823 (1982)

Ashall F., Branwell M.E., Hárris H. A new marker for human cancer cells. I. The Ca antigen and the Ca1 antibody. Lancet ii: 1-6 (1982)

Burchell J., Durbin H., Taylor-Papadimitriou J. Complexity of expression of antigenic determinants, recognized by monoclonal antibodies HMFG-1 and HMFG-2, in normal and malignant human mammary epithelial cells. J. Immunol 131: 508-513 (1983)

Ceriani R.L., Peterson J.A., Lee J.Y., Moncada R., Blank E.W. Characterization of cell surface antigens of human mammary epithelial cells with monoclonal antibodies prepared against human milkfat globules. Somatic Cell Genet. 9: 415-427 (1983)

Colcher D., Horan Hand P., Nuti M., Schlom J. A spectrum of monoclonal antibodies reactive with human mammary tumor cells. Proc. Natl. Acad. Sci. USA 78: 3199-3203 (1981)

Edwards P.A.W., Brooks I.M. Antigenic subsets of human breast epithelial cells distinguished by monoclonal antibodies. J. Histochem. Cytochem. 32: 531-537 (1984)

Finan P.J., Grant R.M., DeMattos C., Takei F., Berry P.J., Lennox E.S., Bleehen N.M. Immunohistochemical techniques in the early screening of monoclonal antibodies to human colonic epithelium. Br. J. Cancer 46: 9-17 (1982)

Foster C.S., Dinsdale E.A., Edwards P.A.W., Neville A.M. Monoclonal antibodies to the human mammary gland. II. Distribution of determinants in breast carcinomas. Virchows Arch. (Pathol. Anat.) 397: 295-305 (1982a)

Foster C.S., Edwards P.A.W., Dinsdale E.A., Neville A.M. Monoclonal antibodies to the human mammary gland. I. Distribution of determinants in non-neoplastic mammary and extra mammary tissues. Virchows Arch. (Pathol. Anat.) 394: 279-293 (1982b)

Gatter K.C., Abdulaziz Z., Beverly P., Corvalan J.R.F., Ford C., Lane E.B., Mota M., Nash J.R.G, Pulford K., Stein H., Taylor-Papadimitriou J., Woodhouse C., Mason D.Y. Use of monoclonal antibodies for the histopathological diagnosis of human malignancy. J. Clin. Pathol. 35: 1253-1267 (1982)

Gooi H.C., Uemura K.I., Edwards P.A.W., Foster C.S., Pickering N., Feizi T. Two mouse hybridoma antibodies against human milk fat globules recognize the I(Ma) antigenic determinant β-D-Galp (1→4)-β-D-GlcpNAc-(1→6). Carbohydr. Res. 120: 293-302 (1983)

Hackett A.J., Smith H.S., Springer E.L., Owens R.B., Nelson-Rees W.A., Riggs J.L., Gardner M.B. Two syngeneic cell lines from human breast tissue: the aneuploid mammary epithelial (Hs578T) and the diploid myoepithelial (Hs578Bst) cell lines. J. Natl. Cancer Inst. 58: 1795-1806 (1977)

Hilkens J., Buijs F., Hilgers J., Hageman Ph., Sonnenberg A., Koldowsky K., Karande K., Van Hoeven R.P., Feltkamp C., Van de Rijn J.M. Monoclonal antibodies against human milkfat globule membranes detecting differentiation antigens of the mammary gland. In: Protides of the Biological Fluids (Ed. H. Peeters) Vol. 29: 813-816 (1981)

Hilkens J., Buijs F., Hilgers, J., Hageman Ph., Calafat J., Sonnenberg A., Van der Valk M. Monoclonal antibodies against human milkfat globule membranes detecting differentiation antigens of the mammary gland and its tumors. Int. J. Cancer 34: 197-206 (1984)

Heyderman E., Steele K., Ormerod G. A new antigen on the epithelial membrane: its immunoperoxidase localization in normal and neoplastic tissue. J. Clin. Pathol. 32: 35-39 (1979)

Horan Hand P., Nuti M., Colcher D., Schlom J. Definition of antigenic heterogeneity and modulation among human mammary carcinoma cell populations using monoclonal antibodies to tumor-associated antigens. Cancer Res. 43: 728-735 (1983)

Imam A., Tokes Z.A. Immunoperoxidase localization of a glycoprotein on plasma membrane of secretory epithelium from human breast. J. Histochem. Cytochem. 29: 581-584 (1981)

Koprowski H., Steplewski Z., Mitchell K., Herlyn M., Fuhrer P. Colorectal carcinoma antigens detected by hybridoma antibodies. Som. Cell Genet. 5: 957-979 (1979)

Kohler G., Milstein C. Continuous cultures of fused cells secreting antibody of predefined specificity. Nature 256: 495 (1975)

Lane E.B. Monoclonal antibodies provide specific intramolecular markers for the study of epithelial tonofilament organization. J. Cell Biol. 92: 665-673 (1982)

Loop S.M., Nishiyama K., Hellstrom I., Woodbury R.G., Brown J.P., Hellstrom K.E. Two human tumor-associated antigens, P115 and p210 detected by monoclonal antibodies. Int. J. Cancer 27: 775-781 (1981)

Mariani-Costantini R., Colnaghi M.I., Leoni F., Menard S., Cerasoli S., Rilke F. Immunohistochemical reactivity of a monoclonal antibody prepared against human breast carcinoma. Virchows Archiv. (Pathol. Anat.) 402: 389-404 (1984)

Miller F.R. Intratumor immunologic heterogeneity. Cancer Metastasis Reviews 1: 319-334 (1982)

McGee J.O'D., Woods J.C., Ashall F., Bramwell M.E., Harris H. A new marker for human cancer cells. 2: Immunohistochemical detection of the Ca antigen in human tissues with the Ca1 antibody. Lancet ii: 7-11 (1982)

Menard S., Tagliabue E., Canevari S., Fossati G., Colnaghi M.I. Generation of monoclonal antibodies reacting with normal and cancer cells of human breast. Cancer Res. 43: 1295-1300 (1983)

Neville A.M. Monoclonal antibodies and human tumor pathology. Hum. Pathol. 13: 1067-1081 (1982)

Nuti M., Teramoto Y.A., Mariani-Costantini R., Horan Hand P., Colcher D., Schlom J. A monoclonal antibody (B 72.3) defines patterns of distribution of a novel tumor-associated antigen in human mammary carcinoma cell populations. Int. J. Cancer 29: 539-545 (1982)

Oi V.T., Herzenberg C.A. In: Selected methods in Cellular Immunology Eds. Michell B.B., Shiigi S.M. (Freeman, San Francisco, CA): 351-372 (1980)

Papsidero D.L., Croghan G.A., O'Connell J.M., Valenzuela L.A., Nemoto T., Chu M.T. Monoclonal antibodies (F36/22 and M7/105) to human breast carcinoma. Cancer Res. 43: 1741-1747 (1983)

Rogers G.T. Carcinoembryonic antigens and related glycoproteins. Molecular aspects and specificity. Biochem. Biophys. 695: 227-249 (1983)

Schlom J., Wunderlich D., Teramoto Y.A. Generation of human monoclonal antibodies reactive with human mammary carcinoma cells. Proc. Natl. Acad. Sci. USA 77: 6841-6845 (1980)

Sloane J.P., Ormerod M.G. Distribution of epithelial membrane antigen in normal and neoplastic tissues and its value in diagnostic tumor pathology. Cancer 47: 1786-1795 (1981)

Soule H.R., Linder E., Edgington T.S. Membrane 126 kilodalton phosphoglycoprotein associated with human carcinomas identified by a hybridoma antibody to mammary carcinoma cells. Proc. Natl. Acad. Sci. USA 80: 1332-1336 (1983)

Stramignoni D., Bowen R., Atkinson B.F., Schlom J. Differential reactivity of monoclonal antibodies with human colon adenocarcinomas and adenomas. Int. J. Cancer 33: 543-552 (1983)

Taylor-Papadimitriou J., Lane E.B., Chang S.E. Cell lineages and interactions in neoplastic expression in the human breast. In: Proceedings, Breast Cancer Research Conference, Denver: (1983)

Taylor-Papadimitriou J., Peterson J.A., Arklie J., Burchell J., Ceriani R.L., Bodmer W.F. Monoclonal antibodies to epithelium-specific components of the human milkfat globule membrane: production and reaction with cells in culture. Int. J. Cancer 28: 17-21 (1981)

Teramoto Y.A., Mariani R., Wunderlich D., Schlom J. The immunohistochemical reactivity of a human monoclonal antibody with tissue sections of human mammary tumors. Cancer 50: 241-249 (1982)

Thompson C.H., Jones S.L., Whitehead R.H., McKenzie I.F.C. A human breast tissue-associated antigen detected by a monoclonal antibody. J. Natl. Cancer Inst. 70: 409-419 (1983)

White C.A., Dulbecco R., Allen R., Bowman M., Armstrong B. Two monoclonal antibodies selective for human mammary carcinoma. Cancer Res. 45: 1337-1343 (1985)

ACKNOWLEDGEMENTS
We gratefully acknowledge Greet van Doornewaard, Douwe Atsma, Dick Schol and Femke Buijs, The Netherlands Cancer Institute, Amsterdam and Judith Osztafin, Research Institute of Oncopathology, Budapest, for their excellent technical assistance. We also thank Dr. Arnoud Sonnenberg, Netherlands Cancer Institute, Amsterdam for profitable suggestions, Dr. Jozef Toth, Research Institute Oncopathology, Budapest, for providing mammary tissues. Dr. Henny J. Daams, Netherlands Cancer Institute, Amsterdam is thanked for his drawings.

IMMUNOCHEMICAL EVALUATION OF ESTROGEN RECEPTOR AND PROGESTERONE RECEPTOR IN BREAST CANCER

Geoffrey L. Greene and Michael F. Press

The Ben May Institute and Department of Pathology
The University of Chicago, 5841 S. Maryland Avenue
Chicago, Illinois 60637

INTRODUCTION

Recent advances in the preparation of monoclonal antibodies to human estrogen receptor (ER) and progesterone receptor (PR) have led to the development of new quantitative and histochemical immunoassays for these proteins in reproductive tissues and related cancers [1-6]. Such assays make use of very specific and sensitive probes that do not depend upon the ability of receptor protein to bind its cognate radiolabeled hormone in tissue extracts. In addition, these antibodies can be used to detect and quantify ER and PR directly in fixed tissue sections and cell dispersions, thereby permitting an evaluation of the type, proportion and distribution of cells that contain immunoreactive ER and/or PR. For metastatic breast cancer, a major potential clinical application of receptor immunoassays is the prediction of response to endocrine therapy and assessment of prognosis (disease-free interval and survival). The clinical utility of ER and PR steroid-binding assays for evaluating these parameters in patients with advanced breast cancer has been well documented [7-9]. However, major limitations of current receptor assays are 1) their inability to predict response to endocrine therapy in 30-40% of the breast cancers defined as ER- or PR-rich and in 5-10% of those that are receptor-poor, and 2) the difficulty of performing such assays on small tumors, metastasies and needle biopsies. In addition, assays performed on extracts of breast tumors cannot provide information about the identity, proportion and distribution of receptor-containing cells.

This paper summarizes the preparation and partial characterization of monoclonal antibodies to human ER and PR, and their use in the development of enzyme immunoassays and immunocytochemical assays for these receptors in breast tumors. The specificity, sensitivity and utility of current assay configurations is described, as well as implications concerning receptor-mediated hormone responses in target tissues for estrogens and progestins.

ESTROGEN RECEPTOR STUDIES

Structure and Composition of human ER

During the past several years, substantial progress has been made in the determination of estrogen receptor structure, composition and properties, particularly in human cells. A combination of events has contributed to this progress, including the development of suitable purification protocols [10], the preparation of a number of monoclonal antibodies to human ER [11-13], and the isolation and sequencing of cDNAs corresponding to the entire ER mRNA from MCF-7 human breast cancer cells [14-16]. At the same time, similar results have been obtained for human and rat glucocorticoid receptor [17,18], and more recently for chicken ER [19] and PR [20,21], providing a wealth of comparative information about these steroid receptors. The cytosol form of ER from MCF-7 cells has been purified to virtual homogeneity by sequential selective adsorption to estradiol-Sepharose and heparin-Sepharose, and by immunoadsorption with specific monoclonal antibodies [10]. The highly purified MCF-7 [^{3}H]estradiol-receptor complex (E*R_c) has properties that are similar to, if not the same as, the activated steroid-receptor complex found in high salt nuclear extracts of MCF-7 cells. Thus, the purified cytosol E*R binds DNA and sediments as a 5.3 S species in sucrose gradients containing 400 mM KCl. In addition, an apparent molecular weight of 140,000, calculated from a Stokes radius of 5.74 A and the 5.3 S sedimentation coefficient, is consistent with the formation of a homodimer of two 65K (4 S) monomers. Chemical crosslinking experiments and dense amino acid labeling of unpurified nuclear MCF-7 ER also indicate that activated E*R is a homodimer [22]. Interestingly, the purified E*R_c has lost its ability to form an 8-9 S complex in low-salt gradients and sediments as a 5.9 S species in 10 mM KCl, indicating that the factors, or factor, responsible for the formation of these larger complexes in cytosols are removed during purification. In fact, if purified receptor is added to receptor-depleted MCF-7 cytosol, a 7-8 S complex is observed in 10 mM KCl. When highly purified receptor is analyzed by SDS-gel electrophoresis under reducing conditions, one major silver-stained band, M_r 65,000, is seen. The same band can be visualized by autoradiography if bound E* is exchanged with [^{3}H]tamoxifen aziridine, a specific covalent tag for estrogen receptor [23]. When incubated with ^{32}P-ATP in the presence of a purified cytosolic calcium/calmodulin-dependent protein kinase isolated from rat brain (by Howard Schulman, Stanford University), human E*R_c was efficiently labeled, indicating that this receptor can serve as a substrate for this enzyme in vitro. There is increasing evidence that steroid receptors, including calf [24] and chicken [25] ER, mouse glucocorticoid receptor [26], and avian [27,28] and rabbit progesterone receptor, are phosphorylated in vivo.

The isolation of cDNA clones corresponding to human ER mRNA from MCF-7 cells has been achieved [14]. ER sequences were identified in randomly-primed λgt10 and λgt11 MCF-7 cDNA libraries by screening either with monoclonal ER antibodies or with synthetic oligonucleotides corresponding to two peptide sequences obtained from purified MCF-7 ER. Among the cDNA clones isolated by oligonucleotide hybridization was a 2.1 kb cDNA (OR8) which contained the entire translated portion of ER mRNA. This cDNA was sequenced and then expressed in chinese hamster ovary (CHO-K1) cells to give a functional protein [15]. An open reading frame of 1785 nucleotides in the cDNA corresponded to a polypeptide of 595 amino acids and M_r 66,200, which is in good agreement with published values of 65-70 kDa for ER. Homogenates of transformed CHO cells contained a protein which bound [^{3}H]estradiol and sedimented as a 4 S complex in salt-containing sucrose gradients and as a 8-9 S complex in the absence of salt. This E*R complex reacted with a monoclonal antibody (D75P3γ) which is specific for primate ER, confirming the identity of the expressed cDNA as human estrogen receptor. Interestingly, although CHO cells do not normally express estrogen receptor, the human E*R expressed by OR8 cDNA in these cells forms a 8-9 S complex in low salt gradients, suggesting either that this complex is a multimer of steroid-binding subunits or that associated non-steroid-binding components are present in nontarget cells. Amino acid sequence comparisons have revealed significant regional homologies among human ER, human and rat glucocorticoid receptor, chicken ER and PR, rabbit PR, and the putative v-erb-A oncogene product, indicating that steroid receptor genes and the avian erythroblastosis viral oncogene are derived from a common primordial gene [15-21]. The cysteine/lysine/arginine-rich homologous region appears to represent the DNA-binding domain of this family of proteins.

Monoclonal Antibodies to ER

To produce monoclonal antibodies to human ER, male Lewis rats were immunized with MCF-7 E^*R_c eluted from the estradiol-Sepharose column (5-10% pure). Fusion of splenic lymphocytes from immunized animals with two different mouse myeloma lines yielded three cloned hybridomas (D58, D75, D547) [11], each of which secretes a unique idiotype of antibody that recognizes a distinct region of the ER molecule. Subsequent fusions, carried out both in our own laboratory [12] and at Abbott Laboratories [13], have produced a total of 13 monoclonal antibodies, all of which (with one possible exception) recognize distinct regions of the receptor molecule. These antibodies have high affinity ($K_d=10^{-9}-10^{-10}$M) for both steroid-occupied and unoccupied estrogen receptor and recognize nuclear as well as cytosol forms of the receptor molecule. Although they vary in their cross reactivity with estrogen receptors from various animal species, each antibody appears to be completely specific for the 65,000-dalton steroid-binding subunit of the estrogen receptor complex, as judged by extensive sucrose gradient and immunoblot analyses (Fig. 1A) of cytosol and nuclear extracts from a variety of tissues and cell lines. Cross reactivity patterns [12] indicate both sequence homology and heterogeneity among mammalian and nonmammalian ERs. Some epitopes (eg. H222 and H226) are common to all tested estrogen receptors, whereas others (eg. D547 and D58) are present only in mammalian receptors, and one (D75) appears to be restricted to primate ER.

In ongoing studies to map the location of various epitopes in relation to each other and to the steroid- and DNA-binding domains, the relative positions of nine unique epitopes have been determined by density gradient analysis of antibody-E*R interaction after limited proteolysis of MCF-7 cytosol E*R with trypsin, chymotrypsin, or papain [12]. Epitopes for three of the monoclonal rat antibodies (D75, D547, H226) are susceptible to selective cleavage by one or more of the enzymes tested. Six other antibodies are capable of binding the smallest (2.6 S) steroid-binding fragment remaining after cleavage with trypsin. When tested for their ability to associate with 0X174 double-stranded DNA in sucrose density gradients, none of the E*R fragments was able to bind DNA, whereas the intact 5 S nuclear receptor co-sedimented with the DNA. Interestingly, the epitopes that are most well conserved across all tested species are located either near the steroid-binding domain (H23, H142, H165, H221, H222) or the DNA-binding domain (H226). These results are consistent with the variable regional homologies found in amino acid sequences derived from cDNAs for human and chicken ER.

Immunoassays for ER

Three monoclonal ER antibodies (D547, D75, H222) have been used to devise simple immunoradiometric (IRMA) [4] and immunocolorimetric (EIA) [5] sandwich assays for estrogen receptor in reproductive tissues and tumors. Polystyrene beads coated with D547 adsorb either occupied or unoccupied receptor present in a tissue or tumor extract. Radiolabeled (IRMA) or peroxidase-conjugated (EIA) D75 or H222 is then used to measure the amount of receptor bound to the bead. When tumor cytosols from 18

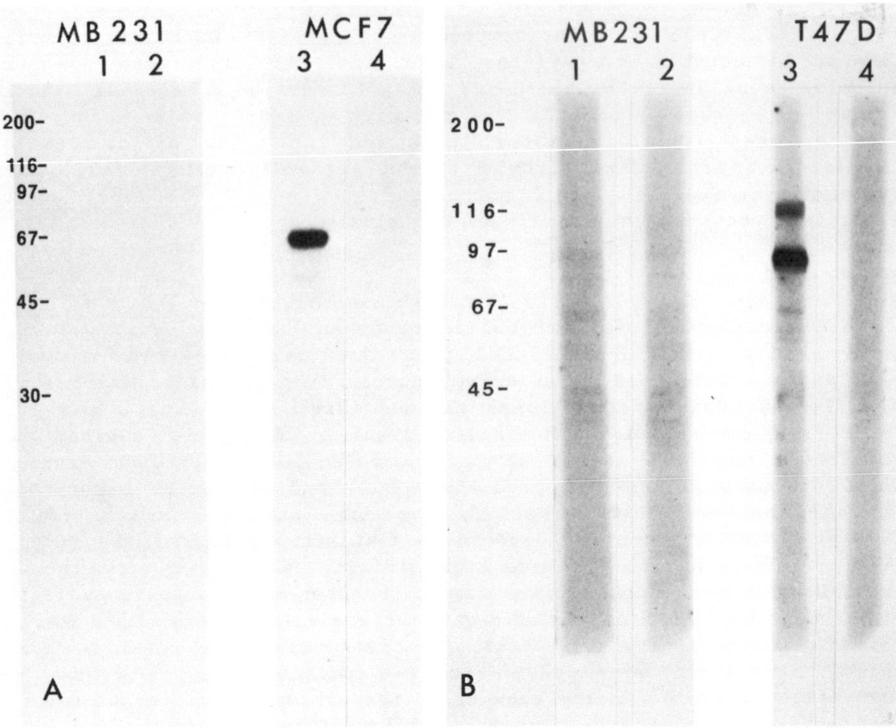

Fig. 1. (A) Immunoblot analysis of H222 (ER) IgG specificity. Cytosols from MCF-7 (6 pmol E*R/ml) and MDA MB-231 (0 pmol E*R/ml) cells were electrophoresed (about 15 µl per lane) under reducing conditions in 15% SDS acrylamide gels. Proteins were electrotransferred onto a nitrocellulose membrane and the membrane was saturated with milk proteins. The blocked membrane was then cut into strips and incubated either with H222 IgG (Lane 1) or with polyclonal IgG from a nonimmunized rat (Lane 2). Successive incubations were with rabbit antibody to rat IgG and ^{125}I-protein A. Dried strips were exposed to Kodak X-Omat XAR 5 film. Marker proteins were electrophoresed in adjacent lanes and visualized colorimetrically. Their relative molecular weights are shown.
(B) Immunoblot analysis of JZB39 (PR) IgG specificity. Cytosols from T47D (2 pmol P*R/ml) and MDA MB-231 (0 pmol P*R/ml) cells were electrophoresed (about 40 µl per lane) under reducing conditions in 10% SDS acrylamide gels. Proteins were electrotransferred to nitrocellulose and strips were incubated either with JZB39 IgG (Lane 1) or with polyclonal IgG from a nonimmunized rat (Lane 2). Subsequent steps were as above.

human breast cancers were analyzed for receptor content by the IRMA method (^{125}I-D75) and the results were compared with ER content determined by specific [^{3}H]estradiol binding to receptor on sucrose density gradients, a linear correlation (m=0.94, r=0.98) was obtained. This sandwich assay has since been modified to an immunocolorimetric assay (ER-EIA) at Abbott Laboratories and tested against more than 500 additional breast cancer cytosols with equally good results. A concordance of 90% between ER-EIA and steroid-binding results has been observed over a broad range of ER levels in tumor cytosols [6]. The sensitivity of the D547/H222 combination is about 2 fmol of ER per milliliter of cytosol (0.2 fmol/mg protein). A commercial version of the ER-EIA diagnostic kit that is simple, rapid, and does not depend on the binding of estradiol to its receptor is now available.

The major disadvantage of all quantitative receptor assays performed on tissue extracts is their inability to provide information about the inter- and intracellular distribution of receptor. As part of our ongoing effort to understand the dynamics of ER and PR in target tissues in the presence and absence of estrogens and antiestrogens, we have developed immunocytochemical assays for visualizing these proteins directly in tissues and cells. Five monoclonal antibodies (D547, D58, D75, H222, H226) were used individually to localize ER by an indirect immunoperoxidase technique in frozen, fixed sections of human breast tumors, human uterus, rabbit uterus, and in other mammalian reproductive tissues, as well as in fixed MCF-7 cell cultures [1-3]. Specific immunoperoxidase staining for receptor in estrogen-sensitive tissues was confined to the nucleus of all stained cells, regardless of hormone status, as shown in Fig. 2A for an infiltrating ductal breast carcinoma known to be ER-rich by DCC assay. Staining was absent in nontarget tissues, such as colon epithelium, and in receptor-negative cancers (Table 1); in addition, it was abolished by the addition of highly purified receptor to primary antibody. Heterogeneous staining was observed in MCF-7 cells as well as in receptor-poor and receptor-rich breast cancers, possibly reflecting either variations in cell cycle or the presence of estrogen-sensitive and insensitive cells. Little or no cytoplasmic staining for ER has been observed in any of the tissues or tumor cells examined thus far, including those deprived of exogenous estrogens. To confirm that ER monoclonal antibodies should be able to recognize unoccupied receptor, regardless of subcellular location, density gradient analyses of MCF-7 ER-antibody interactions were performed in the absence of steroid. As shown in Fig. 3 for D547 and H222 IgGs, the formation of immune complexes could be demonstrated by post-labeling fractions with E*; recovery of E*R was greater than 90%.

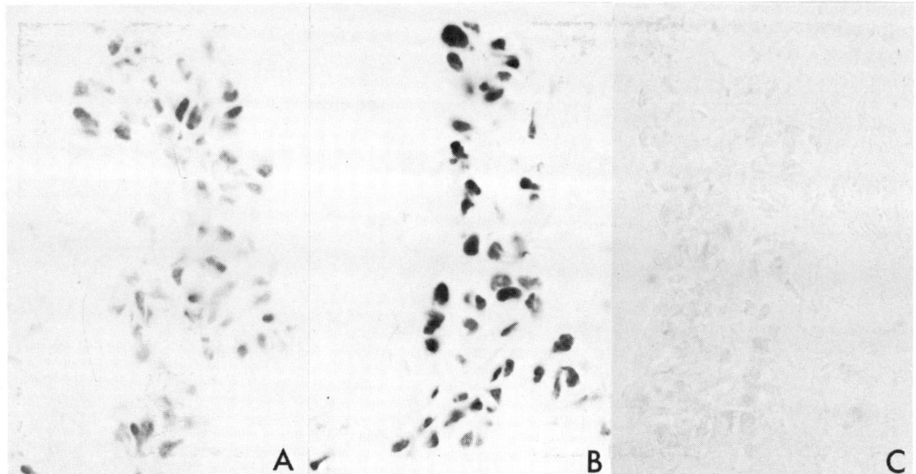

Fig. 2. Immunocytochemical stainining of an ER- and PR-rich breast tumor section. Serial 8-μm frozen sections of a tumor from a postmenopausal patient were fixed in picric acid-paraformaldehyde and stained by the indirect immunoperoxidase technique [1-3] with H222 (A), JZB39 (B), or control rat (C) IgG. The cytosolic ER and PR content, as determined by DCC assay, were 76 and 231 fmol/mg cytosol protein, respectively. Orig. mag., x 400; no counterstain.

Table 1. Tissue and tumor specificity of ER-ICA and PR-ICA

	ER-ICA	PR-ICA
	TISSUES	
BREAST	+	+
VAGINA	+	+
CERVIX	+	+
ENDOMETRIUM	+	+
FALLOPIAN TUBE	+	+
LUNG	–	–
COLON	–	–
STOMACH	–	–
SKELETAL MUSCLE	–	–
SPLEEN	–	–
GALL BLADDER	–	–
PANCREAS	–	–
THYROID	–	–
	TUMORS	
BREAST CANCER	+	+
ENDOMETRIAL CANCER	+	+
OVARIAN CANCER	+	+
COLON CANCER	–	–
LUNG CANCER	–	–
MENINGIOMA	–	+
	CELL LINES	
MCF-7	+	+ (induced)
T47D	–	+
MB-231	–	–

In a study of 117 human breast cancers by the ER-ICA method, the presence or absence of specific nuclear staining for ER was significantly associated with the concentration of cytosolic estrogen receptor determined by steroid-binding assay [3]. A more recent analysis of primary breast tumors from postmenopausal patients at high risk for recurrence has shown that several quantifiable features of ER-ICA determinations correlate significantly with ER concentrations measured in cytosols [29]. The two parameters that contribute the most to this correlation are the staining intensity and the proportion of positively stained cells in the cancer. Fig. 4 depicts the correlation of predicted ER values obtained from a best fit equation of these parameters with ER-DCC results; the correlation ($R = 0.82$) is highly significant ($P < 0.001$). The overall ER-ICA status for these breast cancers also differentiated two populations of patients with different disease-free experience and survival. As shown in Fig. 5, the proportion of patients surviving four years after mastectomy is significantly higher ($P = 0.001$)

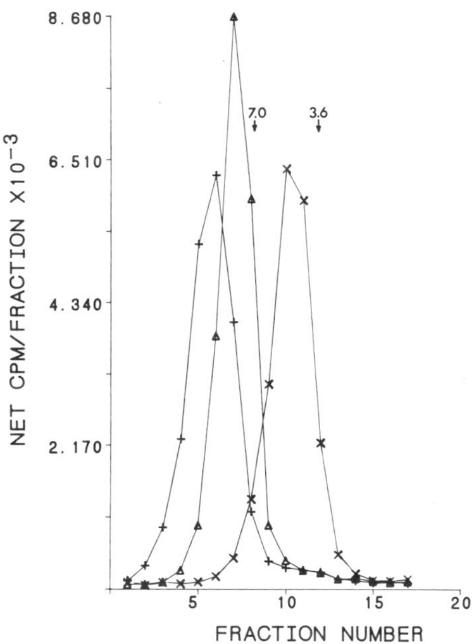

Fig. 3. Interaction of unoccupied MCF-7 ER with D547 and H222 IgGs. Aliquots (150 µl) of unlabeled MCF-7 cytosol ER (0.76 pmol) were incubated with 20 µg each of purified JZB39 (X–X)(control), D547 (Δ–Δ) or D547 + H222 (+–+) for 60 min at 4°C. Incubation mixtures were then layered onto 10-30% sucrose gradients (3.5 ml) containing 10 mM Tris, 400 mM KCL, 1 mM EDTA, 20 mM sodium molybdate, pH 7.4, and centrifuged at 253,000 x g for 15 hr at 2°C. Successive 200-µl fractions were collected in tubes containing 100 µg of ovalbumin and 6 pmol of [^{3}H]estradiol in 50 µl of the same buffer, and the mixtures were incubated for 60 min at 4°C. The E*R content of each fraction was then determined by measuring the specific binding of E*R to Controlled-Pore glass beads. The recoveries of postlabeled ER as [^{3}H]estradiol-receptor complex (E*R) were 0.68 pmol (90%) for JZB39 (4.9 S), 0.73 pmol (96%) for D547 (8.1 S), and 0.72 pmol (95%) for D547/H222 (9.5 S). ^{14}C-labeled ovalbumin (3.6 S) and bovine IgG (7.0 S) were used as external markers in a separate gradient.

for ER-ICA positive tumors than for ER-ICA negative tumors. Although some of this difference may be related to the improved prognosis of patients who received adjuvant tamoxifen therapy, patients with ER-ICA positive lesions have a better prognosis whether treated with tamoxifen or not.

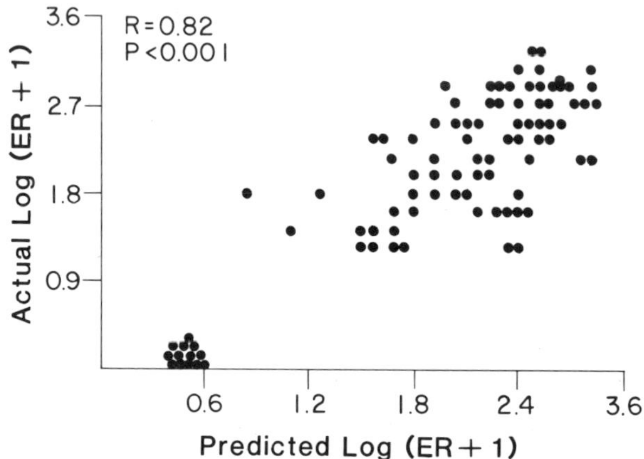

Fig. 4. Regression analysis of ER-ICA and ER-DCC. Relationship of the ER content calculated by the regression equation based on ER-ICA intensity and distribution to the actual (measured by DCC) ER. The correlation coefficient (R) relates to the fit of the calculated results to the actual data. Log(ER + 1) = 0.515 + 0.25(intensity) + 0.015(%ER-ICA positive). Reproduced from [29].

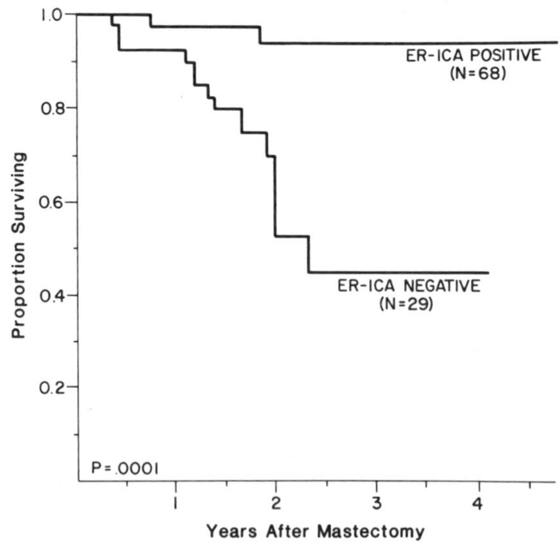

Fig. 5. Patient survival and ER-ICA status. Reproduced from [29].

An additional, and potentially important, clinical application of ER-ICA would be the ability of this assay to identify breast cancer patients with advanced disease who are likely to respond to endocrine therapy. Thus far, four independent studies with clinical response data have been published [30-33]. The results of the correlations between ER-ICA status and hormonal response for patients with metastatic breast cancer are summarized in Table 2. Overall, approximately 74% (56/76) of ER-ICA positive patients responded objectively to endocrine manipulation (complete remission or arrested disease), whereas only 8% (5/66) of ER-ICA negative patients responded. It is of interest that the results among the four unrelated groups are very similar despite the use of different, and subjective, criteria for interpretation of ER-ICA status. Clearly, the number of patients for which response data and ER-ICA evaluations are available is still very low. However, the data suggest that ER-ICA status, and possibly one or more semiquantifiable features of immunocytochemical staining for ER, may be a useful predictor of response to endocrine therapy for patients with advanced breast cancer.

Table 2. Clinical Correlation of Breast Cancer Remissions to Endocrine Therapy and ER-ICA Results

	RESPONDERS (CR and PR)	
INVESTIGATOR	$ER\text{-}ICA^{+}$ (%)	$ER\text{-}ICA^{-}$ (%)
COOMBES [30]	21/29 (72)	1/27 (4)
JONAT [31]	6/11 (55)	1/9 (11)
McCARTY [32]	13/14 (93)	1/9 (11)
PERTSCHUK [33]	16/22 (73)	2/21 (10)
TOTAL	56/76 (74)	5/66 (8)

PROGESTERONE RECEPTOR STUDIES

Structure and Composition of Human PR

During the past few years, significant progress has been made toward establishing a simple and rapid purification sequence for human progesterone receptor. The primary source of PR has been T47D human breast cancer cells [34], a cell line that is rich in progesterone receptor but deficient in estrogen receptor. Also, in contrast to the chicken oviduct, rabbit uterus and MCF-7 cells, progesterone receptor expression in T47D cells is not under estrogen control [35]. The human PR complex appears to consist of two dissimilar subunits that can be photoaffinity labeled specifically with the synthetic progestin ^{3}H-R5020 and visualized on autoradiograms of reducing SDS gels at 95 kDa (A subunit) and at 120 kDa (B subunit) [36]. At this point it is not clear whether these two proteins represent different gene products or whether A is derived from B by proteolysis or possibly by an RNA splicing mechanism.

In the chicken oviduct, A is reported to have a high affinity for DNA and B a high affinity for one or more nonhistone proteins in chromatin [37]. However, rabbit uterine PR exists only in the larger form (110K) when proper precautions are taken during homogenization [38]. We have observed both forms, in agreement with published results, in cytosol and nuclear extracts of T47D cells and MCF-7 cells.

The cytosol and nuclear forms of PR from T47D cells have been partially purified either by selective adsorption to deoxycorticosterone coupled to Sepharose, followed by ion exchange chromatography, or by immunoadsorption to a monoclonal PR antibody (JU601) coupled to Sepharose 4B. Receptor obtained by affinity and ion exchange chromatography is generally 2-10% pure, whereas material obtained by immunopurification is 30-60% pure. Purified PR consists of the expected two steroid-binding components which, when photoaffinity-labeled with ^{3}H-R5020, migrate at 120 kDa (B) and 95 kDa (A) in reducing SDS gels.

Monoclonal Antibodies to PR

We have prepared more than 14 monoclonal antibodies to the A and B steroid-binding components of the PR complex. Of these, 13 recognize epitopes shared by the A and B components. One antibody, KC 146, is specific for the B component. Like the ER monoclonal antibodies, the PR antibodies have high affinity for steroid-occupied as well as unoccupied receptor and recognize both nuclear and cytosol forms. Three of the PR antibodies cross react with rabbit PR, but not with calf, rat or chicken PR. However, the mouse monoclonal antibody which is specific for human B (KC 146) also recognizes the B component in calf uterine, chicken oviduct, and rat uterine cytosol. The specificity of one of the rat IgGs (JZB39) is shown in Fig. 1B. Only the B (120 kDa) and A (95 kDa) components of human PR are recognized by this antibody on a western blot of T47D cytosol after fractionation by SDS gel electrophoresis. These components are absent in MDA MB-231 cell cytosol, consistent with the reported absence of PR in these cells.

Immunoassays for PR

In regard to the development of quantitative immunoassays for PR, an enzyme immunoassay similar to the one developed for ER (PR-EIA) is being developed for PR analysis in extracts of hormone-responsive cancers. Several combinations of antibodies have been tested on polystyrene beads and at least two combinations appear to have the necessary sensitivity and specificity for accurate PR measurement. When 28 human breast tumor cytosols were analyzed by a prototype PR-EIA, the results correlated well (R = 0.96) with values determined by the NEN progestin receptor assay kit [39]. The sensitivity of the PR-EIA was 2-3 fmol of PR per ml of extract.

For immunocytochemical localization of PR in various tissues and tumors, the JZB39 and KD68 IgGs have proved most useful. As shown in Fig. 2B for JZB39, specific nuclear staining for PR is observed, under the same fixation conditions and with the same reagents used for ER-ICA, in a serial section from an ER- and PR-rich breast carcinoma. The overall tissue specificity for this antibody is shown in comparison with ER-ICA in Table 1. Several studies are in progress to evaluate these antibodies as probes for PR in breast tumors, especially in comparison to biochemically determined PR in cytosols and to ER measurement and localization with the ER-ICA method. In a preliminary evaluation of 20 breast tumors by the PR-ICA method, a good correlation was observed between measured PR in tumor cytosols and the presence or absence of specific nuclear staining for PR in frozen, fixed tumor sections (Table 3).

Table 3. Correlation of ER-ICA and PR-ICA with DCC Assays for 20 Breast Cancers

Case	Prop.+ Tumor	ER-ICA° H222	ER*	PR-ICA° JZB39	PR*
1.	0.90	-(0)	1	-(0)	2
2.	1.00	++/+++(.90)	413	++++(.98)	1423
3.	0.75	-(0)	2	-(0)	1
4.	0.87	++/+++(.54)	109	++(.49)	286
5.	0.40	++/+++(.84)	226	+/++(.41)	111
6.	0.44	++/+++(.72)	92	-(0)	0
7.	0.76	-(0)	23	-(0)	5
8.	0.60	++/+++(.84)	383	+(.27)	107
9.	0.69	++(.67)	325	-(0)	4
10.	0.97	+++(.68)	247	++(.32)	275
11.	0.05	-(0)	0	-(0)	4
12.	0.45	++(.52)	90	wk+(.18)	30
13.	0.33	-(0)	15	+(0.33)	22
14.	0.10	+++(0.33)	138	++	270
15.	0.80	wk+(.30)	14	+(.37)	21
16.	0.23	++(.78)	31	-(0)	1
17.	0.38	-(0)	2	-(0)	9
18.	0.40	++(0.71)	116	-(0)	6
19.	0.29	+(0.35)	122	+/++(0.37)	149
20.	0.31	+(0.52)	90	+(0.38)	1

+proportion of tissue that is tumor
*fmol/mg cytosol protein
°average intensity of specific nuclear staining
Numbers in parentheses refer to the proportion of tumor cells with specific nuclear staining.

DISCUSSION

Correlations of patient responses to endocrine therapies with th estrogen receptor and progesterone receptor content of breast cancers hav clearly established the clinical utility of biochemical ER and PR assays While only 25 to 30% of unselected breast cancer patients obtain objectiv remission of metastatic disease following various endocrine therapies, more than 75% of the patients whose cancers contain both ER and PR benefi [7], whereas there is a 33% response rate when only one of the tw receptors is present [8]. Moreover, patients whose primary cancers are ER/PR-rich are more likely to have a longer disease-free interval than those whose lesions lack either receptor [9]. Recent data from several clinical studies [40] indicate that progesterone receptor, as an end product of estrogen action, is an even better marker than estrogen receptor for favorable prognosis and endocrine responsiveness in breast cancer. All of these results were obtained with biochemical radioligand assays. Despite the value of current ER and PR assays, there is a need to improve the accuracy of response and prognosis predictions.

From the results described in this paper, it is clear that immunochemical evaluations of ER and PR content and distribution in breast lesions are feasible and informative. The quantitative sandwich enzyme immunoassays are simple, rapid, sensitive and less likely to be affected by chemical and conformational changes in receptor than steroid-binding assays. Monoclonal antibodies prepared against both ER and PR have been shown to be completely specific for their corresponding receptor, with the exception of two PR antibodies that recognize epitopes present on nuclear proteins present in nontarget tissues. In addition, all ER and PR antibodies used in these assays recognize occupied as well as unoccupied receptor, permitting measurement of total receptor in cytosol as well as nuclear extracts of tumors. In a recent European multicenter study involving eight laboratories and more than 500 breast cancers, a comparison of ER-EIA results with steroid-binding results revealed an excellent correlation over a broad range of ER concentrations [41]. For seven of these studies, the slope of the correlation line was very close to 1.0, and the Y intercept was not significantly different from zero in five laboratories. Inter- and intralaboratory variation coefficients were low, probably due to the standardization of the ER-EIA. Although further testing is warranted, the ER-EIA should provide an accurate and sensitive means of measuring ER in tumors from pre- and postmenopausal women. Preliminary studies with prototype PR-EIAs suggest that this assay will be equally useful for measurement of PR in tumor extracts.

As a complementary, and possibly alternative, approach to receptor assessment in breast cancers, direct localization of ER and PR in tumor cells by immunoperoxidase staining offers several advantages. First, it is possible to distinguish ER- and/or PR-containing tumor cells from negative tumor cells and normal tissue. In addition, cytological preparations from primary tumors or from metastases at different sites can be readily evaluated for ER or PR on relatively few cells. Problems with sample storage and handling are also minimized since no homogenization is required. Finally, as already shown for ER-ICA, several quantifiable features of immunoperoxidase staining, including staining intensity and the proportion of tumor cells stained, correlate with the ER content, patient prognosis for recurrence and length of survival, and response of patients with metastatic breast cancer to hormone therapy. Although clinical data is not yet available for PR-ICA, the results shown in Table 3 and unpublished data from this and other laboratories indicate that immunocytochemical evaluations of PR in breast cancers correlate well with the PR content of these tumors. It is not clear yet whether the ER-ICA and PR-ICA will provide information that is more useful than current steroid-binding assays for ER and PR. However, the direct assessment of ER and PR in frozen, and possibly paraffin, sections of tumors as well as in needle aspirates of lesions will certainly simplify tumor evaluation and repeat sampling. Finally, if tumor heterogeneity is an indicator of cancers that are less likely to respond to hormone therapy, due to the presence of autonomous, ER- and/or PR-negative neoplastic cells, the ability to identify such cells may be important in determining the appropriate therapy and course of the disease.

In view of the exclusively nuclear localization of specific immunoperoxidase staining for ER and PR in all hormone-sensitive tissues and cells studied thus far, it appears that both cytosol and nuclear forms of these receptors may reside in the nuclear compartment in the presence and absence of steroid. We have seen little or no increase in nuclear staining intensity for ER in MCF-7 cells and in uteri from immature rabbits or from postmenopausal women following short-term exposure of cells or tissue to estradiol. A notable exception is the increase in nuclear staining intensity observed by McClellan et al. [42] in monkey endometrium following in vitro exposure to 100nM estradiol. By immunoelectron microscopy, ER was localized in the euchromatin, but not in the marginated heterochromatin or nucleoli of MCF-7 nuclei and epithelial and stromal nuclei of postmenopausal human endometrium [43]. These observations suggest that the majority of the unoccupied receptor actually resides in the nucleus, rather than in the cytoplasm as previously thought. Thus, hormone action may involve binding of the steroid directly to receptor loosely associated with nuclear components, followed by conversion of the steroid-receptor complex to an activated form which becomes more tightly associated with chromatin. This hypothesis is supported by the observations of Welshons et al. [44] and Gurpide [45] that cytochalasin-induced enucleation of ER-, PR- and GR-containing cells leads to partitioning of unoccupied receptor almost exclusively into the nucleoplast fraction. Also, progesterone receptor has been localized to the nuclei of hormone-responsive cells in chick oviduct [46] and in rabbit uterus [47] with polyclonal and monoclonal antibodies, respectively. In contrast, immunoreactive glucocorticoid receptor has been observed both in the cytoplasm and in the nucleus of target cells [48]. The reasons for this discrepancy are not clear at this time. However, thus far no one has been able to demonstrate conclusively the hormone-induced translocation of any steroid receptor from the cytoplasm to the nucleus of a target cell.

Rapid advances are occurring in the utilization of new technologies to study gene regulation by steroid hormones in normal and neoplastic tissues. Much of the current focus is on the use of immunochemical and recombinant DNA techniques to probe the structure, composition and dynamics of the intracellular receptor proteins in target tissues. An understanding of structure-function relationships is beginning to emerge from these studies, in part from mutagenic analyses of ER, PR and GR coupled with immunochemical identification of receptor fragments produced by expression of cloned cDNAs and/or controlled proteolytic cleavage of receptor proteins. The same probes will facilitate investigations of the interaction of these receptors and their altered forms with cloned enhancer elements of hormone-responsive genes. Finally, it is now possible to begin to look at the regulation of expression of ER and PR in responsive tissues and cancers by northern blot analysis and by in situ hybridization techniques, as well as to look for altered genes or possibly gene rearrangements in neoplastic cells. As the molecular aspects of receptor-mediated steroid responses are elucidated, it is likely that the nature of hormone regulation in breast cancer and other hormone-dependent neoplasms will be better understood.

ACKNOWLEDGEMENTS

These studies were supported by Abbott Laboratories, the American Cancer Society (BC-86), the NCI (CA-02897) and by the Women's Board of the University of Chicago Cancer Research Foundation.

REFERENCES

1. W. J. King and G. L. Greene, Monoclonal antibodies localize estrogen receptor in the nuclei of target cells, Nature 307:745 (1984).

2. M. F. Press and G L. Greene, An immunocytochemical method for demonstrating estrogen receptor in human uterus using monoclonal antibodies to human estrophilin, Lab. Invest. 50:480 (1984).

3. W. J. King, E. R. DeSombre, E. V. Jensen and G. L. Greene, Comparison of cytochemical and steroid-binding assays for estrogen receptor in human breast cancer, Cancer Res. 45:293 (1985).

4. G. L. Greene and E. V. Jensen, Monoclonal antibodies as probes for estrogen receptor detection and characterization, J. Steroid Biochem. 16:353 (1982).

5. C. Nolan, L. W. Przywara, L. S. Miller, V. Susuikis and J. Tomita, A sensitive solid-phase enzyme immnoassay for human estrogen receptor, in Current Controversies in Breast Cancer," F. C. Ames, G. R. Blumansheim, and E. D. Montague, eds., Univ. of Texas Press, Austin, (1984).

6. Cancer Res. Suppl. 46:4231s (1986).

7. E. R. DeSombre, P. P. Carbone, E. V. Jensen, W. L. McGuire, S. A. Wells, J. L. Wittliff and M. B. Lipsett, Special report: steroid receptors in breast cancer, N. Engl. J. Med. 301:1011 (1979).

8. E. R. DeSombre, Steroid receptors in breast cancer, in "The Breast", R. W. McDivitt, H. A. Oberman, L. Ozzello and N. Kaufman, eds., Williams & Wilkins, Baltimore (1984).

9. C. K. Osborne, M. G. Yochmowitz, W. A. and W. L. McGuire, The value of estrogen and progesterone receptors in the treatment of breast cancer, Cancer 46:2884 (1980).

10. G. L. Greene, Application of immunochemical techniques to the analysis of estrogen receptor structure and function, in "Biochemical Actions of Hormones", Vol 11, G. Litwack, ed., Academic, New York (1984).

11. G. L. Greene, C. Nolan, J. P. Engler and E. V. Jensen, Monoclonal antibodies to the human estrogen receptor, Proc. Natl. Acad. Sci. USA 77:5115 (1980).

12. G. L. Greene, N. B. Sobel, W. J. King and E. V. Jensen, Immunochemical studies of estrogen receptors, J. steroid Biochem. 20:51 (1984).

13. L. S. Miller, I. I. E. Tribby, M. R. Miles, J. T. Tomita and C. Nolan, Hybridomas producing monoclonal antibodies to human estrogen receptor, Fedn. Proc. 41:520 (1982).

14. P. Walter, S. Green, G. Greene, A. Krust, J. M. Bornert, J. M. Jeltsch, A. Staub, E. Jensen, G. Scrace, M. Waterfield and P. Chambon, Cloning of the human estrogen receptor cDNA, Proc. natl. acad. Sci. USA 82:7889 (1985).

15. G. L. Greene, P. Gilna, M. Waterfield, A. Baker, Y. Hort and J. Shine, Sequence and expression of human estrogen receptor complementary DNA, Science 231:1150 (1986).

16. S. Green, P. Walter, V. Kumar, A. Krust, J.-M. Bornert, P. Argos and P. Chambon, Human oestrogen receptor cDNA: sequence, expression and homology to v-erb-A, Nature 320:134 (1986).

17. S. M. Hollenberg, C. Weinberger, E. S. Ong, G. Cerelli, A. Oro, R.

Lebo, E. B. Thompson,m M. G. Rosenfeld and R. M. Evans, Primary structure and expression of a functional human glucocorticoid receptor cDNA, Nature 318:635 (1985).

18. R. Miesfeld, S. Rusconi, P. J. Godowski, B. A. Maler, S. Okret, A. C. Wikstrom, J. A. Gustafsson, and K. R. Yamamoto, Genetic complementation of a glucocorticoid receptor deficiency by expression of cloned receptor cDNA, Cell 46:389 (1986).

19. A. Krust, S. Green, P. Argos, V. Kumar, P. Walter, J. M. Bornert and P. Chambon, The chicken oestrogen receptor sequence: homology with v-erbA and the human oestrogen and glucocorticoid receptors, EMBO J. 5:891 (1986).

20. O. M. Conneely et all, Molecular cloning of the chicken progesterone receptor, Science 233:767 (1986).

21. J. M. Jeltsch, Z. Krozowski, C. Quirin-Stricker, H. Gronemeyer, R. J. Simpson, J. M. Garnier, A. Krust, F. Jacob and P. Chambon, Cloning of the chicken progesterone receptor, Proc. natl. acad. Sci. USA 83:5424 (1986).

22. M. A. Miller, A. Mullick, G. L. Greene and B. S. Katzenellenbogen, Characterization of the subunit nature of nuclear estrogen receptors by chemical cross-linging and dense amino acid labeling, Endocrinology 117:515 (1985).

23. J. A. Katzenellenbogen, K. E. Carlson, D. F. Heiman, D. W. Robertson, L. L. Weill and B. S. Katzenellenbogen, Efficient and highly selective covalent labeling of the estrogen receptor with [^{3}H]tamoxifen aziridine, J. biol. Chem. 258:3487 (1983).

24. A. Migliaccio, A. Rotondi and F. Auricchio, Calmodulin-stimulated phosphorylation of 17β-estradiol receptor on tyrosine, Proc. natn. acad. Sci. U.S.A. 81:5921 (1984).

25. W. J. Raymoure, R. W. McNaught and R. G. Smith, Reversible activation of non-steroid binding oestrogen receptor, Nature 314:745 (1985).

26. P. R. Housley and W. B. Pratt, Direct demonstration of glucocorticoid receptor phosphorylation by intact L-cells, J. biol. Chem. 258:4630 (1983).

27. N. L. Weigel, J. S. Tash, A. R. Means, W. T. Schrader and B. W. O'Malley, Phosphorylation of hen progesterone receptor by cAMP dependent protein kinase Biochem. biophys. Res Commun. 102:513 (1981).

28. J. J. Dougherty, R. K. Puri and D. O. Toft, Polypeptide components of two 8S forms of chicken oviduct progesterone receptor, J. biol. Chem. 259:8004 (1984).

29. E. R. DeSombre, S. M. Thorpe, C. Rose, R. R. Blough, K. W. Andersen, B. B. Rasmussen and W. J. King, Prognostic usefulness of estrogen receptor immunocytochemical assays for human breast cancer, Cancer Res. 46:4256s (1986).

30. R. A. McClelland, U. Berger, L. S. Miller, T. J. Powles, E. V. Jensen and R. C. Coombes, Immunocytochemical assay for estrogen receptor: relationship to outcome of therapy in patients with advanced breast cancer, Cancer Res. 46:4241s (1986).

31. W. Jonat, H. Maass and H. E. Stegner, Immunohistochemical measurement of estrogen receptors in breast cancer tissue samples, Cancer Res. 46:4296s (1986).

32. K. S. McCarty Jr. et al, Use of a monoclonal anti-estrogen receptor antibody in the immunohistochemical evaluation of human tumors, Cancer Res. 46:4244s (1986).

33. L. P. Pertschuk, K. B. Eisenberg, A. C. Carter and J. G. Feldmann, Immunohistologic localization of estrogen receptors in breast cancer with monoclonal antibodies, Cancer (Phila.) 55:1513 (1985).

34. K. B. Horwitz, D. T. Zava, A. K. Thilagar, E. M. Jensen and W. L. McGuire, Steroid receptor analyses of nine human breast cancer cell lines, Cancer Res. 38:2434 (1978).

35. K. B. Horwitz, M. B. Mockus and B. A. Lessey, Variant T47D human breast cancer cells with high progesterone-receptor levels despite estrogen and antiestrogen resistance, Cell 28:633 (1982).

36. K. B. Horwitz and P. S. Alexander, In situ photolinked nuclear progesterone receptors of human breast cancer cells: subunit molecular weights after transformation and translocation, Endocrinology 113:2195 (1983).

37. B. W. O'Malley, Steroid hormone action in eukaryotic cells, J. Clin. Invest. 74:307 (1984).

38. H. Loosfelt, F. Logeat, M. T. V. Hai and E. Milgrom, The rabbit progesterone receptor. Evidence for a single steroid-binding subunit and characterization of receptor mRNA, J. Biol. Chem. 259:13196 (1984).

39. R. A. Weigand, C. Nolan, R. J. Kinders, L. W. Przywara, D. L. Cotter, R. Dunn, B. S. Moore, V. V. Suduikis and G. L. Greene, Measurement of progesterone receptor in human breast tumors by monoclonal enzyme immunoassays, 68th Annual meeting of the Endocrine Society, Anaheim, Abstr. 1005 (1986).

40. G. M. Clark, W. L. McGuire, C. A. Hubay, O. H. Pearson and J. S. Marshall, New Engl. J. Med. 309:1343 (1983).

41. G. Leclercq et al, Abbott monoclonal enzyme immunoassay measurement of estrogen receptors in human breast cancer: a European multicenter study, Cancer Res. 46:4233s (1986).

42. M. C. McClellan, N. B. West, D. E. Tacha, G. L. Greene and R. M Brenner, Immunocytochemical localization of estrogen receptors in the Macaque reproductive tract with monoclonal antiestrophilins, Endocrinology 114:2002 (1984).

43. M. F. Press, N. A. Nousek-Goebl and G. L. Greene, Immunoelectron microscopic localization of estrogen receptor with monoclonal estrophilin antibodies, J. Histochem. Cytochem. 33:915 (1985).

44. W. V. Welshons, B. M. Krummel and J. Gorski, Nuclear localization of unoccupied receptors for glucocorticoids, estrogens, and progesterone in GH_3 cells, Endocrinology 117:2140 (1986).

45. A. Gravanis and E. Gurpide, Enucleation of human endometrial cells: nucleo-cytoplasmic distribution of DNA polymerase α and estrogen

46. J. M. Gasc, J. Renoir, C. Radanyi, I. Joab, P. Tuohimaa and E. E. Baulieu, Progesterone receptor in the chick oviduct: an immunohistochemical study with antibodies to distinct receptor components, J. Cell. Biol. 99:1193 (1984).

47. M. Perrot-Applanat, F. Logeat, M. T. Groyer-Pickard and E. Milgrom, Immunocytochemical study of mammalian progesterone receptor using monoclonal antibodies, Endocrinology 116:1473 (1985).

48. K. Fuxe, A.-C. Wikstrom, S. Okret, L. F. Agnati, A. Harfstrand, Z.-Y. Yu, L. Granholm, M. Zoli, W. Vale and J.-A. Gustafsson, Mapping of glucocorticoid receptor immunoreactive neurons in the rat tel- and diencephalon using a monoclonal antibody against rat liver glucocorticoid receptor, Endocrinology 117:1803 (1985).

APPLICABILITY OF MONOCLONAL ANTIBODIES AGAINST ESTROGEN AND PROGESTERONE RECEPTORS IN THE IMMUNOCYTOCHEMICAL EVALUATION OF BREAST CARCINOMAS

L. Ozzello, C.M. DeRosa, and D.V. Habif

Arthur Purdy Stout Laboratory of Surgical
Pathology and Department of Surgery
College of Physicians and Surgeons
Columbia University, New York, N.Y. 10032

INTRODUCTION

The development of monoclonal antibodies against receptor proteins for estrogen (ER) and progesterone (PR) has opened a new perspective in the endocrinological evaluation of breast cancer patients. Indeed, a great deal of information can be obtained by applying these antibodies to tissue sections, including information that cannot be provided by steroid-binding assays. Of particular interest is the assessment of the percentage of receptor-positive cells in any given tumor, which can be easily evaluated in stained sections, but cannot be estimated by biochemical assays on tissue homogenates. Basic research in this field has been done on frozen sections which have proved to be quite reliable as documented by several reports presented at a recent symposium on Estrogen Receptor Determination with Monoclonal Antibodies (Cancer Res. Suppl. 46: 4231-4314, 1986). However, for the purpose of using immunocytochemistry for the practical assessment of the ER and PR status of breast cancer patients it should be realized that tissue for frozen sections is not always available and for this reason it is important to be able to apply these techniques to paraffin embedded tissues or to cytological preparations.

During the past few years we have been interested in establishing technical procedures by which monoclonal antibodies against ER and PR can be used to generate diagnostic information in the setting of a Surgical Pathology service. By testing several modalities we have found that different anti-ER and anti-PR antibodies react optimally under particular conditions, and that through the proper selection of antibodies it is possible to obtain valid information in all kinds of cases. Pertinent observations are described below.

MONOCLONAL ANTIBODIES

For the visualization of ER we mostly used 2 antibodies: D75-P3γ prepared and given to us by Dr. G.L. Greene[3], and H222-Spγ developed by Dr. L.S. Miller and supplied by Abbott Laboratories. Antibodies JZB-39 for the immunostaining of PR was kindly made available to us by Dr. G.L. Greene.

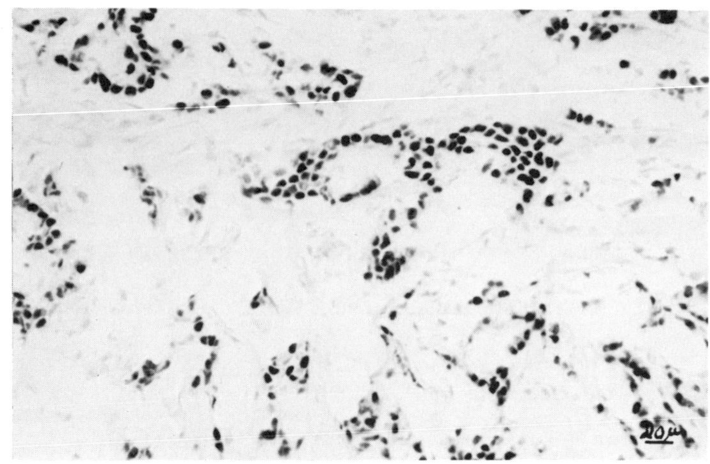

Fig. 1. Positive nuclear immunoreactivity in an infiltrating ductal carcinoma (49 year-old woman, DCC 650 fmol/mg). ER-ICA.

IMMUNOSTAINING OF ESTROGEN RECEPTOR

Frozen sections

Our work on frozen sections of breast carcinomas has been done using H222 antibody. It was first carried out in collaboration with Abbott Laboratories as part of preliminary testing of the ER-ICA kit.[5] Subsequently, we have continued to use the same technique and obtained consistently reproducible results which are described below.

The technique, an adaptation of the peroxidase-anti-peroxidase (PAP) technique, is that suggested by the manufacturer for the ER-ICA assay.[5] Briefly, cryostat sections 4-6 µ thick are cut from tissue samples frozen at -80°C. Two adjacent sections from each specimen are fixed in 3.7% formaldehyde at room temperature and then passed through cold methanol and cold acetone. Following incubation with blocking reagent (normal goat serum), one section is incubated with H222 monoclonal antibody for 30 minutes at room temperature, while the other section is exposed to control antibody (normal rat IgG). All sections are then incubated with bridging antibody (goat anti-rat antibody) and with PAP complex (rat anti-PAP in Tris buffer). Diaminobenzidine is used as chromogen and Harris hematoxylin as nuclear counterstain. MCF-7 cells attached to glass slides serve as ER-positive controls and are processed simultaneously with the diagnostic sections. A quantitative assay for ER (dextran-coated charcoal analysis, DCC) is performed on every tumor in another laboratory.

A positive reaction is characterized by brown staining of the nuclei of the carcinoma cells (Fig. 1.). The intensity of the reaction varies among the nuclei of any one case as does the number of positive nuclei. Therefore, sections are evaluated as to the overall intensity of the reaction and to the percentage of positive nuclei. In terms of correspondence with DCC results, however, we regard the number of positive nuclei as the more reliable semiquantitative criterion of the two since in previously studied material it was found to correlate with the DCC assay in a statistically significant manner ($p < 0.01$) whereas the intensity of the staining did not.[5]

Table 1. Comparison of immunostaining with DCC assay values for 62 breast carcinomas (ER-ICA, frozen sections)

Nuclear staining	fmol/mg cytosol protein		
	<3	3-50	>50
Negative	8	2	0
Borderline	3	2	0
Positive			
<1/3 cells	0	6	2
>1/3 cells	1	11	27

Table 1 summarizes the results for 62 breast carcinomas. Of 10 tumors with no nuclear staining, 8 had no ER by DCC assay, but 2 had borderline or low DCC values and were regarded as probable false negatives. Among the 47 carcinomas with nuclear ER-staining 46 had positive DCC values, the largest number of those with more than 1/3 of positive cells having DCC values above 50 fmols. One case with more than 1/3 of positive nuclei had a negative DCC value which in retrospect was found to result from an error in the latter. In 5 cases with questionable (borderline) nuclear staining, 3 were negative by DCC and 2 had borderline or low DCC values. These findings confirm that immunostaining of frozen sections using H222 antibody according to the ER-ICA technique is reliable and can be effectively used for a semiquantitative assessment of the ER status of breast carcinomas.

In some patients, however, the tumors are very small so that the entire tissue must be processed for histological diagnosis. Under these circumstances we have used 2 alternate techniques: one is to prepare cytological touch preparations (imprints) from the cut surface of the tumor, and the other is to use frozen sections from the block of tissue used for the histological diagnosis. These imprints and frozen sections can be stained with the ER-ICA kit either immediately or after storage at -80°C. Preliminary results (Fig. 2) suggest that these techniques are promising in terms of ER evaluation and of utilizing a minimal amount of tissue without jeopardizing the histological work-up. The technique for the touch preparations is comparable to that for cytological smears obtained through fine needle biopsies,[6] but offers the advantage of being feasible even in tumors that cannot be properly sampled by fine needle aspiration because they are too small or are difficult to localize through the intact skin.

Paraffin sections

Earlier attempts at staining ER in sections of breast cancers routinely processed and embedded in paraffin were carried out in this laboratory using monoclonal antibodies D75 alone or in combination with D547 visualized either with the PAP or the avidin-biotin (ABC) techniques. In two separate studies[7,8] concordance with the DCC assay ranged from 67 to 90% among tumors with positive ER immunoreactivity and from 29 to 83% for tumors with negative immunostaining. It was apparent that in these patients

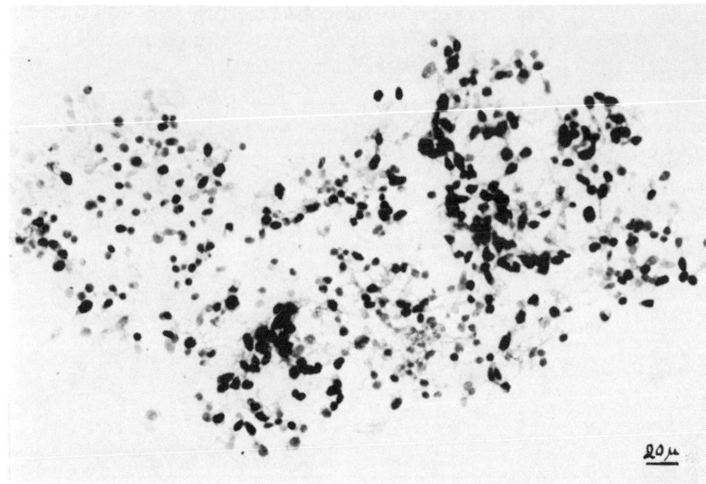

Fig. 2. Imprint from an infiltrating ductal carcinoma stained with H222 antibody. Frozen sections of the same tumor stained with ER-ICA were equally positive (58-year-old woman; inadequate sampling for DCC).

the largest proportion of positively stained specimens and the largest number of positive nuclei were found in ER-rich tumors, but a number of carcinomas with low DCC values were missed by the immunocytochemical staining.

Successful staining of paraffin sections of breast cancers using H222 antibody was reported recently by two separate groups. Shimada et al.[9] used biopsy material especially fixed in cold formalin for 24 hours and stained with H222 (10 μg/ml for 30 minutes at 37°C) using the ABC technique. They achieved a concordance with the DCC assay of 83.7% for the positively stained tumors and of 80.3% for the negative ones. The other study was reported by Anderson et al.[10] who stained paraffin sections of breast cancers that had been routinely fixed in formalin and stored for 1 to 5 years. Following trypsinization, they incubated the sections with H222 for 16 hours at 4°C and stained them with the ABC method. All of their cases with nuclear staining were also positive by DCC assay, but of the 18 that showed no immunoreactivity 5 had DCC values ranging from 28 to 101 fmols.

A major drawback in using material routinely processed in a surgical pathology laboratory is that routine handling and preparation of tissues is not uniform especially in laboratories processing a large number of cases received from different sources such as operating rooms, clinics and surgeon's private offices. Under these circumstances the time interval between excision and fixation can vary considerably as do the type, duration and temperature of fixation, all variables that can affect the immunoreactivity of the tissue. Therefore, in an attempt to improve and standardize the results of immunostaining of ER on paraffin sections we compared several fixation parameters.

The tumors were obtained fresh at the time of surgery and, except for the fixation, they were processed in the same manner. They were fixed within 10 minutes of excision, embedded in paraffin and stained with the D75 antibody (25μg/ml for 40 minutes at room temperature) using the ABC

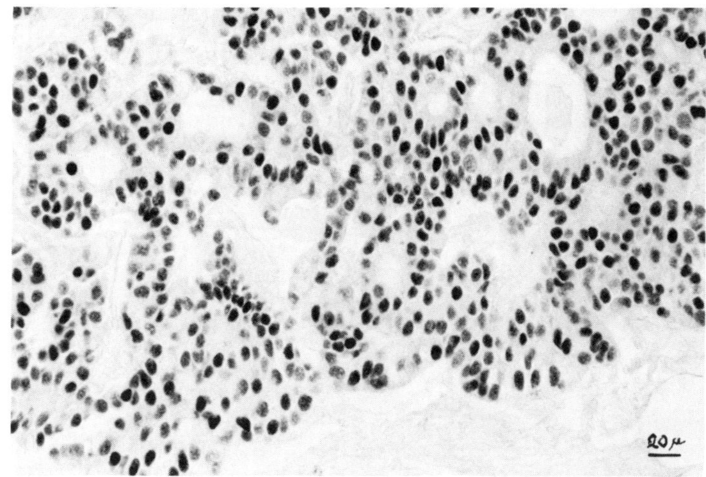

Fig. 3. Strong ER-immunoreactivity in a paraffin section of an infiltrating ductal carcinoma fixed in Bouin's for 2 hours at room temperature (80 year-old woman, DCC 614 fmol/mg). ABC technique, D75 antibody.

technique. In a series of experiments we compared Bouin's with buffered formalin, the two commonest fixatives in routine diagnostic practice, used at different temperatures (room temperature and 4°C) and for different lengths of time ranging from 30 minutes to 24 hours.

With Bouin's the best results were obtained at room temperature for 1 to 2 hours. Longer fixation times (4-24 hours) were also effective and provided information as to whether or not a tumor contained ER-positive cells, but in many specimens the staining was weaker in both intensity and extent. Formalin was found to be most effective when used at 4°C for 1 or 2 hours.

As with other techniques the staining was localized to the nuclei of carcinoma cells (Fig. 3,4). Cytoplasmic staining was noticeable in about 50% of the specimens fixed in Bouin's for 4 to 24 hours, whereas it was negligible with shorter fixation times.

The correspondence with the DCC assay values proved to be very good (Tables 2 and 3). With 1-2 hours fixation in Bouin's at room temperature or cold formalin the correspondence was 93.0% and 87.5% respectively for the ER-positive tumors. All the carcinomas with no ER staining had DCC values below 3 fmol/mg of cytosol protein.

Monoclonal antibody H222 gave less constant and much weaker staining reactions than D75 when applied in the same manner to corresponding paraffin sections of the same specimens.

IMMUNOSTAINING OF PROGESTERONE RECEPTOR

In this laboratory monoclonal antibody JZB-39 (Dr. G.L. Greene) has been used to stain progesterone receptor on frozen and paraffin sections of breast carcinomas from the same specimens prepared for ER-staining described above.

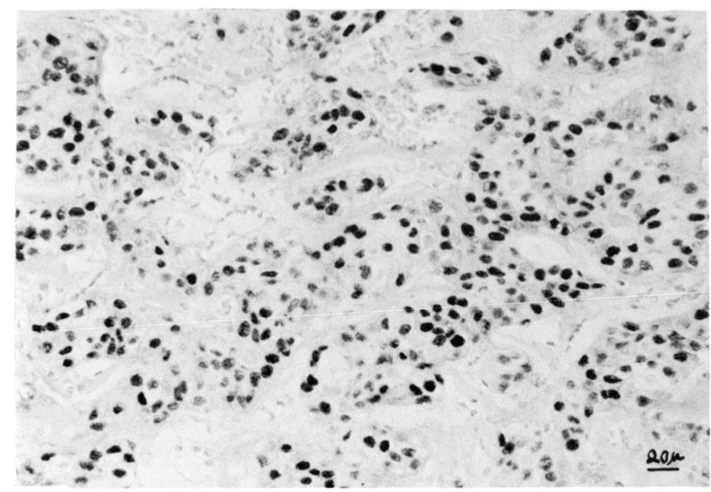

Fig. 4. Moderate ER-staining in a paraffin section of an infiltrating ductal carcinoma, fixed in cold formalin for 2 hours (72-year-old patient, DCC 27 fmol/mg). ABC technique, D75 antibody.

Table 2. Comparison of DCC assay values with immunostaining of paraffin sections of 21 breast carcinomas fixed in Bouin (1-2 hours at room temperature)

Nuclear staining	fmol/mg cytosol protein		
	<3	3-50	>50
Negativc	4	0	0
Borderline	1	0	0
Positive			
<1/3 cells	0	2	0
>1/3 cells	1	6	7

Table 3. Comparison of DCC assay values with immunostaining of paraffin sections of 21 breast carcinomas fixed in cold formalin (1-2 hours)

Nuclear staining	fmol/mg cytosol protein		
	<3	3-50	>50
Negative	4	0	0
Borderline	0	1	0
Positive			
$<1/3$ cells	2	2	3
$>1/3$ cells	0	3	6

On frozen sections this antibody was applied at the concentration of 10 µg/ml using the same reagents and the same technique as for the ER-ICA assay. Paraffin sections were stained with 25 µg/ml of primary antibody and the ABC technique. Positive PR-immunoreactivity was found to be localized to the nuclei of carcinoma cells and displayed varying degrees of heterogeneity in the intensity of the staining and in the number of stained nuclei.

Preliminary results indicate that PR-immunostaining can be performed with the same techniques utilized for ER and provides a high degree of correspondence with DCC assay values.

CONCLUSIONS

It is apparent that monoclonal antibodies to ER and PR can be effectively used to evaluate the ER and PR status of breast cancers. They can be applied to samples of mammary carcinomas prepared in different ways including frozen sections, paraffin sections and cytological preparations. Therefore, by appropriate adaptations, the techniques can be applied to different kinds of samples according to the type and amount of material available. The versatility of these techniques is of great practical interest since it can provide valuable information on the receptor status of specimens even when the latter cannot be processed for the conventional steroid binding assays.

AKNOWLEDGEMENTS

This work was supported in part by the Milstein Medical Research Foundation, Columbia University Research in Surgery Gift, and Mr. and Mrs. G.M. Shapiro. The authors wish to thank Dr. Geoffery L. Greene of the University of Chicago and Abbott Laboratories for providing antibodies and other immunocytochemical reagents.

REFERENCES

1. W. J. King, and G. L. Greene, Monoclonal antibodies localize oestrogen receptor in the nuclei of target cells, Nature (Lond.) 307: 745 (1984).
2. W. J. King, E. R. DeSombre, E. V. Jensen and G. L. Greene, Comparison of immunocytochemical and steroid-binding assays for estrogen receptor in human breast tumors, Cancer Res. 45: 293 (1985).
3. G. L. Greene, C. Nolan, J. P. Engler and E. V. Jensen, Monoclonal antibodies to human estrogen receptor, Proc. Natl. Acad. Sci. USA 77: 5115 (1980).
4. L. S. Miller, I. I. E. Tribby, M. R. Miles, J. T. Tomita, and C. Nolan, Hybridomas producing monoclonal antibodies to human estrogen receptor, Fed. Proc. 41: 520 (1980).
5. L. Ozzello, C. M. DeRosa, J. G. Konrath, J. L. Yeager and L. S. Miller, Detection of estrophilin in frozen sections of breast cancers using an estrogen receptor immunocytochemical assay. Cancer Res. 46: 4303 (1986).
6. J. L. Flowers, G. V. Burton, E. B. Cox, K. S. McCarty Sr., G. A. Dent, K. R. Geisinger, and K. S. McCarty Jr., Use of monoclonal anti-estrogen receptor antibody to evaluate estrogen receptor content in fine needle aspiration breast biopsies, Ann. Surg. 203: 250 (1986).
7. H. S. Poulsen, L. Ozzello, W. J. King, and G. L. Greene, The use of monoclonal antibodies to estrogen receptors (ER) for immunoperoxidase detection of ER in paraffin sections of human breast cancer tissue, J. Histochem. Cytochem. 33: 87 (1985).
8. L. Ozzello, C. DeRosa, D. V. Habif, and R. Lipton, Immunostaining of estrogen receptors in paraffin sections of breast cancers using anti-estrophilin monoclonal antibodies, in: "Monoclonal Antibodies and Breast Cancer," R. L. Ceriani, ed., Martinus Nijhoff Publishing, Boston (1985).
9. A. Shimada, S. Kimura, K. Abe, K. Nagasaki, J. Adachi, K. Yamaguchi, M. Suzuki, T. Nakajima, and L. S. Miller, Immunocytochemical staining of estrogen receptor in paraffin sections of human breast cancer by use of monoclonal antibody: Comparison with that in frozen sections, Proc. Natl. Acad. Sci. USA 82: 4803 (1985).
10. J. Anderson, T. Orntoft, and H.S. Poulsen, Semiquantitative oestrogen receptor assay in formalin-fixed paraffin sections of human breast cancer tissue using monoclonal antibodies, Br. J. Cancer 53: 691 (1986).

HETEROGENEITY VS. ASYNCHRONY OF RECEPTOR EXPRESSION IN BREAST CANCER AS DETERMINED BY MONOCLONAL ANTIBODIES.

L.B. Kinsel*, J.L. Flowers,* J. Konrath,**,
G.S. Leight*,G.L. Greene**, and K.S. McCarty*

*Duke University Medical Center, Durham, N. C.
**University of Chicago, Chicago, IL

ABSTRACT

The availability of monoclonal antibodies directed against estrogen and progesterone receptor proteins have made immunohistochemical study of these proteins in human breast tissue possible. Semiquantitative immunohistochemical analyses for estrogen receptor (ER) using H222 Sp correlated with quantitative biochemical receptor analyses. Two different monoclonal antibodies against progesterone receptor (PgR), B39 and KD68 were compared. Both were found to correlate with biochemical quantitation. Heterogeneity within breast tumors was investigated by comparing receptor expression with tumor histology and studying the effect of administered steroid hormone on receptor content. Both estrogen and progesterone receptor content was found to correlate with histologic grade. Within a given specimen, receptor expression often varied between different tumor components. A shift toward more homogeneous expression of PgR was observed in some tumors with estrogen pretreatment.

INTRODUCTION

Sex steroid receptor content has become widely used in the evaluation of breast cancers. Since conventional ligand assays use homogenization techniques, the distribution of ER in the tissue cannot be determined. This has been suggested to contribute to the limitation of the predictive value of these analyses. Histochemical techniques for visualizing ER distribution have been developed to complement the information derived from quantitative biochemical ligand assays.

Early autoradiographic techniques were cumbersome and histochemical techniques, using fluoresceinated estrogens, lacked specificity and failed to correlate with biochemical analysis or predict clinical response (1-3). The availability of highly specific monoclonal antibodies to the estrogen receptor protein permitted the development of an ER immunohistochemical assay (4). Numerous centers have reported that this assay correlates well with biochemical assays and reasonably predicts clinical response to hormone therapy (5-16).

In addition to the evaluation of ER, progesterone receptors (PgR) have been recognized as an indicator of a functioning ER system (17-20).

Studies using biochemical assays for PgR have shown that PgR levels are a useful addition in the evaluation of tumor hormone responsiveness. With the purification of PgR and the preparation of monoclonal antibodies to this protein, an immunohistochemical assay has been developed. Immunohistochemical visualization of PgR using two antibodies, B39 and KD68, are compared with the biochemical PgR assay.

An important potential application of immunohistochemical techniques is their use in evaluating tumor heterogeneity. Steroid receptor content differs between various components of a tumor (i.e. intraductal vs. invasive) and between the cells within a component. Two processes may play a role in this pattern of expression: 1) Tumors may develop multiple clones which differ in their ability to differentiate and express receptors, or 2) tumor cells may be equally capable of expressing receptors but cyclic ER changes are asynchronous within cell populations. We explored this issue by comparing receptor content with tumor cellularity and histologic grade, and determined if relative cellular receptor content can be synchronized in breast cancers with estrogen administration given 72 hours prior to mastectomy.

MATERIALS AND METHODS

Patient Populations/Tissue Storage:

Seven cohorts of patients were studied (Table 1):

1. Seventy-two cases of Stage I primary breast carcinoma which represented the first 10 cases accessioned in each year from 1976 to 1983. Eight cases from the initial 80 cases were excluded due to loss of either the primary or the control sections. These tissues were quick frozen after being washed in 0.005M 4-(2-hydroxy- ethyl)- 1-piperazine ethanesulfonic acid-0.010M Tris-0.0015 mEDTA-0.01 M thioglycerol-0.02% NaN_3 buffer, pH 7.4, and were maintained at -70°C in airtight liquid nitrogen capsules from the time of excision until sectioning for histochemical receptor localization.

2. Sixty-two primary breast carcinomas from 1983 which were acquired in the fresh state immediately prior to routine pathological sectioning for immunohistochemical receptor assay.

3. Two hundred sixty-two cases of primary breast carcinoma were accessioned from 1976-1980. These cases represented all the primary breast cancer specimens received by this laboratory for biochemical analysis for which sufficient cancerous tissue remained for immunohistochemical analysis. These specimens were from Duke University Medical Center, and Cabarrus Memorial Hospital.

4. Twenty-three cases of metastatic breast cancer. This cohort was restricted to patients treated only with primary hormone therapy for whom objective measures of disease status and response to therapy were documented.

5. Thirty-three fine needle aspirations of breast cancers, representing 28 primary breast cancers and 5 metastases to regional lymph nodes. Of 41 consecutive cases seen between April 1984 and January 1985, eight were excluded due to either inadequate tissue or paucity of malignant cells.

6. One hundred and two cases of primary breast carcinoma accessioned from 1977-1985. These represented 10 cases selected per year and 5 cases per month from January through November 1985 from a pool of tissues with previously determined biochemical ER and PgR values and H222 evaluation. Forty-three cases were rejected for inadequate residual tumor tissue from the original 145 cases pulled. This population was used for analysis of PgR using monoclonal antibodies B39 and KD68.

7. Tissue from sixteen patients with palpable primary breast cancer, seen at Duke University Medical Center in 1985, were evaluated for the effects of estrogen administration _in vivo_ on receptor distribution. Of the sixteen patients, seven completed the full protocol and provided adequate tissue for both immunohistochemical analysis (ER and PgR) and controls. After full IRB Review, informed consent was obtained from each patient and at the time of initial examination a tru-cut needle biopsy was performed. Three days prior to mastectomy, patients were placed on ethinyl estradiol 2mg.p.o./day. Immediately following surgery, tissue was obtained for ER and PgR analyses.

Table 1. Tumors Evaluated with H222 and/or B39/KD68

No. of Cases	Year(s) accessioned
Primary breast carcinoma	
72 (Cohort I)	1976-1983
62 (Cohort II)	1983
262 (Cohort III)	1976-1980
Metastatic Breast Carcinoma	
23 (Cohort IV)	1976-1985
Fine Needle Aspiration Biopsies	
33 (Cohort V)	1984-1985
Primary Breast Cancer	
102 (Cohort VI)	1977-1980
Primary Breast Carcinoma Treated With Ethinyl Estradiol	
7 (Cohort VII)	1985

Biochemical Receptor Analysis

For each case, biochemical estrogen and progesterone receptor analyses were performed at the time that the tissue was first obtained. The methods used have been described previously (21). Multiconcentration titration analysis (dextran-coated charcoal analysis) and/or sucrose density gradient analysis of estrogen and progesterone binding were used.

Tissue Preparation

Cryostat sections of fresh frozen tissue were utilized in all cases except from needle aspirations when the biopsy material was placed directly on slides. The sections were fixed in 3.7% formaldehyde 0.1M phosphate buffered saline at 25°C for 10 minutes, followed by immersion in 100% methanol at -10°C to -25°C for 4 minutes and acetone at -10°C to -25°C for 1 minute.

Selection and Use of H222, B39 and KD68 Monoclonal Antibodies

The monoclonal antibody H222 Spγ was selected because it recognizes a stable and well conserved determinant that is close to the steroid binding site of human estrogen receptor (4). This binding location was chosen since it is thought to correlate the most closely to conventional estrogen binding assays. Monoclonal antibodies B39 and KD68 were developed by Greene and associates and are reported to have high specificity and affinity for the human progesterone receptor.

Immunohistochemical Staining Procedure

The peroxidase anti-peroxidase method for immunocytochemical localization was performed as described by Sternberger (22). Normal goat serum was used as the blocking reagent. The primary antibodies H222 Spγ, B39 and KD68 were used at concentrations of 0.1, 4.3, and 16.3 ug/ml, respectively. The bridging antibody was goat anti-rat immunoglobulin and the PAP complex was of rat origin. Control slides consisted of sections of cancers adjacent to those used as test slides; however, normal rat immunoglobulin was used in place of the primary monoclonal antibodies. The slides were treated with poly-L-lysine to improve adhesion of tissue. Localization of antigen-antibody complexes with peroxidase was developed using diaminobenzidine-H_2O_2.

Scoring of Assays

Biochemical Receptor Analyses: Results were expressed as fmol of estrogen or progesterone binding per mg of cytosol protein.

Immunohistochemical Analyses: Localization of estrogen and progesterone receptors was scored in a semiquantitative fashion incorporating both the intensity and the distribution of specific staining. The evaluations were recorded as percentages of positively stained target cells in each of four intensity categories which were denoted as 0 (no staining), 1+ (weak but detectable above control), 2+ (distinct), 3+ (strong, with minimal light transmission through stained nucleus). For each tissue, a value designated the histologic score, HSCORE, was derived by summing the percentages of cells staining at each intensity multiplied by the weighed intensity of staining.

$$\text{HSCORE} = \sum P_i \ (i+1)$$

when i=1,2,3 and P_i varies from 0 to 100%. Component HSCOREs were generated in addition to the total tissue HSCORE, for the 262 patients in Cohort III. These component HSCOREs were determined by assessing the percentage of target cells comprising the various morphological patterns such as tubules, nests, intraductal elements, etc. The component HSCOREs for a given specimen were each multiplied by the percentage of cells of that particular component, and the products were summed to give a total HSCORE.

Histological Grading of Tumors

Nuclear and histological grading was performed on Cohort III (262 primary cancers) according to the method of Fisher et al. (23), with modification. Nuclear grades consisted of 1 (poorly differentiated), 2 (moderately differentiated) and 3 (well differentiated). The category described by nuclear Grade 2 was further subdivided into 2A and 2B, with 2A representing a higher level of differentiation than 2B. Histological grade was based on a scale of 0-3, with 0 being intraductal elements only and 3 being poorly differentiated. Each morphologic component was assigned a nuclear grade. The grade indicating the best differentiation was used in determining the overall nuclear and histological grade for the tumor.

Data Management and Analysis

Clinical data were evaluated by a nurse clinician under the supervision of Dr. Cox. Clinical response was defined by the Breast Cancer Task Force criteria for objective response. Clinical data, biochemical assay values, and histochemical assay values were coded separately in a blinded fashion and maintained as independent files in the Time Oriented Record for Oncology (TORO) System of the Duke Cancer Center Database until completion of each phase of the study. Record identification numbers were used to match samples for the analysis.

Comparison of intra- and interobserver variation for ER analysis was performed with replicate double-blind scoring of the histological slides no less than 4 days apart. Each observer recorded two independent interpretations of the slide and the corresponding HSCOREs were calculated. Differences between observers were settled by consensus evaluation. The sensitivities and specificities were determined as described. (24) Evaluation of intra- and interobserver variation and biochemical and HSCORE values was done by correlation analysis. The significance of two-way tables was determined by chi-square test or Fisher's exact test, as appropriate.

RESULTS

Histochemical Evaluation of ER Using Monoclonal Antibody H222

As reported earlier, immunohistochemical evaluation of ER with H222 revealed nuclear staining of tumor cells. Estrogen receptor content estimated with the HSCORE had excellent intraobserver reliability ($r=0.96$, $p<0.0001$) and interobserver variation ($r=0.91$, $p<0.0001$).

Table 2 shows the sensitivity and specificity of H222 ER determination when compared to dextran-coated charcoal or sucrose density gradient analysis in Cohorts I-III and V. It should be noted that Cohort III made use of the sum of component HSCOREs whereas the other cohorts used a simple total HSCORE made with one determination. This may account for the lower specificity and sensitivity seen in Cohort III. Table 3 compares the H222 determined ER content with the hormone responsiveness of metastatic breast cancers (Cohort IV) (see reference 6 for further description).

Table 2. Sensitivity and Specificity of H222 on Cohorts I-III and V

	Cohort I	II	III	Fine Needle Asp. (V)
Sensitivity (%)	88	95	86	80
Specificity (%)	94	86	74	89

Table 3. Comparison of H222 with Hormone Response in Cohort IV

HSCORE	RESPONDER	NONRESPONDER
≥ 75	13	1
< 75	1	8
Biochemical (fmol/mg protein)		
≥ 10	10	2
< 10	4	7

Evaluation of PgR Content: Comparison of Monoclonal Antibodies B39 and KD68

Staining of PgR using either B39 or KD68 was located in the nucleus of tumor cells. B39 and KD68 were found to have a similar relationship to the biochemical assay results. There was a linear correlation between the biochemical results and B39 HSCORE (r=0.68) A linear correlation was also obtained with KD68 (r=0.67). Table 4 compares the sensitivity and specificity of B39 and KD68 when each are compared to the biochemical assay.

Table 4. Comparison of B39 and KD68 PgR Assay: Sensitivity and Specificity.

	B39	KD68
Sensitivity	72%	76%
Specificity	85%	73%

Heterogeneity vs. Asynchrony:

ER and PgR content determined with H222 and B39 did not correlate with tumor cellularity. A correlation was noted between histological grade and ER/PgR HSCOREs. (Figures Ib and IIb). The separation between groups was not as distinct when histological grade was compared with the biochemical values for ER and PgR (Figures Ia and IIa). Similar relationships were seen between nuclear grade and ER/PgR HSCORE. The well differentiated tumors tend to contain more steroid receptors than poorly differentiated tumors.

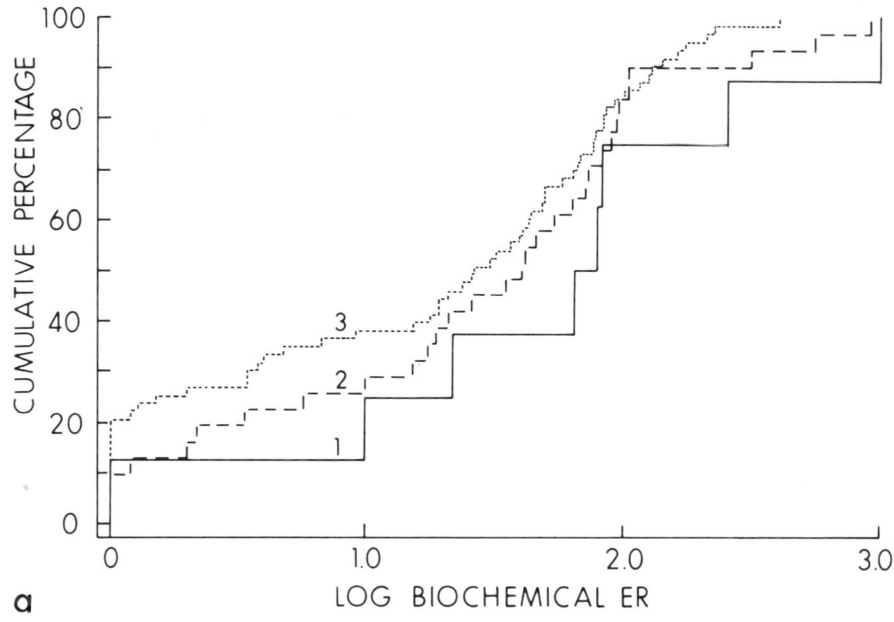

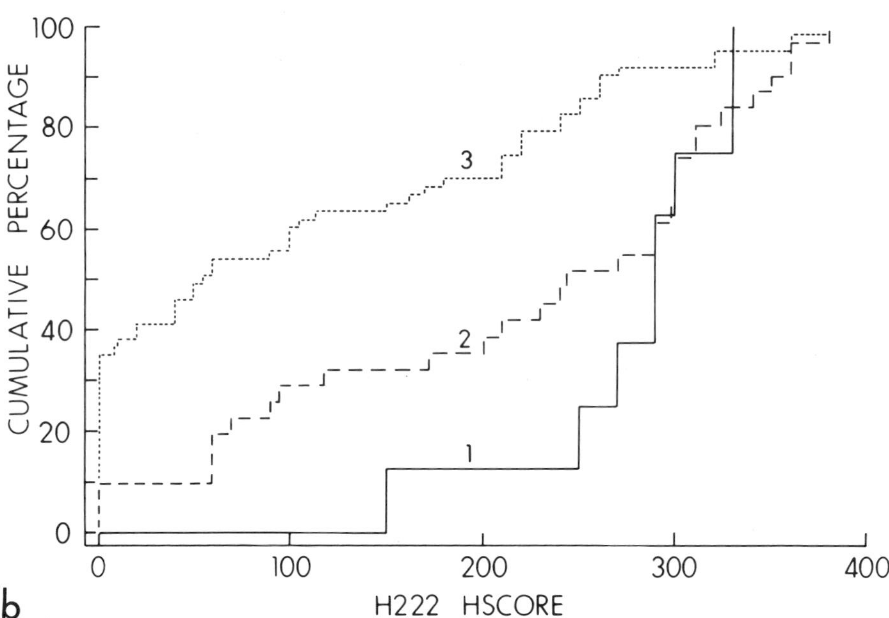

Figure 1. Comparison of histological grade with a) Log of the biochemically determined ER content and b) ER HSCORE using H222 in 102 breast cancer specimens (Cohort VI).

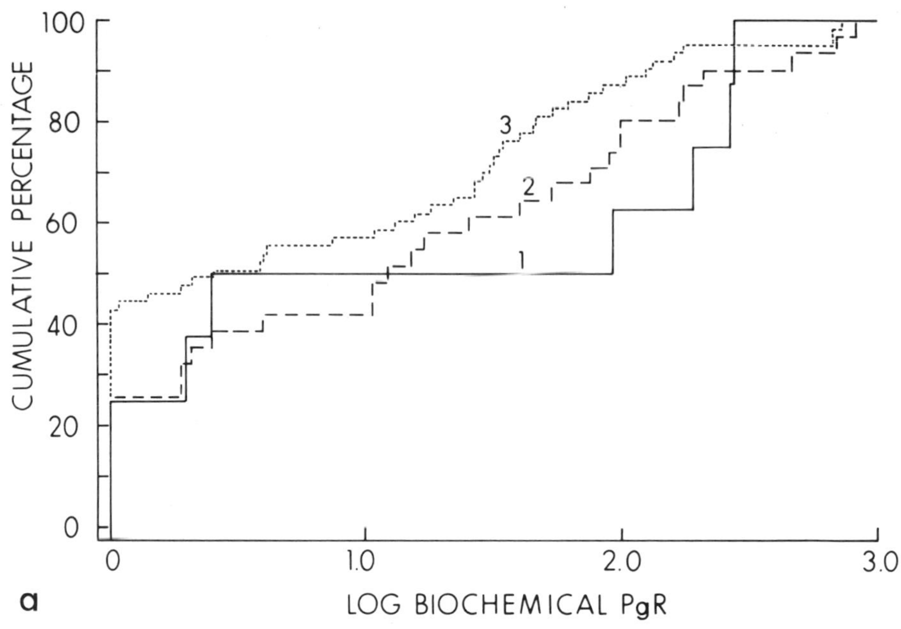

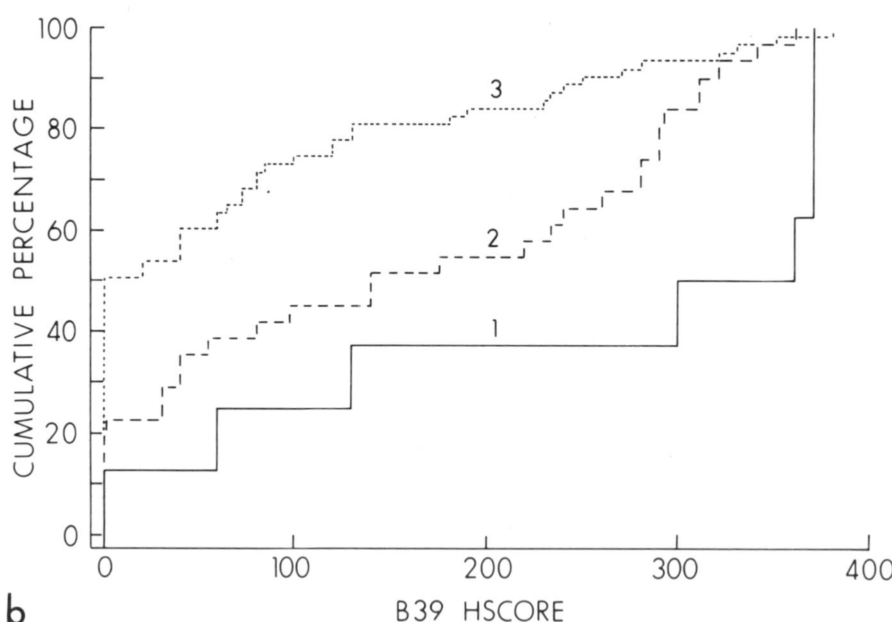

Figure 2. Comparison of histological grade with a) Log of the biochemically determined PgR and b) PgR HSCORE using B39 in 102 breast cancer specimens (Cohort VI).

Of the seven patients given ethinyl estradiol before mastectomy (Cohort VII), five showed profound decreases (range 8-100%, average 58%) in measurable ER content with a striking shift to homogeneity of the receptor expressed as compared to pretreatment values. One case showed no change and only a single example showed an increase. Progesterone receptor similarly showed a shift to greater homogeneity of the population expressed with four of the five patients showing an increase in PgR (at least 2-7 times the pre-value) with two remaining unchanged and only a single example showing a decrease (both pre and post treatments were significantly positive and uniform in intensity).

DISCUSSION

Determination of estrogen receptor (ER) content and distribution using immunohistochemical techniques has been shown to be an important component of breast tumor evaluation (5-16). Immunohistochemical evaluation correlates with the standard biochemical assays, provides information regarding distribution of receptor among tissue components, and predicts a tumor's hormone responsiveness as does biochemical analysis.

Some investigators have suggested the use of paraffin sections as a source of material for immunohistochemical analysis. It has been our experience that the use of such material leads to markedly lowered sensitivity. Data from other laboratories tend to corroborate this. Shimada, et al. (1985), reported that they had a lower agreement percentage when using paraffin sections than when using frozen sections (agreements of 82% and 86% respectively) with the main problem being a loss of sensitivity (25). Andersen (1986) reported an agreement of 86% when comparing immunohistochemical analysis of paraffin sections with DCC analysis (after modifying the staining method of Poulsen) (26,27). Both Shimada and Andersen's methods require overnight incubations and additional steps in the procedure to assure minimal background staining. Rigorous fixation control is also required.

Immunohistochemical techniques are particularly useful for fine needle aspirates, although the need for specimen quality control and sample handling by defined protocol is amplified. Though we see a lower sensitivity with this method, it offers the opportunity to obtain receptor data in situations where tissue may not otherwise be available.

Evaluating individual tumor component HSCOREs appears to provide additional information regarding distribution of receptor. Such component scoring lowers the agreement with the biochemical method but appears to enhance correlation with the biologic behavior of the tumor. Immunohistochemistry has certain disadvantages. The determination of the HSCORE is semiquantitative and subjective. It is subject to a number of procedural handling artifacts. Only tumor cells should be counted toward the HSCORE, thus the observer must be adequately trained in breast histopathology to make the distinction between tumor and normal breast tissue. Also, the technique does not determine if the receptor antigen is functional with regard to steroid binding capacity nor transcriptional regulation.

Analysis of progesterone receptor (PgR) quantity and distribution is an additional indicator of tumor hormone responsiveness and differentiation (17-20). The monoclonal antibodies to progesterone receptor, B39 and KD68, appear to be sensitive and specific.

Heterogeneity within individual tumors is an important consideration in the evaluation and treatment of breast cancer. Nilsson and Osborne (1986) suggest the use of monoclonal antibodies in determining the basis of heterogeneity (29,30). A positive correlation between the histologic grade and immunohistochemically determined receptor content confirms earlier studies using biochemical methods (31-33). We also noted differences in receptor expression between cell populations contained in various components of a tumor. Interestingly, many morphologically heterogeneous tumors contained intraductal cell populations which were ER negative even if the invasive component was ER positive. Podhajcer et al. (1986) sorted breast tumor cells by density and characterized three populations: 1) an intermediate density population of proliferating cells which were ER negative, 2) a high density, non-proliferating small cell population which were strongly ER positive, and 3) a low density non-proliferating population which had scarce ER activity (34). This supports the thought that ER expression is a relatively late step in differentiation (not seen in highly proliferating, poorly differentiated "stem"-type cells) and that cell populations within one tumor vary in their capacity to differentiate. Additional studies are needed to confirm this.

Host factors, however, may also influence the heterogeneous expression of steroid receptors. Normal breast tissue exhibits cyclic receptor changes (35). Breast cancer receptor expression in well differentiated tumors also may be influenced by endogenous hormonal changes. The recruitment of homogeneous PgR expression with the suppression of ER in cancers exposed to ethinyl estradiol indicates that asynchrony may be a source of heterogeneous receptor expression in some tumors.

ACKNOWLEDGEMENTS

The authors wish to thank Dr. Ed Cox for his assistance with data analysis. We are also deeply grateful to Ms. Donna Silva for her assistance in preparing the manuscript. This work is supported by NIH 1 R01 CA39635-01A2, 5R01 CA38989-02, and Laura Kinsel is supported by the Eugene Stead Nicewonder Fellowship.

REFERENCES

1. K.S. McCarty, Jr., et al., Cytochemistry of Sex Steroid Receptors: a critique, Breast Cancer Res. and Treat. 1: 315-325, (1981).
2. K.S. McCarty, Jr., et al. Clinical Response to Hormone Therapy Correlated with Estrogen Receptor Analysis, Arch. Pathol. Lab. Med. 108: 24-26, (1984).
3. Ton F.P.M. DeGoeij, et al., Determination of Steroid Hormone-Dependency of Tumours Utilizing Tissue Sections. Survey of Histochemical Techniques and Their Application in Surgical Pathology, J. Pathol. 149: 163-172, (1986).
4. G.L. Greene, et al., Immunochemical Studies of Estrogen Receptors, J. Steroid Biochem. 20: 51-56 (1984).
5. K.S. McCarty, Jr., et al., Estrogen Receptor Analysis. Correlation of Biochemical and Immunohistochemical Methods Using Monoclonal Antireceptor Antibodies, Arch. Pathol. Lab. Med. 109: 716-721 (1985).
6. K.S. McCarty, Jr., et al., Monoclonal Antibodies Against Estrogen Receptor: Specificity, Sensitivity and Potential Applications, Dev. in Oncology 35: 190-202 (1985).

7. K.S. McCarty, Jr., et al. Use of Monoclonal Anti-Estrogen Receptor Antibody in the Immunohistochemical Evaluation of Human Tumors, Cancer Res. (Suppl.) 46: 4244s-4248s (1986).
8. L.P. Pertschuk, et al., Immunohistologic Localization of Estrogen Receptors in Breast Cancer with Monoclonal Antibodies, Cancer 55: 1513-1518 (1985).
9. W.J. King, et al., Comparison of Immunocytochemical and Steroid-Binding Assays for Estrogen Receptor in Human Breast Tumors, Cancer Res. 45: 293-304, (1985).
10. R.A. Hawkins, et al., Histochemical Detection of Oestrogen Receptors in Breast Carcinoma: A successful technique, Br. J. Cancer 53: 407-410 (1986).
11. R.A. McClelland, et al., Immunocytochemical Assay for Estrogen Receptor: Relationship to Outcome of Therapy in Patients with Advanced Breast Cancer, Cancer Res. (Suppl.) 46: 4241s-4243s (1986).
12. C. Charpin, et al., Estrogen Receptor Immunocytochemical Assay (ER-ICA): Computerized Image Analysis System, Immunoelectron Microscopy, and Comparisons with Estradiol Binding Assays in 115 Breast Carcinomas, Cancer Res. (Suppl.) 46: 4271s-4277s (1986).
13. W. Jonat, et al., Immunohistochemical Measurement of Estrogen Receptors in Breast Cancer Tissue Samples, Cancer Res. (Suppl.) 46: 4296s-4298s (1986)
14. E.R. DeSombre, Prognostic Usefulness of Estrogen Receptor Immunocytochemical Assays for Human Breast Cancer, Cancer Res. et al. (Suppl.) 46: 4256s-4264s (1986).
15. L. Ozzello, et al. Detection of Estrophilin in Frozen Sections of Breast Cancers Using an Estrogen Receptor Immunocytochemical Assay, Cancer Res. (Suppl.) 46: 4303s-4307s (1986).
16. A. Heubner, et al. Comparison of Immunocytochemical Estrogen Receptor Assay, Estrogen Receptor Enzyme Immunoassay, and Radioligand Estrogen Receptor Assay in Human Breast Cancer and Uterine Tissue, Cancer Res. (Suppl.) 46: 4291s-4295s (1986).
17. K.B. Horwitz, et al., Progestin Action and Progesterone Receptor Structure in Human Breast Cancer: A Review, Rec. Prog. in Horm. Res. 41: 249-316 (1985).
18. S.C. Brooks, et al., Relation of Tumor Content of Estrogen and Progesterone Receptors with Response of Patient to Endocrine Therapy, Cancer 46: 2775-2778 (1980).
19. G.A. Degenshein, et al., The Value of Progesterone Receptor Assays in the Management of Advanced Breast Cancer, Cancer 46: 2789-2793 (1980).
20. W.L. McGuire, et al., Role of Steroid Hormone Receptors as Prognostic Factors in Primary Breast Cancer, NCI Monographs 1: 19-23 (1986).
21. K.S. McCarty, Jr., et al. Correlation of Estrogen and Progesterone Receptors with Histologic Differentiation in Endometrial Adenocarcinoma. Am. J. Pathol. 96: 171-183 (1979).
22. L.A. Sternberger, "Immnocytochemistry ", Prentice-Hall, Inc., Englewood Cliffs, N. J. (1974).
23. E.R. Fisher, et al., The Pathology of Invasive Breast Cancer. Syllabus Derived from Findings of the National Surgical Adjuvant Breast Project (Protocol No. 4), Cancer 36: 1-85 (1975).
24. R.S. Galen and S.R. Gambino, "Beyond Normality: The Predictive Value and Efficiency of Medical Diagnosis", John Wiley and Sons, Inc., New York, N.Y. (1975).
25. A. Shimada, et al., Immunocytochemical Staining of Estrogen Receptor in Paraffin Sections of Human Breast Cancer by Use of Monoclonal Antibody: Comparison with that in Frozen Sections, Proc. Natl. Acad. Sci. USA 82: 4803-4807 (1985).
26. J. Andersen, et al. Semiquantitative Oestrogen Receptor Assay in Formalin-fixed Paraffin Sections of Human Breast Cancer Tissue Using Monoclonal Antibodies, Br. J. Cancer 53: 691-694 (1986).

27. H.S. Poulsen, et al., The Use of Monoclonal Antibodies to Estrogen Receptors (ER) for Immunoperoxidase Detection of ER in Paraffin Sections of Human Breast Cancer Tissue, J. Histochem. Cytochem. 33: 87-92 (1985).
28. J.L. Flowers, et al., Use of Monoclonal Antiestrogen Receptor Antibody to Evaluate Estrogen Receptor Content in Fine Needle Aspiration Breast Biopsies, Ann. Surg. 203: 250-254 (1986).
29. K. Nilsson, Toward the Use of Monoclonal Antibodies in the Analysis of Tumor Progression and Cellular Heterogeneity of Human Breast Cancer, Acta. Chir. Scand. (Suppl.) 519: 15-18 (1984).
30. C.K. Osborne, Heterogeneity in Hormone Receptor Status in Primary and Metastatic Breast Cancer, Seminars in Oncology 12: 317-326 (1985).
31. K.S. McCarty, Jr., et al. Correlation of Estrogen and Progesterone Receptors with Histologic Differentiation in Mammary Carcinoma, Cancer 46: 2851-2858 (1980).
32. J.S. Silva, et al. Biochemical Correlates of Morphologic Differentiation in Human Breast Cancer, Surgery 92: 443-449, (1982).
33. R.H. Mohammed, et al. Estrogen and Progesterone Receptors in Human Breast Cancer. Correlation With Histologic Subtype and Degree of Differentiation, Cancer 58: 1076-1081 (1986).
34. O.L. Podhajcer, et al., Determination of DNA Synthesis, Estrogen Receptors and Carcinoembryonic Antigen in Isolated Cellular Subpopulations of Human Breast Cancer, Cancer 58: 720-729 (1986).
35. J.S. Silva, et al., Menstrual Cycle-Dependent Variations of Breast Cyst Fluid Proteins and Sex Steroid Receptors in the Normal Human Breast, Cancer 51: 1297-1302 (1983).

IMMUNOAFFINITY PURIFICATION AND STRUCTURAL ANALYSIS OF HUMAN BREAST CANCER PROGESTERONE RECEPTORS

Dean P. Edwards, Patricia A. Estes, Dorraya El-Ashry,
Eric Suba, and Janet Lawler-Heavner

Department of Pathology
University of Colorado Health Sciences Center
Denver, Colorado 80262

INTRODUCTION

Progesterone receptors (PR) are well established as an important clinical marker in breast cancer in predicting patient response to adjuvant endocrine therapies[1] and as markers of disease aggressiveness.[2] Development of antibodies specific for human PR and methods for their use in the immunocytochemical detection of receptors in breast tumors would be of value clinically in providing a number of advantages over the biochemical ligand binding assays that are currently in use for routine PR determinations. Immunocytochemistry for example, will make PR screening accessible to most pathology laboratories, is possible to perform with cellular aspirates and very small tissue samples, and will provide information on cellular heterogeneity and PR content in individual cells which itself may be of diagnostic value.

Receptor specific antibodies are potentially valuable as well for fundamental studies of receptor structure and function. As probes which recognize receptor protein directly, independent of hormone binding activity, antibodies will be useful for purification and structural analysis of the receptor molecule, for molecular studies of receptor biosynthesis, covalent modification, receptor activation mechanisms, and for immunocytochemical localization in the presence and absence of hormone.

This paper describes immunoaffinity purification and structural analysis of human PR by use of an anti-chick receptor monoclonal antibody (MAb) which cross reacts with human PR.[3,4] Also described are the production and characterization of three monoclonal antibodies to purified human PR and application of these MAbs for the immunocytochemical detection of receptors in breast cancer cells.

Experimental System

T47D human breast cancer cells[5] were used as the tissue source for receptor purification and structural analysis. This is an ideal model for these studies since T47D cells have an unusually high PR content[6] (i.e. ≈ 250,000 sites/cells) and contain functional receptors since a number of biological responses to progestins have been described. Growth of T47D cells has been reported to be inhibited by the synthetic progestin R5020[7] and progestins have been described to induce the synthesis of specific intracellular as well as secreted proteins.[8,9] PR in T47D cells are also functional by several other parameters including their ability to undergo transformation and acquire tight nuclear binding in response to binding hormone, and receptors are down regulated to low levels after prolonged exposure to progestins.[10]

Cross Reaction of Anti-Chick Receptor MAb with Human Progesterone Receptors

The human progesterone receptor is composed of two hormone binding proteins termed A and B with apparent molecular weights respectively of 94,000 and 120,000. These can be identified by photoaffinity labeling with the progestin analog [^{3}H]R5020 and SDS-gel electrophoresis followed by autofluorography as described by Horwitz et al.[11] In crude cytosol of T47D cells, [^{3}H]R5020 binds with proteins of 120 kDa (which migrate as doublets) and 94 kDa, as illustrated in Figure 1. Each of these proteins represents receptors since [^{3}H]R5020 binding is displaceable with excess cold hormone. The PR-6 monoclonal antibody, raised by Toft and co-workers[3] against chick oviduct PR was tested for cross reaction with human PR by immunoblot assay[12] of these same T47D cytosols. This antibody reacts strongly with human B receptors, but has no apparent affinity for A receptors (Figure 1, left panel). PR-6, therefore, is a B receptor specific antibody.

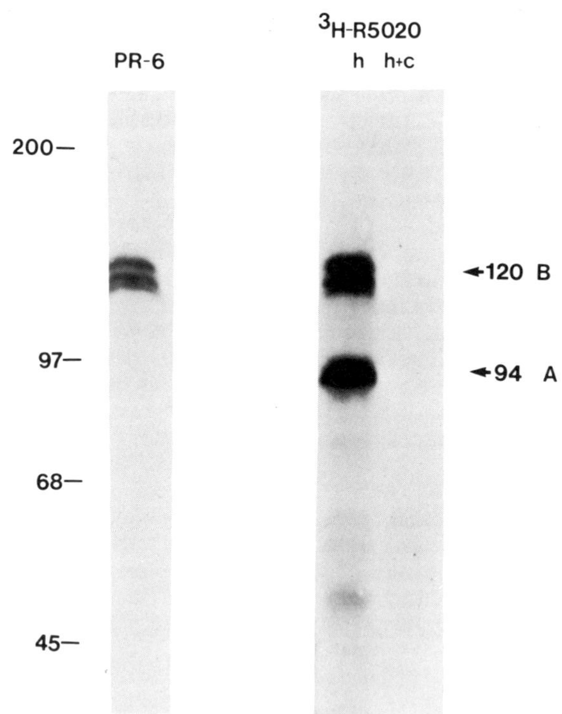

Fig. 1. Cross reaction of PR-6 with human B receptors. T47D cytosol progesterone receptors were photoaffinity labeled with [^{3}H]R5020(h) or [^{3}H]R5020 + cold hormone (h+c) and analyzed by SDS-gel electrophoresis and fluorography (right). The same cytosol was immunoblotted with the PR-6 MAb (left). (Further details to be published in Biochemistry.[4])

In addition to reacting with human receptors resolved on denaturing SDS-gels, PR-6 also recognizes and binds with native receptor-hormone complexes since it displaces sedimentation of receptors on sucrose density gradients. Moreover, it is equally reactive with different molecular forms of receptors (Figure 2). By contrast with a control antibody, addition of PR-6 shifts the sedimentation of 8S cytosol receptors on low salt gradients to a heavier form. It also shifts 4S cytosol receptors on salt containing sucrose gradients, and displaces the sedimentation of 4S salt extractable nuclear receptors. With each molecular form, PR-6 complexes with and shifts the sedimentation of ≈ 40-45% of receptors which is expected since this is a B specific antibody capable of detecting at most, half of the total cellular receptors.

PR-6 is also capable of immunoprecipitating native receptor-hormone complexes by use of a secondary anti-mouse IgG and protein A Sepharose as an immunoabsorbent. A maximum of 45% of total cytosol receptors can be precipitated with PR-6 (which represents 90% of B receptors). By keeping the antibody as the constant and varying the concentration of receptors we have determined that PR-6 binds human receptors with a Kd of 1.2×10^{-8} M.

Immunoaffinity Purification and Structural Analysis of Human Progesterone Receptors

Since PR-6 reacts efficiently with native receptors and has a receptor binding affinity (Kd = 10^{-8} M) ideal for antigen purification, we sought to use this MAb for immunoaffinity purification of human B receptors. We first prepared an immunomatrix by chemically cross linking PR-6 to protein A

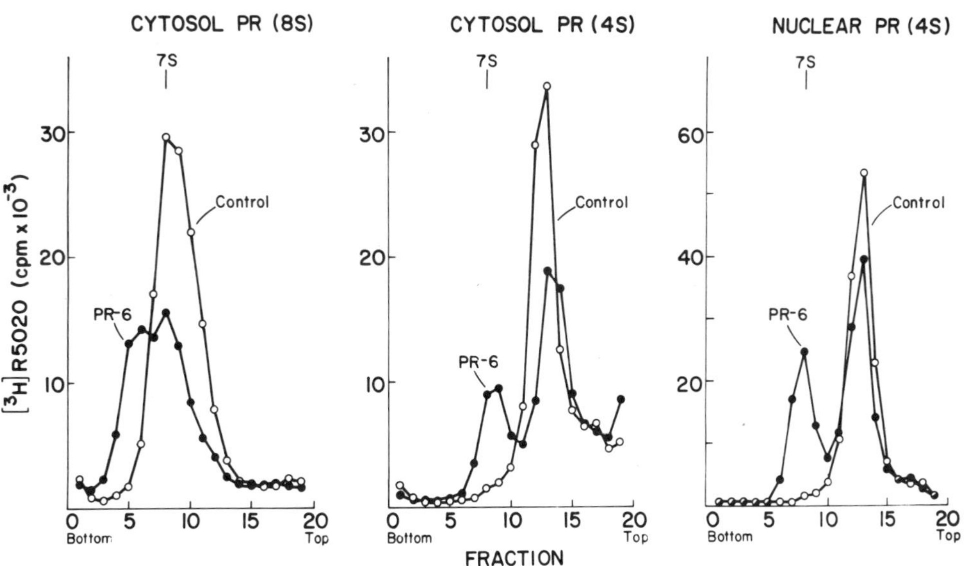

Fig. 2. PR-6 effect on sucrose gradient sedimentation of different molecular forms of human PR. (Further details to be published in Biochemistry.[4])

Sepharose beads as described by Schneider et al.[13] Approximately 5 mg of MAb were coupled/ml of beads and the matrix has a receptor binding capacity of ≈ 250 pmol/ml. For routine purifications we start with 80 ml of concentrated cytosol receptor-[^{3}H]R5020 complexes prepared from T47D cells which are absorbed to the immunomatrix in a column. The column is washed extensively with alternating high and low salt containing buffers and absorbed receptor-hormone complexes are eluted with alkaline pH buffers. Eluted receptors are immediately neutralized. Alkaline pH elution is a relatively mild condition which releases receptors largely in native form still capable of binding hormone. This allows a second step purification by DEAE chromatography. Purifications were performed in the absence of sodium molybdate (Mo) for isolation of transformed PR and in presence of 20 mM Mo to stabilize receptors in the 8-10S non-transformed state. All buffers used in purification, including homogenization buffers, contained a mixture of proteolysis inhibitors to protect receptors from degradation. This included leupeptin, aprotinin, pepstatin A and bacitracin as described by Loosfelt et al.[14]

Single step purification in the absence of Mo results in enrichment of B receptors from 0.71 pmol/mg protein in cytosol to a specific hormone binding activity of 1,915 pmol/mg protein. This represents a ≈ 2,700 fold purification over the starting cytosol (Table 1). Based on a maximal theoretical specific activity of 8,352 pmol/mg protein for homogeneity, receptors are obtained by this single step in 23% purity with a 27% yield. SDS-gel electrophoresis and silver staining of the purified product reveals a predominant doublet band at 120 kDa which represents B receptors since it is reactive by immunoblotting with the PR-6 MAb (Figure 3, left panel) and also binds [^{3}H]R5020 by photoaffinity labeling (not shown). In addition, three other silver stained bands are detected at 58-, 62- and 76 kDa which are not reactive by immunoblotting with PR-6 and do not bind [^{3}H]R5020.

The purity of the B receptor doublets as judged by gel electrophoresis (Figure 3) and densitometric scanning is in close agreement to that estimated by hormone binding activity (Table 1). Thus, we can account for most of the 120 kDa doublet as having hormone binding capacity which indicates that the purification product cannot contain an abundant non-hormone binding contaminant of identical size to the 120 kDa B receptors. We have determined in a number of separate experiments that the three lower molecular weight bands obtained are not receptor fragments but rather are non-receptor proteins. The two smaller sized bands (58- and 62 kDa) appear to be abundant cellular contaminants that bind the immunomatrix non-specifically since they purify in the same amounts from receptor negative cytosols and they separate from B receptors by a second step purification with DEAE ion-exchange chromatography (not shown). The 76 kDa protein in the purification product, however, appears to require the presence of receptors, since this protein is nearly absent in mock immunoaffinity purifications of receptor negative cytosols. Furthermore, the 76 kDa protein co-fractionates with B receptors by second step DEAE chromatography. This two step purification (immunoaffinity chromatography + DEAE), therefore, yields highly purified receptors that are ≈ 50% pure and contain only the 120 kDa receptor doublets and the 76 kDa protein. Receptors isolated under these conditions (-Mo) are in the transformed state since they bind strongly to DNA-cellulose and require high salt elution for their release (not shown). These immunoaffinity purification data therefore indicate that transformed receptors may complex with a 76 kDa non-steroid binding protein. Gustafsson et al.[15] recently reported that transformed glucocorticoid receptors isolated by comparable immunoaffinity purification methods remained associated with a 72 kDa non-hormone binding protein obtained in amounts equal to that of the receptor protein. As a result they proposed that transformed glucocorticoid receptors may be a heterodimer composed of one molecule of the hormone binding receptor protein and one molecule of the 72 kDa protein.

Table 1: Purification of Human B Receptors by Single Step Immunoaffinity Chromatography

	Protein		B Receptors			
	mg/ml	Total mg	pmol[1]	yield	Sp. Act. pmol/mg	%purity[2]
Cytosol	14.40	1,152.0	814	---	0.71	
pH eluate	0.021	0.132	221[3]	27.1%	1,915	23%

[1] B receptors in starting cytosol (estimated to be 50% of total receptors) were measured by DCC ligand binding assay.
[2] Theoretical purity for B receptors based on M_r of 120,000 = 8,352 pmol/mg protein.
[3] Receptor-hormone binding of the purified product was measured by hydroxylapatite assay with inclusion of 1% carrier albumin since the protein concentration is very low. Non-specific binding was determined with carrier albumin alone. Values are average determinations from three separate purifications.

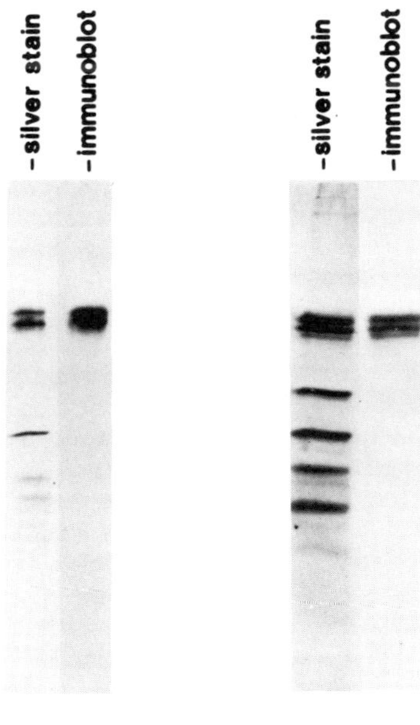

Fig. 3. Analysis of single step immunoaffinity purification performed in the absence (-Mo) or presence (+Mo) of sodium molybdate. Alkaline pH eluates were analyzed by silver staining of SDS-electrophoresis gels and by immunoblotting with PR-6. (Further details to be published in Biochemistry.[4])

Since sodium molybdate stabilizes PR in the 8S untransformed state,[16] immunoaffinity purifications were also performed in the continuous presence of 20 mM Mo which was included in the homogenization buffers and in all subsequent wash and elution buffers. The single step purification product obtained under these conditions contains the same protein components as purified transformed receptors plus an additional 90 kDa protein which is not detectable in the absence of Mo. This is illustrated by silver stained SDS electrophoresis in the right panel of Figure 3. Also shown is an immunoblot of this same preparation with PR-6 which identifies the 120 kDa doublets as B receptors. A non-hormone binding 90 kDa protein has been described to be associated with 8S molybdate stabilized chick PR and with 8S forms of other steroid receptors.[17-18] This polypeptide has been identified as a 90 kDa heat shock protein (hsp)[19,20] and is thought to be a component of 8S non-transformed receptors. Using the AC-88 MAb produced by Toft and co-workers[21] against the chick receptor associated-90 kDa hsp, we have been able to confirm the identity of the 90 kDa protein isolated with Mo stabilized human PR as an hsp (not shown). Thus, human progesterone receptors appear also to complex with a 90 kDa hsp in the molybdate stabilized state.

Since the 90 kDa protein is a heat shock protein, we wondered if the 76 kDa component associated with both receptor forms might also be an hsp. Heat shock proteins are a group of highly conserved polypeptides which

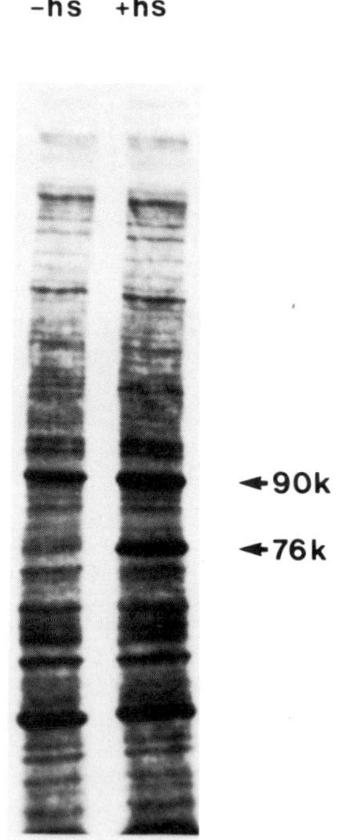

Fig. 4. Effect of heat shock on protein synthesis in T47D cells. Cell cultures maintained at 37°C (-hs) and shocked for 2.5 hr at 42°C (+hs) were pulse-labeled with ^{35}S-methionine and total cell extracts analyzed by SDS-gel electrophoresis and autoradiography.

undergo dramatic increases in synthesis in response to heat as well as other cellular stresses, and they serve a protective function for the cell.[22] T47D cell cultures maintained at their normal temperature of 37°C or stressed by exposure to 42°C for 2.5 hr, were metabolically labeled with ^{35}S-methionine and total radiolabeled extracts from each group of cells were analyzed by SDS-gel electrophoresis and autoradiography. Increased synthesis of two proteins of 90- and 76 kDa occurred in response to heat shock (Figure 4). The 90 kDa protein is synthesized constitutively in substantial amounts at normal temperature and is elevated to even higher levels after heat shock. By contrast, the 76 kDa protein is not readily detectable as a major cellular component at physiological temperature and appears to undergo dramatic induction in response to heat shock. We have immunoprecipitated these ^{35}S-methionine labeled protein extracts from control and heat shocked cells with the PR-6 MAb using protein A Sepharose as an immunoabsorbent. Immunoprecipitations were performed under conditions which isolate transformed receptors (-Mo). The protein A Sepharose beads were washed extensively with high salt containing buffers as well as 0.2% Triton X-100 and absorbed immune

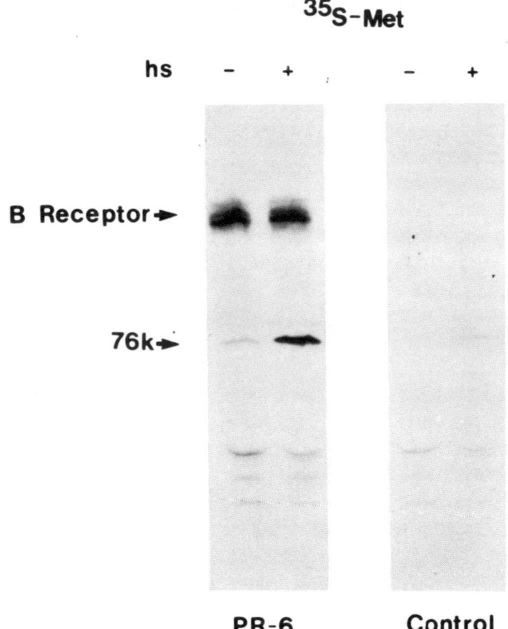

Fig. 5. Immunoprecipitation of ^{35}S-methionine labeled proteins from control (-hs) and heat shocked (+hs) T47D cell cultures with PR-6 and a control antibody. Immunoprecipitations were in the absence of molybdate (-Mo) and analysis of the precipitates was by SDS-gel electrophoresis and autoradiography.

Table 2: Monoclonal Antibodies to Human PR

MAb	A(94K)	B(120K)[1]	Type
A/B-52	+	+	IgG_1
B-30	-	+	IgG_1
B-64	-	+	IgG_1

[1]Reactivity with A or B receptors was determined by immunoblotting assay. (Further details to be published in Biochemistry[4])

complexes were extracted with SDS sample buffer and analyzed by SDS-gel electrophoresis and autoradiography (Fig. 5). Equivalent amounts of ^{35}S-labeled 120 kDa B receptors were precipitated by PR-6 from control (-hs) and heat shocked cells (+hs). The receptor specific MAb also precipitates a labeled 76 kDa protein and radiolabeling of this molecule was greatly increased in the heat shocked cells. By contrast, little or no labeled B receptors or 76 kDa proteins were precipitated with a control antibody (Fig. 5). The increased radiolabeling of a 76 kDa protein in cytosol and in PR-6 immunoprecipitates of heat shocked cells indicates that the 76 kDa molecule associated with highly purified receptors (Fig. 3) is a heat shock protein.

Production of Monoclonal Antibodies to Purified Human Progesterone Receptors

B receptors purified by single step immunoaffinity chromatography (see Figure 3) in the absence of Mo, to obtain transformed PR, were used as immunogen in mice for production of three MAbs against human PR. Further details of immunizations, hybridoma procedures and screening strategies for production and isolation of these MAbs have been previously described.[4] We chose to immunize with transformed PR to avoid production of antibodies to the 90 kDa hsp. The identification code, mouse immunoglobulin subtype and reactivity of each MAb with A or B receptors are given in Table 2. Monospecificity of these antibodies for human receptors was established by a number of criteria. Each MAb is capable of immunoprecipitating native receptor-hormone complexes by use of a secondary antimouse IgG and protein A Sepharose as an absorbant. They displace the sedimentation of 4S receptors on salt containing sucrose gradients and by immunoblot assay of crude cytosols they react only with receptor polypeptides. Two of the MAbs (B-30 and B-64) react only with B receptors and the third (A/B-52) recognizes both A and B receptors. Further proof of antibody specificity for receptors is provided by the fact that A/B-52 which reacts by immunoblotting with both A and B proteins, immunoabsorbs twice the number of receptors as the B specific antibodies, B-30 and B-64 (not shown). Although mice were injected with B receptors only, production of A/B-52 which recognizes both A and B, provides evidence that these two proteins share regions of structural homology. Gronemeyer et al.[23] obtained similar results using chicken A and B receptors purified separately from SDS-gels and used as immunogens in rabbits. Polyclonal antisera reactive with both A and B receptors were obtained in each case. Partial proteolytic peptide mapping studies of photoaffinity labeled human PR in T47D cells also indicate that A and B proteins are structurally related.[11] These MAbs produced against human PR are valuable reagents for further studies of human receptor structure and function, and for clinical immunodetection of PR in breast tumors.

Immunocytochemical Localization of Progesterone Receptors in Breast Cancer Cells

Methods were developed for immunocytochemical detection of PR in breast cancer cells using each of the above described MAbs. Studies were performed with human breast cancer cell lines grown as monolayers on cover slips. Cells were fixed for 15 min with 3.7% buffered formalin and were permeabilized by incubation for another 5 min with 1% Triton X-100. Immunocytochemistry was performed by the indirect avidin-biotin immunoperoxidase method using diaminobenzidine as the chromagen as previously described.[24] Since receptors are low abundant cellular proteins, it is important to establish that the immunochemical staining obtained is not in any part contributed to by cross reaction with other cellular antigens.

Each MAb was titrated to find the optimal concentration range which gives the strongest staining with minimal non-specific background. For PR-6 the optimal concentration range was 1-2 ug/ml and for the other MAbs was in the range of 7-10 ug/ml. Typical immunoperoxidase staining of fixed T47D cells with PR-6 is shown in Figure 6. Peroxidase staining is predominantly nuclear and we observe cell to cell heterogeneity in intensity. Some nuclei stain strongly, others moderately and some nuclei react weakly. We also observe weak cytoplasmic staining which is above background seen with control antibodies. The other three MAbs give a similar predominantly nuclear staining pattern (not shown). Control incubations were performed by the same procedures except that the anti-receptor antibody was replaced with a MAb of the same subtype and concentration, but reactive with an antigen not found in breast cancer cells. No staining of either nuclei or cytoplasm was observed with this control antibody. Omitting either secondary biotinylated antibody or the avidin biotin-complex also gave no staining reaction.

To more rigorously test specificity of the immunocytochemical reaction for receptors we attempted to block immunostaining of T47D cells by preincubation of the anti-receptor antibody with highly purified human PR, and we have performed immunocytochemistry with a series of breast cancer cell lines that have different PR contents by hormone binding assay.[25] Preincubation with purified receptors completely blocked immunostaining of T47D cells and immunoreactivity with the different cell lines correlated with their receptor status. Three PR positive cell lines, T47D, MCF-7 and ZR-75.1 each gave nuclear peroxidase staining. Moreover, in MCF-7 and ZR-75.1, which are cell lines in which PR is inducible by estrogen, weak staining was observed in estrogen withdrawn cells while staining intensity increased in cells grown with estrogen containing medium. No immunoreactivity was detected with the PR negative cell lines, MDA-231, MDA-330 and HBL-100. We conclude, therefore, that the immunoperoxidase staining obtained with these MAbs is specific for receptors.

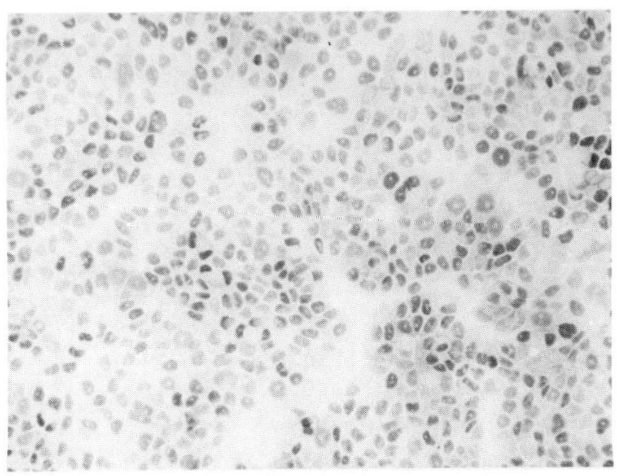

Fig. 6. Immunocytochemistry of formalin fixed T47D cell cultures with PR-6.

The immunocytochemical reaction shown in Figure 6 is that obtained with cells grown in hormone free medium so that receptors are unoccupied. Under these conditions we find that receptor localization is predominantly nuclear. Other investigators working with MAbs to human estrogen receptors[26,27] and Milgrom and co-workers[28] working with MAbs to rabbit uterine PR, have also observed predominantly nuclear immunocytochemical localization of unoccupied receptors. Thus, unoccupied human progesterone receptors appear to reside largely in the nucleus of breast cancer cells suggesting that receptors, at least in part, are capable of translocation from their sites of synthesis in the cytoplasm to the nucleus in a hormone independent manner.

SUMMARY

By use of immunoaffinity chromatography, we have been able to obtain highly purified human B receptors in intact native form. Isolated receptors were maintained as undegraded 120 kDa doublets and they retained their hormone and DNA binding capacities. Under conditions which promote receptor transformation *in vitro*, immunoisolated receptors remained associated with a 76 kDa non-steroid binding protein. In the presence of sodium molybdate, which stabilizes PR in the 8S non-transformed state, an additional 90 kDa protein was associated with immunoisolated PR. Based on these immunoaffinity purification data, we propose the following working model for human PR structure. In the non-transformed 8S state, receptors are complexed with two different non-steroid binding proteins of 76- and 90 kDa, identified as hsps. Transformation results from dissociation of the 90 kDa component, exposing DNA binding sites masked in the 8S receptors. Transformed 4S receptors which bind tightly to DNA, therefore, may be heterodimers composed of the steroid binding protein and the 76 kDa protein. The functional significance of receptor association with these other proteins is not known as yet. Since receptor association with hsps is different in transformed vs. non-transformed state, one logical connection to make is that associated hsps may modulate receptor-DNA binding capacity and may in part explain mechanisms of receptor transformation. An important unanswered question is whether receptor association with these hsps is artifactual occurring only *in vitro* after cell lysis or whether these interactions occur *in vivo*. At the very least, receptor association/dissociation with these other cellular proteins may account for the different molecular forms (8S and 4S) of PR observed in crude cell extracts. Under no conditions have we been able to co-precipitate A receptors with the PR-6 B specific antibody. This strongly suggests that A and B receptors do not form dimers but are likely to exist as separate molecules. Although our work so far has been with B receptors, we would expect that A receptors also complex with hsps to form separate 8S molecules.

We have been able to produce three MAbs directly against purified human B receptors. Two are specific for B (B-30 and B-64) and the third (A/B-52) recognizes epitopes on A and B proteins. These MAbs will be valuable reagents for further structural and functional studies of human PR. By their use in immunoaffinity chromatography it will now be possible to purify human A and B receptors separately or together and begin to answer questions regarding functional roles of A vs. B receptors. By use of the immunocytochemical methods described here, these MAbs may also be useful for clinical immunocytochemical detection of PR in breast tumors.

Acknowledgments. We are indebted to Dr. David Toft at the Mayo Clinic for generously providing the PR-6 monoclonal antibody. This work was supported by American Cancer Society Grant BC 391A and NIH Grant CA 41386.

References

1. C. K. Osborne, M. D. Michael, G. Yochmowitz, W. A. Knight and W. L. McGuire. The value of estrogen and progesterone receptors in the treatment of breast cancer. Cancer 37:2884 (1980).
2. G. M. Clark, W. L. McGuire, C. A. Hubay, O. H. Pearson and M. D. Marshall. Progesterone receptors as a prognostic factor in stage II breast cancer. New Engl. J. Med. 309:1343 (1983).
3. W. P. Sullivan, T. G. Beito, J. Proper, C. T. Krco and D. O. Toft. Preparation of monoclonal antibodies to avian progesterone receptors. Endocrinology 119:1549 (1986).
4. P. A. Estes, E. J. Suba, J. Lawler-Heavner, D. El-Ashry, L. L. Wei, D. O. Toft, W. P. Sullivan, K. B. Horwitz and D. P. Edwards. Immunologic analysis of human breast cancer progesterone receptors: Immunoaffinity purification and production of monoclonal antibodies. Biochemistry, in press (1987).
5. I. Keydar, L. Chen, S. Karby, F. R. Weiss, J. Delarea, M. Radu, S. Chaitcik and H. J. Brenner. Establishment and characterization of cell line of human breast carcinoma origin. Eur. J. Cancer 15:659 (1979).
6. K. B. Horwitz, M. B. Mockus and B. A. Lessey. Variant T47D human breast cancer cells with high progesterone receptor levels despite estrogen and antiestrogen resistance. Cell 28:633 (1982).
7. K. B. Horwitz and G. R. Freidenberg. Growth inhibition and increase of insulin receptors in antiestrogen-resistant T47D human breast cancer cells by progestins. Implications for endocrine therapies. Cancer Res. 45:167 (1985).
8. D. Chalbos and H. Rochefort. Dual effects of the progestin R5020 on proteins released by the T47D human breast cancer cells. J. Biol. Chem. 259:1231 (1984).
9. D. Chalbos and H. Rochefort. A 250 kilodalton cellular protein is induced by protestins in two human breast cancer cell lines MCF-7 and T47D. Biochem. & Biophys. Res. Commun. 121:421 (1984).
10. M. B. Mockus and K. B. Horwitz. Progesterone receptors in human breast cancer. Stoichiometric translocation and nuclear receptor processing. J. Biol. Chem. 258:4778 (1983).
11. K. B. Horwitz, M. D. Francis and L. L. Wei. Hormone-dependent covalent modification and processing of human progesterone receptors in the nucleus. DNA 4:451 (1985).
12. H. Towbin, T. Staehlin and J. Garclan. Electrophoretic transfer of proteins from polyacrylamide to nitrocellulose sheets. Proc. Natl. Acad. Sci., USA 76:4350 (1979).
13. C. Schneider, D. Newman, R. Sutherland, U. Asser and M. F. Greaves. A one step purification of membrane proteins using a high efficiency immunomatrix. J. Biol. Chem. 257:10766 (1982).
14. H. Loosfelt, F. Logeat, M. T. B. Hai and E. Milgrom. The rabbit progesterone receptor: Evidence for a single steroid binding subunit and characterization of receptor mRNA. J. Biol. Chem. 259:14196 (1984).
15. J.-A. Gustafsson, O. Bakke, K. Carlstsdt-Duke, A. Fuxe, S. Harfstrand, S. Okret, L. Poellinger and A.-C. Wikstrom. Purification, oligomerism, regulation and localization of the glucocorticoid receptor, in: "Advances in Gene Technology: Molecular Biology of the Endocrine System," vol. 4, D. Preutt et al., eds, Cambridge University Press (1986).
16. R. K. Puri, P. Grandics, J. J. Dougherty and D. O Toft. Purification of "nontransformed" avian progesterone receptors and preliminary characterization. J. Biol. Chem. 257:10831 (1982).
17. I. Joab, C. Radanyi, M. Renoir, T. Buchou, M.-G. Catelli, N. Binart, J. Mester and E.-E. Baulieu. Common non-hormone binding component in non-transformed chick oviduct receptors of four steroid hormones. Nature 308:850 (1984).

18. P. R. Housley, E. R. Sanchez, H. M. Wesphal, M. Beato and W. B. Pratt. The molybdate-stabilized L-cell glucocorticoid receptor isolated by affinity chromatography or with a monoclonal antibody is associated with a 90-92-kDa nonsteroid-binding protein. J. Biol. Chem. 260:13810 (1985).
19. M. G. Catelli, N. Binart, I. J. Testat, J. M. Renoir, E.-E. Baulieu, J. R. Feramisco and W. J. Welch. The common 90-kd protein on non-transformed steroid receptors is a heat shock protein. EMBO J. 4:3131 (1985).
20. S. Schuh, Yonemoto, J. Brugge, V. Bauer, R. Riehl, W. Sullivan and D. O. Toft. A 90,000- dalton binding protein common to both steroid receptors and the Rous Sarcoma Virus transforming protein, $pp60^{v-src}$. J. Biol. Chem. 260:14292 (1985).
21. W. P. Sullivan, B. T. Vroman, V. J. Bauer, R. K. Puri, R. M. Riehl, G. R. Pearson and D. O. Toft. Isolation of steroid receptor binding protein from chicken oviduct and production of monoclonal antibodies. Biochemistry 24:4214 (1985).
22. R. H. Burdan. The human heat-shock protein: Their induction and possible intracellular functions, in: "Heat Shock From Protein to Man," M. J. Schlesinger, M. Ashburner and A. Tissieres, eds. Cold Spring Harbor Symposium (1982).
23. H. Gronemeyer, M. Govindan and P. Chambon. Immunological similarity between the chick oviduct progesterone receptor forms A and B. J. Biol. Chem. 260:6916 (1985).
24. D. P. Edwards, K. T. Grzyb, L. G. Dressler, R. E. Mansel, D. T. Zava, G. W. Sledge, Jr. and W. L. McGuire. Monoclonal antibody identification and characterization of a Mr 43,000 membrane glycoprotein associated with human breast cancer. Cancer Res. 46:1306 (1986).
25. K. B. Horwitz, D. T. Zava, K. T. Arulasanam, E. M. Jensen and W. L. McGuire. Steroid receptor analysis of nine human breast cancer cell lines. Cancer Res. 38:2434 (1978).
26. W. J. King and G. L. Greene. Monoclonal antibodies localize estrogen receptor in nuclei of target cells. Nature 307:745 (1984).
27. S. Madhabananda. Application of avidin-biotin complex technique for the localization of estradiol-receptor in target tissues using monoclonal antibodies, in: "Techniques in Immunocytochemistry," vol. 3, G. R. Bollock and P. Petrusz, eds., Academic Press (1985).
28. M. P. Applanat, F. Logeat, M. T. Picard-Groyer and E. Milgrom. Immunocytochemical study of mammalian progesterone receptors using monoclonal antibodies. Endocrinology 116:1473 (1985).

SESSION IV

ANALYSIS OF THE HUMORAL IMMUNE REPERTOIRE IN PATIENTS WITH CANCER

Richard J. Cote, Donna M. Morrissey, Alan N. Houghton, Herbert F. Oettgen and Lloyd J. Old

Memorial Sloan-Kettering Cancer Center
1275 York Avenue
New York, NY 10021

In the mid-1950's Foley (1), and later Prehn (2), showed that mice could respond to antigens expressed by chemically-induced tumors in a biologically significant way. Prehn also found that each tumor expressed completely unique tumor-specific antigens, even if the tumors were developed in the same animal.

In the mid-1970's Old, Oettgen and their colleagues began investigating the human immune response to tumors. The focus of their investigation was the search for tumor-specific antigens analogous to the antigens first described by Foley and Prehn. More generally, they were interested in whether humans could respond to their tumors, and the nature of the antigenic stimulus initiating that response. The method developed to study these questions is known as autologous typing (3). It involves testing the serum from a tumor-bearing patient against cultured autologous and allogeneic malignant and non-malignant cell lines, in order to find antibodies reactive with antigens expressed by the autologous tumor, and the distribution of the antigens (Fig. 1). Using this method, 3 classes of antigens expressed by tumors and recognized by the host were described (3). Class 1 antigens are only expressed by the autologous tumor, and are not expressed by normal autologous cells, or allogeneic normal and malignant cells. Seven examples have been described so far in melanoma and leukemia (4-9). Biochemical analysis of these antigens has indicated that most are proteins/glycoproteins, again, analogous to the tumor-specific antigens of methylcolanthrene induced tumors (9,10). Class 2 antigens are expressed only by autologous and allogeneic tumors, or their expression is restricted to cells of a particular differentiation pathway (6,11,12). Class 3 antigens are expressed by a wide variety of tumors and normal cells (3). The critical feature of all of these antigens is that they are autoimmunogenic and can be recognized by the host.

Although a large number of antigens were defined, these

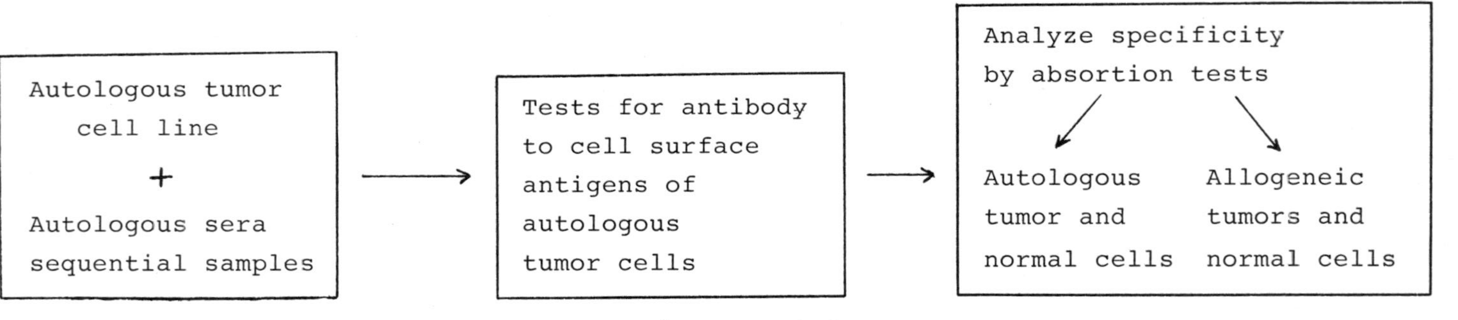

Fig. 1. Essentials of autologous typing

studies strained the limits of conventional serology. Among the major problems were the low titer of antibodies, the presence of a heterogeneous population of antibodies, and the limited quantities of serum available. The development of the mouse hybridoma (13) and then the Epstein-Barr virus (EBV) tranformation technology (14,15) suggested methods which could extend and expand these studies.

Our initial efforts were to develop the hybridoma technology so that human monoclonal antibodies could be reliably and reproducibly obtained. This work has been described elsewhere (16-19). We have used drug marked human myelomas (20), human lymphoblastoid (21,23), and mouse myeloma lines (24) as fusion partners (Table 1) for the generation of human immunoglobulin secreting hybridomas, and have explored EBV-transformation of lymphocytes (14,15). The human drug-marked cell lines can be difficult to work with, and fusion efficiency is generally poor, especially when compared with human lymphocyte-mouse myelona fusions. We found that, contrary to the prejudice of the time, stable human-mouse hybrids could be reliably and reproducibly obtained at resonably high frequency (16-19).

We have generated over 8000 human hybridomas, many through fusions with the mouse myeloma NS-1. Approximately 50% produce detectable levels of immunoglobulin, (greater than 500ng/ml culture supernatent) regardless of the fusion-partner (Table 2). The examination of antibody reactivity has focused on cultured malignant cells, since we are interested in antibodies which might be important in tumor immunity. We have found that a significant proportion of the immunoglobulin-secreting clones (5-10%) produce antibody reactive with cellular antigens (16,19). We further observed that the majority of these antibodies are directed against intracellular antigens, and that most are broadly distributed or are epitopes shared by multiple antigens. Antibodies reactive with cell surface antigens are uncommon (Table 2). The reasons for this are not clear, but may be in part due to a general prohibition against the development of autoantibodies to cell surface antigens due to immunological tolerance (16,19,25).

Hybridomas derived from lymphocytes of patients with cancer, autoimmune disease, or normal individuals yield similar results; the proportion of clones secreting antibody reactive with cellular antigens is comparable in normal and disease states (16,19). There does not appear to be selection for a subpopulation of lymphocytes in our system; all of the fusion partners studied appear to fuse with representative population of lymphocytes (16). We have tentatively concluded that a significant proportion of the human B cell repertoire (between 5 10% of the evaluable clones) is directed to the production of antibodies reactive with cellular antigens. Antibodies directed against cell surface antigens are uncommon, indicating that these clones are rare in the repertoire.

The finding of antibodies reactive with cellular antigens is not unexpected; sera from patients with tumors and autoimmune disease commonly contain such reactivities (3,26). In addition, antibodies from patients with monoclonal gammopathies, such as multiple myeloma or Waldenstom's macroglobulinemia, have been reported to react with cellular

Table 1

CHARACTERISTICS OF DRUG-MARKED MYELCMA AND LYMPHOBLASTOID LINES STUDIED

Cell line	Karyotype	Heavy chain	Light chain	Cell doubling time (hr)	Comments
LICR-LON-HMy-2	Human	γ	κ	24	$EBNA^{+*}$
SKO-007	Human	ε	λ	35	Mycoplasma-free
UC729-6	Human	μ	κ	24	$EBNA^{+}$
GM4672	Human	γ	κ	30	$EBNA^{+}$
NS-1	Mouse	--	κ	24	--

*EBNA: Epstein-Barr virus nuclear antigen

Table 2

GENERATION OF HYBRIDOMAS SECRETING HUMAN MONOCLONAL ANTIBODY

RESULTS OF FUSIONS

HYBRIDOMAS	
NUMBER OBSERVED	8,000
SECRETING Ig	4,000
REACTING WITH CELLULAR ANTIGENS	200
CELL SURFACE ANTIGENS	9
INTRACELLULAR ANTIGENS	194

antigens (for eg, see 27,28). However, to our knowledge, our studies were the first to suggest that lymphocytes capable of secreting antibody to cellular antigens comprise a significant proportion of the normal humoral repertoire (16,19). Further, it appears that this proportion is not dramatically changed in disease states (except of course in the case of hematopoietic disorders); rather, there is a change in the secretory state of these clones either through activation or disregulation.

Examination of the data from other groups involved in the generation of human monoclonal antibodies has revealed that, regardless of the fusion partner, assay system, or patient population studied, approximately 10% of the immunoglobulin secreting hybrids produce antibody reactive with cellular antigens (Table 3) (28-36). Lymphocytes from patients with tumors and autoimmune diseases, and both human and mouse fusion partners, were used. Avrameas and his collegues examined sera from normal individuals and patients with monoclonal gammopathies, and found that 5 to 10% of these sera contained monoclonal antibody reactive with cellular antigens in their assays (28,29,37). The antigens detected by all of these groups are for the most part broadly distributed and intracellular. Thus, using a number of lymphocyte sampling techniques and a variety of lymphocyte sources, the results are consistant with our findings. Finally, fusions with splenocytes from non-immunized mice show similar results (Table 4) (38-41); between 5 to 10% of the evaluable B cells secrete antibody reactive with broadly distributed intracellular antigens, perhaps indicating that a significant proportion of the mammalian B cell repertoire is directed to the production of autoreactive antibodies. When looked for, reactivities to cell surface antigens are rare (41).

Since normal individuals, as well as patients with cancer or with autoimmune disease, have lymphocytes with the capacity to produce antibodies to cellular antigens, the relationship of these antibodies to the development of a significant anti-tumor response is unclear. Activation of a clone, determined either by secretion of antibody into the serum or an immunoglobulin class switch, could be interpreted as a response, whether or not it is biologically effective (i.e. affects the growth of the tumor). In addition, patients with cancer may produce antibodies which react against a different range of determinants than antibodies from non-tumor bearing individuals. In order to further assess this, we have examined the distribution and biochemical nature of the antigens recognized by human monoclonal antibodies.

Human monoclonal antibodies produced in our laboratory have been shown to react against a wide range of cellular structures, including cell surface, cytoplasmic, cytoskeletal, nuclear and nucleolar determinants (16-19).

Analysis of antibodies reactive with cell surface antigens has revealed that, while these antibodies are rare, they react with a heterogeneous group of antigens (16-19). The distribution of the antigens can be divided into three categories (Table 5). Antigens with highly restricted distribution have been described, including one (GXM1) which is expressed by the autologous melanoma cell line (i.e., derived from the patient from which the hybridoma was produced) (42).

Table 3

PROPORTION OF Ig^+ CLONES SECRETING HUMAN MONOCLONAL ANTIBODY TO CELLULAR ANTIGENS

Author	Year	Patient Population	% Clones Secreting Human Monoclonal Antibody to Cellular Antigens
Dighiero *et al.*[28,29]	1982-1983	Monoclonal Ig (serum)	8.1%/5.8%*
Shoenfeld *et al.*[30,31]	1982-1983	SLE	9.7%
Satoh *et al.*[32]	1983	Autoimmune	5.7%
Olsson *et al.*[33]	1984	AML	8.5%
Haspel *et al.*[34]	1985	Colon Cancer	15.0%
Mitchell *et al.*[35]	1986	Melanoma	11.3%
Rauch *et al.*[36]	1986	SLE, RA	6.5%

*% of patients with monoclonal Ig spike that had antibody reactive with cellular antigens

Abbreviations; Ig: immunoglobulin, SLE: Systemic Lupus Erythematosus, AML: Acute myelogenous leukemia, RA: rheumatoid arthritis

Table 4

PROPORTION OF CLONES FROM NON-IMMUNIZED MICE SECRETING MOUSE MONOCLONAL ANTIBODY TO CELLULAR ANTIGENS

Author	Year	Mouse Strain	% Clones Secreting Mouse Monoclonal Antibody to Cellular Antigens
Dighiero *et al*.[38,39]	1983-84	BALB/c BALB/c x C57BL/6	6.3%
Prabhakar *et al*.[40]	1984	SJL/J BALB/c	12.2%
Underwood *et al*.[41]	1985	BALB/c	9.8% (.04% surface reactive)

The antibody also reacts weakly with one other melanoma cell line, but not with any other malignant or normal cells, including autologous B cells. This antigen could be considered analogous to the Class 1 antigens defined by autologous typing.

A second group of cell surface antigens have intermediate distributions, including several which show differentiation related expression. Two of the antigenic systems (Ev248, Ma4) have not been detected on any normal cells tested (17,19). Thus, several antigens in this group could be considered analogous to the Class 2 tumor antigens, either on the basis of a tumor-restricted or differentiation-related distribution.

A group of cell surface antigens which are broadly distributed have been described, including one (Sp909) which is expressed by all cell types tested (19); these antigens are similar to the Class 3 antigens.

A critical feature of the antigens identified by human monoclonal antibodies (along with antigens defined by autologous typing) is that they are potentially autoimmunogenic and can be recognized by the host.

In addition to the similarities in their distribution, antigens defined by autologous typing and human monoclonal antibodies have shown structural similarities as well. The antigen GXM1 is a glycoprotein (42). Class 1 antigens defined by autologous typing have been found, when defined, to be proteins/glycoproteins (9,10), and the unique antigens expressed by methylcolanthrene- induced sarcomas have been found to be proteins as well (3). Biochemical studies have indicated that Ma4, Ev248, HJM1 and 32-27M (antigens which show Class 2 characteristics) are lipids/glycolipids (17,19,42), and many of the Class 2 antigens defined by autologous typing are glycolipids as well (unpublished results). Ev248 and Ma4 appear to be associated with malignant transformation, while Ev248, HJM1 and 32-27M are associated with specific stages of differentiation. Irie and her colleagues have identified antibodies (both in sera and from supernatents of EBV transformed lymphocytes) to Class 2 glycolipid antigens. Hakomori has shown that changes in the carbohydrate structure of cell-surface glycolipids are associated with differentiation and malignant transformation of cells (44). Our laboratory has shown that blood group carbohydrates expressed by epithelial cells undergo characteristic changes in association with malignant transformation (45). Our results indicate that carbohydrate/glycolipid antigens associated with differentiation and malignant transformation may be an important group of autoimmunogenic determinants on tumor cells, thus forming an intriguing link between known antigenic changes that take place on tumor cells and the capacity to respond immunologically to these changes.

A complex array of intracellular antigens are recognized by human monoclonal antibodies produced in our laboratory, and the distribution of many of these has been well described (17,19). While most of the antibodies react with broadly distributed antigens or with epitopes share by multiple antigens, a series of intracellular determinants showing differentiation related or restricted distributions have been identified (Table 6), including several which react with intermediate filament

Table 5

HUMAN MONOCLONAL ANTIBODIES REACTIVE WITH CELL SURFACE ANTIGENS

Distribution	Antibody Designation
Restricted	GXM1
Intermediate	Ma4, Ev248, Ri37, HJM1, 32-27M
Broad	Gr169, DSM1, Sp909

Table 6

HUMAN MONOCLONAL ANTIBODIES REACTIVE WITH INTRACELLULAR ANTIGENS*

Distribution	Antibody Designation
Restricted	Te39, Hu44, Gr431, Ch13, Ch45
Intermediate	Pa24, Hu22, Hu11, M307, M304
Broad	De8, Sm21, Po71

*This is a partial list of over 194 antibodies studied

proteins such as cytokeratin (Pa24) or vimentin (M307) (46).

A number of human monoclonal antibodies which recognize distinct intracellular antigens expressed by only a few cell lines have been identified, including several which have not been found in normal cells so far (19). These antigens are expressed by a subpopulation of epithelial cells, and all of these antibodies were derived from patients with epithelial tumors (breast, colon and lung cancer).

The meaning of the reactivities to intracellular antigens remains problematical. Do these antibodies play any role in an active immune response to tumor cells, or do they simply develop in response to (tumor) cell lysis, as has been previously suggested (47)? We have found several human monoclonal antibodies reactive with intracellular antigens restricted to epithelial cells, including two antibodies to cytokeratin intermediate filament proteins, which are IgA isotype. These antibodies were derived from lymph node lymphocytes of patients with breast cancer, indicating activation of the clones in response to a specific antigenic stimulus. Whether this might have significance in terms of tumor cell recognition or control remains to be established.

Several general points have emerged from the study of human monoclonal antibodies:

- A significant proportion of the evaluable B cell repertoire in patients with cancer, autoimmune disease and in normal individuals is directed to the production of antibodies reactive with cellular antigens.

- The majority of these antibodies react with intracellular antigens; antibodies directed against cell surface antigens are uncommon, indicating that these clones are rare in the repertoire.

- While most antibodies react with widely distributed antigens, or epitopes expressed by multiple antigens, a number of human monoclonal antibodies reactive with antigens which show differentiation related distribution, are highly restricted, or which are transformation-related, have been described.

- Human monoclonal antibodies which recognize cell surface antigens analogous to the Class 1, 2 and 3 antigens defined by autologous typing have been described. Several of the Class 2-related differentiation and transformation associated antigens are glycolipids, indicating that glycolipids may be an important group of autoimmunogenic determinants on tumor cells.

Many questions remain. We do not know the source of the immunogenic signal which elicited the antibodies described by our studies. Are some antibodies generated in direct response to unique tumor antigens, as suggested by the presence of antibodies to Class 1 antigens? Does immune surveillance play a role in tumor recognition, as suggested by the presence of natural antibodies (37,48) and the finding of B cells in non-tumor bearing individuals capable of producing antibodies to Class 2-type antigens? Or, is the immunogenic stimulus not related to cellular antigen expression; the antibodies described here may be fortuitously cross-reactive with cellular antigens. We have gained, however, fundemental insight about the B cell repertoire, which will help to unravel the nature of the immune response in cancer and autoimmune disease.

Acknowledgement: We thank Jannette Rios for her expert assistance in the preparation of this manuscript.

REFERENCES

1. E.J. Foley, Antigenic properties of methylcholanthrene-induced tumors in mice of the strain of origin, Cancer Res., 13:835-837, (1953).

2. R.T. Prehn, J.M. Main, Immunity to methylcholanthrene-induced sarcomas, J. Natl. Cancer Inst., 18:769-778, (1957).

3. L.J. Old, Cancer Immunology: The search for specificity - G.H.A. Clowes Memorial Lecture, Cancer Res. 41: 361-375, (1981).

4. T.E. Carey, T. Takahashi, L.A. Resnick, H.E. Oettgen, and L.J. Old, Cell surface antigens of human malignant melanoma. I: mixed hemadsorption assays for humoral immunity to cultured autologous melanoma cells, Proc. Natl. Acade. Sci. USA 73:3278-3282 (1976).

5. H. Shiku, T. Takahashi, H.F. Oettgen, and L.J. Old, Cell surface antigens of human malignant melanoma II: Serological typing with immune adherence assays and definition of two new surface antigens, J. Exp. Med., 144:873-881, (1976).

6. H. Shiku, T. Takahashi, L.A. Resnick, H.F. Oettgen, and L.J. Old, Cell surface antigens of human malignant melanoma. III: Recognition of autoantibodies with unusual characteristics, J. Exp. Med., 145:784-789, (1977).

7. A.P. Albino, K.O. Lloyd, A.N. Houghton, H.F. Oettgen, and L.J. Old, Heterogeneity in surfce antigen expression and glycoprotein expression of cell lines derived from different metastases of the same patient: Implications for the study of tumor antigens, J. Exp. Med., 154:1764, (1981).

8. T.J. Garrett, T. Takahashi, B.D. Clarkson, and L.J. Old, Detection of antibody to autologous human leukemia cells by immune adherence assays, Proc. Natl. Acad. Sci. USA, 74:4587-4590, (1977).

9. F.X. Real, M.J. Mattes, A.N. Houghton, H.F. Oettgen, and L.J. Old, Class 1 (unique) tumor antigens of human melanoma: Identification of a 90,000 Dalton surface glycoprotein by autologous antibody, J. Exp. Med., 160:1219-1233, (1984).

10. T.E. Carey, K.O. Lloyd, T. Takahashi, L. Travassos, and L.J. Old, AH cell-surface antigen of human malignant melanoma: Solubilization and partial characterization, Proc. Natl. Acad. Sci., USA, 76:2898-2902, (1979).

11. M. Pfreundschuh, H. Shiku, T. Takahashi, R. Ueda, J. Ransohoff, H.F. Oettgen and L.J. Old, Serological analysis of cell surface antigens of malignant human brain tumors, Proc. Natl. Acad. Sci. USA, 75:5122-5126, (1978).

12. R. Ueda, H. Shiku, M. Pfreundschuh, T. Takahashi, L.T.C. Li, W.F. Whitmore, H.F. Oettgen and L.J. Old, Cell Surface antigens of human renal cancer defined by autologous typing, J. Exp. Med., 150:564-579, (1979).

13. G. Kohler and C. Milstein, Continuous cultures of fused cells secreting antibody of predefined specificity, Nature, 236:495-497, (1975).

14. M. Steinitz, G. Klein, S. Koskimies, and O. Makel, EB virus-induced B lymphocyte cell lines producing specific antibody, Nature, 269:420-422, (1978).

15. V.R. Zurawski, E. Haber, and P.H. Black, Continuous human lymphoblastoid cell lines, Science, 199:1439-1441, (1978).

16. R.J. Cote, D.M. Morrissey, A.N. Houghton, E.J. Beattie, H.F. Oettgen, and L.J. Old, Generation of human monoclonal antibodies reactive with cellular antigens, Proc. Natl. Acad. Sci. USA, 80:2026-2030, (1983).

17. A.N. Houghton, H. Brooks, R.J. Cote, M.C. Taormina, H.F. Oettgen, and L.J. Old, Detection of cellular antigens by human monoclonal antibodies, J. Exp. Med., 158:53-65, (1983).

18. R.J. Cote, D.M. Morrissey, H.F. Oettgen, and L.J. Old, Analysis of human monoclonal antibodies derived from the lymphocytes of patients with cancer, Fed. Proc., 43:2465-2469, (1984).

19. R.J. Cote, D.M. Morrissey, A.N. Houghton, T.M. Thomson, M.E. Daly, H.F. Oettgen, and L.J. Old. Specificity analysis of human monoclonal antibodies reactive with cell surface and intracellular antigens, Proc. Natl. Acad. Sci. USA, 83:2959-2963, (1986).

20. L. Olsson, and H.S. Kaplan, Human-human hybridomas producing monoclonal antibodies of predefined antigenic specificity, Proc. Natl. Acad. Sci. USA, 77:5429-5431, (1980).

21. C.M. Croce, A. Linnenbach, W. Hall, Z. Steplewski, and H. Koprowski, Production of human hybridomas secreting antibody to measles virus, Nature, 288:488-489, (1980).

22. P.A.W. Edwards, C.M. Smith, A.M. Neville, and M.J. O'Hare, A human-human hybridoma system based on a fast growing mutant of the ARH-77 plasma cell leukemia-derived line, Eur. J. Immunol., 12:641-648, (1982).

23. M.C. Glassy, H.H. Handley, H. Hagiwara, and I. Royston, UC729-6, a human lymphoblastoid B-cell line useful for generating antibody-secreting human-human hybridomas, Proc. Natl. Acad. Sci. USA, 80:6327-6331, (1983).

24. G. Kohler, and C. Milstein, Derivation of specific antibody-producing tissue culture and tumor cell lines by cell fusion, Eur. J. Immunol., 6:511-519, (1976).

25. G.J.V. Nossal, Cellular mechanisms of immune tolerance, Ann Rev. Immunol., 1:33-62, (1983).

26. P. Miescher, M. Fauconnet, and T. Berand, Experimental immunonucleophagocytosis and the LE phenomenon, Exp. Med. Surg., 11:173, (1953).

27. K. Dellagi, P. Dupoey, J.c. Brouet, A. Billecocg, D. Gomez, J.P. Clauvel, and M. Seligmann, Waldenstrom's macroglobulinemia and peripheral neuropathy: A clinical and immunologic study of 25 patients, Blood, 62:280-285, (1983).

28. G. Dighiero, B. Guilbert, and S. Avrameas, Naturally occurring antibodies against nine common antigens in human sera: II. High incidence of monoclonal Ig exhibiting antibody activity against actin and tubulin and sharing antibody specificities with natural antibodies, J. Immunol., 128:2788-2792, (1982).

29. G. Digniero, B. Guilbert, J-P. Fermand, P. Lymberi, F. Danon, and S. Avrameas, Thirty six human immunoglobulins with antibody activity against cytoskeleton proteins, thyroglobulin, and native DNA: Immunologic studies and clinical correlations, Blood, 62:264-270, (1983).

30. Y. Shoenfeld, S.C. Hsu-Lin, J.E. Gabriels, L.E. Silberstein, B.C. B Furie, B.D. Stollar, and R.S. Schwartz, Production of autoantibodies by human-human hybridomas, J. Clin. Invest, 70:205-208, (1982).

31. Y. Shoenfeld, J. Rauch, H. Massicotte, S.K. Datta, J. Andre-Schwartz, D. Stollar, and R.S. Schwartz, Polyspecificity of monoclonal lupus autoantibodies produced by human-human hybrodomas, NEJM, 308:414-420, (1983).

32. J. Satoh, B.S. Prabhakar, M.V. Haspe, F. Ginsberg-Fellner, A.L. Notkins, Human monoclonal antibodies that react with multiple endocrine organs, NEJM, 309:217-220, (1983).

33. L. Olsson, R.B. Andreaasen, A. Ost, B. Christensen, and P. Biberfeld, Antibody producing human hybridoma: II. Derivation and characterization of an antibody specific for human leukemia cells, J. Exp. Med., 159:537-550, (1984).

34. M.V. Haspel, R.P. McCabe, N. Pomato, N.J. Janesch, J.V. Knowlton, L.C. Peters, H.C. Hoover, and M.G. Hanna, Generation of tumor cell-reactive human monoclonal antibodies using peripheral blood lymphocytes from actively immunized colorectal carcinoma patients, Cancer Res.., 45:3951-3961, (1985).

35. J. Kan-Mitchell, A. Imam, R.A. Kempf, C.R. Taylor and M.S. Mitchell, Human monoclonal antibodies directed against melanoma tumor-associated antigens, Cancer Res. 46:2490-2496, (1986).

36. J. Rauch, H. Tannenbaum, K. Straaton, H. Massicotte, and J. Wild, Human-human hybridoma autoantibodies with both anti-DNA and rheumatiod factor activities, J. Clin. Invest., 77:106-112, (1986).

37. B. Guilbert, G. Dighiero, and S. Aurameas, Naturally occurring antibodies against nine comman antigens in human sera: I. Detection, isolation, and characterization, J. Immunol., 128:2779-2787, (1982).

38. G. Dighiero, P. Lymberi, D. Holmbrg, I. Lundquist, A. Coutinho, and S. Avrameas, High frequency of natural autoantibodies in normal newborn mice, J. Immunol., 134:765-771, (1984).

39. G. Dighiero, P. Lymberi, J-C. Mazie, S. Rouyre, G.S. Butler-Browne, R.G Whalen, and S. Avrameas, Murine hybridomas secreting natural monoclonal antibodies reacting with self antigens, J. Immunol., 131:2267-2272, (1983).

40. B.S. Prabhaker, J. Saegusa, T. Onodera, and A.L. Notkins, Lymphocytes capable of making autoantibodies that react with multiple organs are a comman feature of the normal B cell repertoire, J. Immunol., 133:2815-2817, (1984).

41. J.R. Underwood, J.S. Pedersen, Chalmers, P.J. and B.H. Toh, Hybrids from normal, germ free, nude and neonatal mice produce monoclonal autoantibodies to eight different intracellular structures, Clin. Exp. Immunol., 60:417-426, (1985).

42. H. Yamaguchi, K. Furukawa, S.R. Fortunato, P.O. Livingston, K.O. Lloyd, H.F. Oettgen, and L.J. Old, Cell surface antigens of melanoma recognized by human monoclonal antibodies. Proc. Natl. Acad. Sci. USA, 1987 (in press)

43. R.F. Irie, L.L. Sze, and R.E. Saxton, Human antibody to OFA-I, a tumor antigen, produced in vitro by Epstein-Barr virus-transformed human B-lymphoid cell lines, Proc. Natl. Acad. Sci. USA, 79:5666-5670, (1982).

44. S. Hakamori, and R. Kannagi, Glycosphingolipids as tumor-associated and differentiation markers, J. Natl. Cancer Inst., 71(2):231-251 (1983).

45. C. Cordon-Cardo, K.O. Lloyd, S. Sakamoto, M.E. McGrorty, L.J. Old, and M.R. Melamed, Immunohistologic expression of blood-group antigens in normal human gastrointestinal tract and colonic carcinoma, Int. J. Cancer, 37:667-676, (1986).

46. T.M. Thomson, R.J. Cote, A.N. Houghton, H.F. Oettgen, and L.J. Old, Human monoclonal antibodies recognizing intermediate filament (IF) molecules, Fed. Proc., 43:1513, (1985).

47. P. Grabar, Autoantibodies and the physiological role of immunoglobulins, Immunol. Today, 4:337-340, (1983).

48. A.N. Houghton, M.C. Taormina, H. Ikeda, T. Watanabe, H.F. Oettgen, and L.J. Old, Serological survey of normal humans for natural antibody to cell surface antigens of melanoma, Proc. Natl. Acad. Sci. USA, 77:4260-4264, (1980).

AN IMPROVED METHOD FOR THE RADIOHALOGENATION OF MONOCLONAL ANTIBODIES

Michael R. Zalutsky and Acharan S. Narula
Department of Radiology
Duke University Medical Center
Durham, North Carolina 27710, USA

INTRODUCTION

Radiolabeled monoclonal antibodies directed against human cancer-associated antigens offer a conceptually appealing approach to the more selective identification and treatment of breast and other cancers *in vivo*. Although a few studies, in particular, those employing regional delivery of antibodies, suggest that antibody-mediated delivery of isotopes is a promising technique, most of the results in the literature do not support the belief that radioimmunoscintigraphy and therapy are ready for widespread application in the clinical domain. In general, the absolute magnitude uptake of isotope in the tumor is low[1] and the specificity of localization, determined by comparison to a nonspecific immunoglobulin, has not been documented in clinical studies. While pharmacological factors such as flow and permeability present significant obstacles which must be overcome[2], the successful utilization of radiolabeled monoclonal antibodies requires both the development of antibodies with greater specificity and affinity for tumors and improved labeling methods which decrease the loss of isotope from the antibody *in vivo*. The production and characterization of new antibodies which react more selectively with human breast cancers is described in several chapters in this volume; in this chapter we will discuss our approach to increasing the *in vivo* stability of labeled antibodies.

Currently, monoclonal antibodies are labeled either by radiohalogenation or with metallic isotopes using bifunctional chelates. An advantage of the chelate approach is that a wide variety of metallic isotopes are available with nuclear properties which would be appropriate for a wide range of diagnostic and therapeutic applications. Problems inherent with the labeling of proteins with radioactive metals are the need to exclude metallic impurities from reagents because of their ability to saturate chelation sites and nonspecific and reversible binding of the radiometal to the protein. However, the most significant problem encountered *in vivo* with antibodies labeled with ^{111}In via bifunctional chelates is the accumulation of a large fraction of the injected dose of ^{111}In in the liver[3-6]. In studies comparing ^{111}In-labeled antibodies to those labeled with radioiodine, the fraction of the injected dose taken up by the liver and in some cases the spleen and kidneys is considerably higher using ^{111}In-labeled antibodies[6,7]. The reasons for these differences are unclear. Although dehalogenation, as discussed below, may be a contribuatory factor, loss of label from the antibody via transchelation, resulting in the formation of ^{111}In-labeled ferroproteins such as transferrin, must also be considered[8].

Table 1. Halogen isotopes for antibody labeling

Isotope	Half-life (hr)	Application	Emission	Energy (keV)
^{18}F	1.83	diagnosis	positron	511
^{75}Br	1.63	diagnosis	positron	511
^{76}Br	16.1	diagnosis	positron	511
^{77}Br	57.0	diagnosis	gamma	239
		therapy	Auger	<5
^{123}I	13.0	diagnosis	gamma	159
^{131}I	193	diagnosis	gamma	364
		therapy	beta	607
^{211}At	7.2	therapy	alpha	6786

Alternatively, antibodies can be labeled with halogen isotopes. In Table 1, properties of some of the radiohalogens of potential utility for labeling antibodies are presented. Iodine-131 and ^{123}I have been used for single photon imaging studies. For applications which might require the quantitative capabilities of positron emission tomography, it might be possible to label antibodies with ^{18}F, ^{76}Br or ^{75}Br. With regard to radiotherapeutic applications, ^{211}At is a particularly promising nuclide because it decays by the emission of highly cytotoxic, short range alpha particles. In addition, studies with ^{125}I-labeled iododeoxyuridine[9] suggest that if a monoclonal antibody can be localized in close proximity to the cell nucleus, then Auger electron emitters such as ^{125}I and ^{77}Br could be valuable as antibody labels.

The most significant problem with using radiohalogenated antibodies is that they frequently undergo extensive dehalogenation *in vivo*. Our group has been working on the development of methods for labeling proteins with iodine and astatine which will decrease the loss of radiohalogen from an antibody *in vivo*. Our results labeling proteins using one compound, N-succinimidyl 3-(tri-*n*-butylstannyl) benzoate, an activated, tin-containing ester (ATE) have been very encouraging. The selection of this compound as well as our general approach to antibody radiohalogenation is based on a consideration of the possible nature of the dehalogenation process.

DEHALOGENATION

Following injection of radioiodinated antibodies in animals and patients, significant uptake of radioiodine in both the thyroid and stomach is observed, suggesting that these proteins have undergone dehalogenation *in vivo*. In clinical studies, the cumulative amount of nonprotein-associated activity in the urine is often used as an indicator of loss of iodine from the antibody. The fraction of the injected dose recovered from the urine has been variable ranging between 15% and greater than 50% for the first 24 hr after antibody administration[10,11].

At least three types of processes contribute to the dehalogenation of proteins *in vivo* -- hydrolytic, enzymatic and possibly those mediated by cell binding. Their action is related in part to the nature of the sites of iodine substitution on the protein. Use of oxidants such as chloramine-T or Iodogen affect the substitution of iodine for a hydrogen present in an amino acid residue on the protein with addition ortho to the hydroxyl group on the aromatic ring of tyrosines predominating at neutral pH. Similarly, with the Bolton-Hunter reagent, the iodine is also substituted ortho to a hydroxyl on an aromatic ring.

Loss of radioiodine from proteins can occur *in vitro* as a result of a hydolytic reaction that involves the substitution of a hydrogen atom for the iodine on the aromatic ring. The presence of a hydroxyl group ortho to the halogen decreases the strength of the carbon-iodine bond; however, the rate of dehalogenation of labeled antibodies measured by dialysis is about 1-2% per day, at least 10-fold less than that observed in clinical studies.

Enzymatic processes are generally thought to be responsible for the markedly increased rate of dehalogenation *in vivo*. Iodinated tyrosine residues on antibodies are similar structurally to thyroid hormones which are known to be rapidly dehalogenated in the presence of certain tissues. The differential loss of iodine from D and L iodotyrosine is indicative of the substrate specificity of the dehalogenation process[12]. Results from a number of *in vitro* investigations have demonstrated that there are multiple dehalogenases with varying degrees of specificity for iodotyrosines and both the phenolic and nonphenolic rings of iodothyronines. Dehalogenating enzymes have been found in the microsomal fractions of the liver, kidney and thyroid[13,14] as well as in the kidney plasma membrane[15] and liver cytosol[16].

If the dehalogenation of an antibody occurred at a greater rate in normal versus tumor tissue, then loss of iodine from the protein followed by rapid excretion could be advantageous in that it could increase the therapeutic index. Unfortunately, binding of a labeled antibody to tumor may accelerate the rate of dehalogenation and/or degradation. We and others have observed that the thyroid uptake of ^{125}I in mice injected with ^{125}I-labeled antibody is higher in animals with antigen positive tumors than in animals with antigen-negative tumors or in those with antigen-positive tumors injected with an irrelevant antibody[17,18]. In addition, other radioiodinated proteins have been shown to be degraded rapidly following cell-surface binding and internalization[19-21].

Based on a consideration of these processes, we believe that one approach to decreasing the dehalogenation of labeled antibodies is to develop a method which does not involve the substitution of the halogen ortho to a hydroxyl group on an aromatic ring. The hydroxyl group not only activates the ring towards hydrolytic dehalogenation but also increases the structural similarity between the site of iodination and thyroid hormones.

Our approach attempts to exploit the fact that the regiospecific synthesis of aryl halides can be achieved via tri-alkylstannane intermediates[22]. The compound which we have selected as our model system is N-succinimidyl 3-(tri-n-butylstannyl) benzoate, an activated tin-containing ester designated "ATE". Although conceptually similar to the Bolton-Hunter reagent[23], there are several important differences. First, the aromatic ring does not contain a hydroxyl substituent. Second, halogenation occurs in the meta instead of para position which should decrease the loss of halogen because of the structural and electronic features inherent in meta-substituted halides[24]. And third, ATE lacks the two- carbon spacer between the aromatic ring and the succinimidyl ester.

LABELING PROTEINS WITH THE ATE REAGENT

A detailed discussion of the methods which we have developed for the radioiodination of proteins using the ATE reagent can be found in reference 25. Briefly, synthesis of ATE was accomplished in three steps starting from m-bromobenzoic acid (Figure 1). Following bromine-lithium exchange and conversion of the m-bromobenzoic acid to the dianion, the stannyl ester was produced by quenching the dilithio-anion with $(n\text{-Bu})_3SnCl$. Reaction of this ester with N-hydroxysuccinimide and dicyclohexylcarbodiimide gave the desired product ATE. Purification of ATE was achieved using flash chromatography. The assigned structure of ATE is in agreement with the observed ^1H NMR spectra.

Iodination of ATE was first optimized using stable iodine. A novel method was developed for oxidizing iodine while minimizing the hydrolysis of the N-hydroxysuccinimidyl ester through the use of t-butylhydroperoxide in chloroform-acetic acid (Figure 2). Using this approach, ATE has been labeled with no-carrier-added ^{125}I and ^{131}I in 85-90%

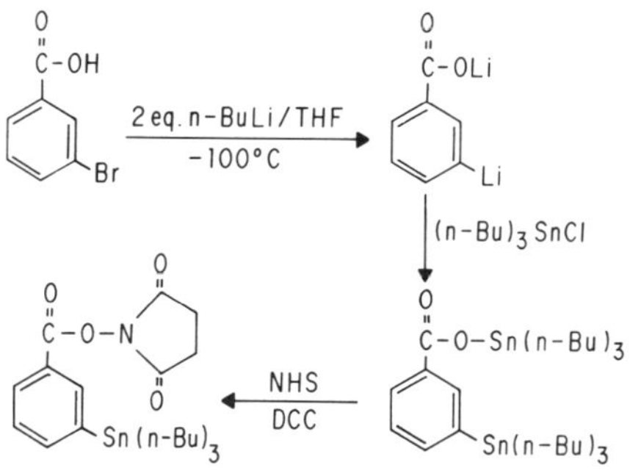

Figure 1. Synthesis of ATE reagent

yield. A Waters silica gel Sep-Pak column was used to isolate the radioiodinated product. The column was first eluted with 40 ml of hexane and approximately 50 ml of 8% ethyl acetate in hexane. Radioiodinated ATE was then isolated by elution with 12-15 ml of 30% ethyl acetate in hexane.

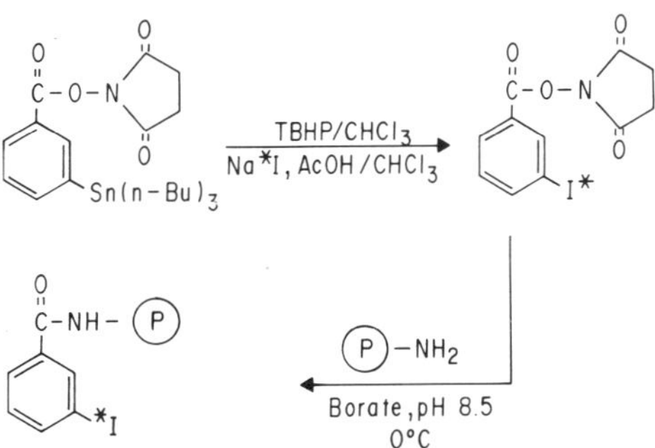

Figure 2. Iodination of proteins using ATE

The utility of 125I-labeled ATE as a protein labeling agent was investigated using goat IgG as the model protein. Initial efforts resulted in variable labeling yields and the retention of significant quantities of 125I activity in the reaction vessel and on pipettes. This behavior was assumed to be related to inadequate separation of the lipophilic ATE starting material from the radioiodinated product. This supposition was confirmed by two methods, mass spectroscopy and the rereaction of the 30% ethyl acetate in hexane fractions with an excess of iodine spiked with 125I. Both methods demonstrated that discarding the first 3 ml of 30% ethyl acetate eluant decreased the amount of unreacted ATE in the product by more than 6-fold. Using this modified isolation procedure, the effective yield of radioiodinated ATE was approximately 80%.

Labeling of goat IgG was accomplished by addition of the protein to the evaporated residue of 125I-labeled ATE in a small conical vial. Following a 30 min. incubation at 4oC on a rotary shaker, the labeled protein was isolated using a Sephadex G-25 column. The efficiency of protein labeling was dependent on the pH and protein concentration. With 50 ug of protein, yields of about 33% were obtained; however if the amount of protein was increased to more than 200 ug, the goat IgG could be labeled in more than 60% yield.

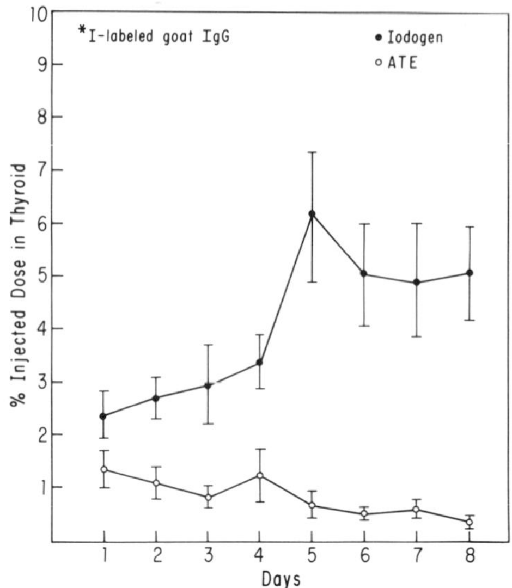

Figure 3. Comparison of thyroid uptake following injection of goat IgG radioiodinated using ATE and Iodogen. Vertical bars represent ± SD.

EVALUATION OF PROTEINS LABELED USING THE ATE METHOD

If proteins labeled via the ATE approach were less succeptible to dehalogenation _in vivo_, one would expect that the accumulation of radioiodine in the thyroid (and to some extent, the stomach) would be less than that observed with proteins labeled using conventional methods. This was investigated by comparing the tissue distribution of 125I and 131I in mice following simultaneous injection of goat IgG labeled with

Table 2. Distribution of radioiodine following injection of radioiodinated goat IgG in normal mice. Values are expressed as mean ± SD.

Tissue	Percent Injected Dose					
	24hr		72hr		120hr	
	ATE	Iodogen	ATE	Iodogen	ATE	Iodogen
blood	26.2±9.9	21.6±7.9	17.4±5.4	14.8±5.2	12.6±3.5	14.4±4.1
liver	6.83±1.21	5.58±1.05	3.84±0.63	3.33±0.43	2.89±0.53	3.33±0.43
lungs	1.50±0.48	1.24±0.28	0.94±0.34	0.82±0.29	0.86±0.17	0.99±0.19
spleen	0.21±0.06	0.19±0.05	0.19±0.07	0.16±0.05	0.15±0.04	0.17±0.05
kidneys	2.16±0.55	1.65±0.39	1.38±0.37	1.18±0.37	1.00±0.27	1.24±0.34
stomach	0.48±0.09	0.87±0.20	0.40±0.06	0.41±0.05	0.17±0.04	0.27±0.05

125I using ATE and 131I using the Iodogen method. Groups of 5 mice were sacrificed daily for 8 days and the uptake of 125I and 131I in the thyroid, blood, liver, lungs, muscle, intestines, spleen, kidneys, stomach, heart and bone determined. As shown in Figure 3, use of the ATE method for protein labeling results in a significant decrease ($p<0.001$, Student's t-test) in the thyroid uptake of radioiodine. With the exception of the stomach, no statistically significant differences in the uptake of 131I and 125I in the other tissues was observed (Table 2 and reference 25).

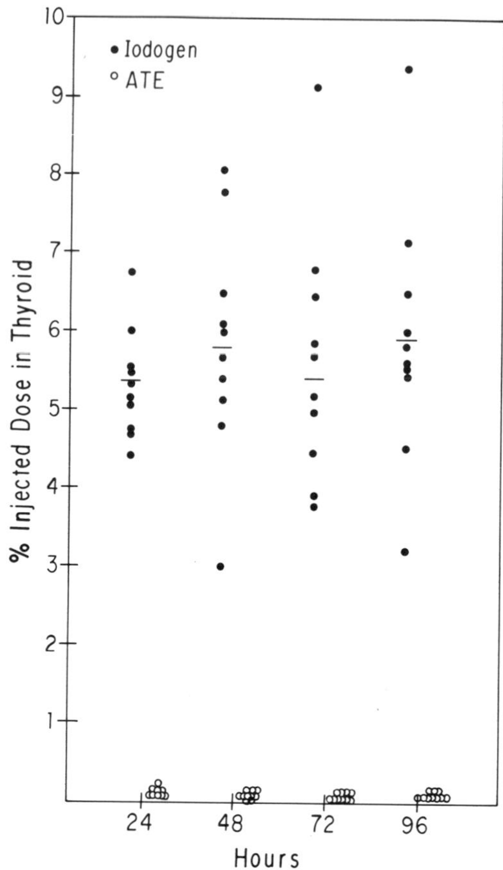

Figure 4. Comparison of the thyroid uptake of radioiodine in mice following injection of radioiodinated OC 125 $F(ab')_2$.

We have also investigated the utility of the ATE reagent as a method for the radiohalogenation of monoclonal antibodies[26]. These studies were performed using OC 125, an antibody directed against a human ovarian carcinoma associated antigen[27], as a model system. One hundred and fifty micrograms of the $F(ab')_2$ fragment of OC 125 were labeled with 900 uCi of ^{125}I in 62% radiochemical yield and the _in vitro_ and _in vivo_ properties of the preperation were compared to those of OC 125 radioiodinated using the Iodogen method.

In order to assess the effect of radiohalogenation on the immunoreactivity of OC 125, the binding of ^{125}I-labeled antibody to CA 125 antigen purified from McDonald ovarian carcinoma cells was determined *in vitro*. Scatchard analyses of the binding data yield affinity constants of $(5.2 \pm 1.0) \times 10^{10}$ M^{-1} and $(2.5 \pm 0.9) \times 10^{10}$ M^{-1} for the $F(ab')_2$ fragment of OC 125 labeled using the ATE and Iodogen methods, respectively. Similarly, use of the ATE procedure for labeling OC 125 IgG resulted in a labeled antibody with a 2-3 fold higher affinity constant. It is interesting to note that when the less stringent isolation method for ^{125}I-labeled ATE was used, the affinity constant of ^{125}I-labeled OC 125 $F(ab')_2$ decreased by as much as 10-fold.

Two sets of paired-label experiments were performed in nude mice bearing OVCAR-3 human ovarian carcinoma xenografts. In the first (Exp. 1), groups of 5 mice were sacrificed 24, 48, 72 and 96 hr following injection of 5 ug of OC 125, half labeled with ^{131}I using Iodogen and half labeled with ^{125}I-ATE purified by the old method. The second experiment was the same as the first except that ^{125}I-labeled ATE isolated using the revised elution procedure was used.

Table 3.

ATE vs. Iodogen: Relative Selectivity Index

Tissue	48 hr		96 hr	
	Exp. 1	Exp. 2	Exp. 1	Exp. 2
Liver	1.3	1.2	2.4	2.9
Spleen	0.7	0.9	0.9	0.9
Lungs	1.2	2.5	3.4	5.1
Heart	2.1	4.5	4.9	3.7
Kidney	1.4	2.9	3.5	6.4
Skin	1.2	2.3	3.5	5.2
Muscle	1.8	2.8	1.7	6.6
Blood	3.1	3.0	4.1	4.2
Intestines	4.0	2.1	4.4	5.0
Stomach	1.9	7.7	6.4	11.8

$$RSI = \frac{(\text{Tumor: Tissue})_{\text{ATE}}}{(\text{Tumor: Tissue})_{\text{Iodogen}}}$$

In Figure 4, thyroid uptake data from the two experiments have been combined. Labeling OC 125 $F(ab')_2$ using the ATE approach reduced the thyroid uptake of radioiodine to less than 0.1% of the injected dose, a level which was more than 100-fold less than that observed with Iodogen-labeled antibodies.

In Table 3, the tumor to tissue ratios obtained with OC 125 $F(ab')_2$ labeled via the Iodogen and ATE methods are compared. With the exception of the spleen, higher tumor to normal tissue ratios were observed with antibodies labeled using the ATE reagent. Differences were most significant in the stomach, intestines and blood pool where 4 to 12-fold improvements were seen 96 hours after injection of antibody. In experiment 1, tumor uptake of radioiodine was the same, despite the fact that the affinity constant of the Iodogen-labeled antibody was about 4 times greater. In experiment 2, tumor uptake of radioiodine was 30 to 50% higher for ATE-labeled OC 125 $F(ab')_2$. The tumor to tissue ratios for blood, liver and muscle which were observed in Experiment 2 are shown in Figures 5-7.

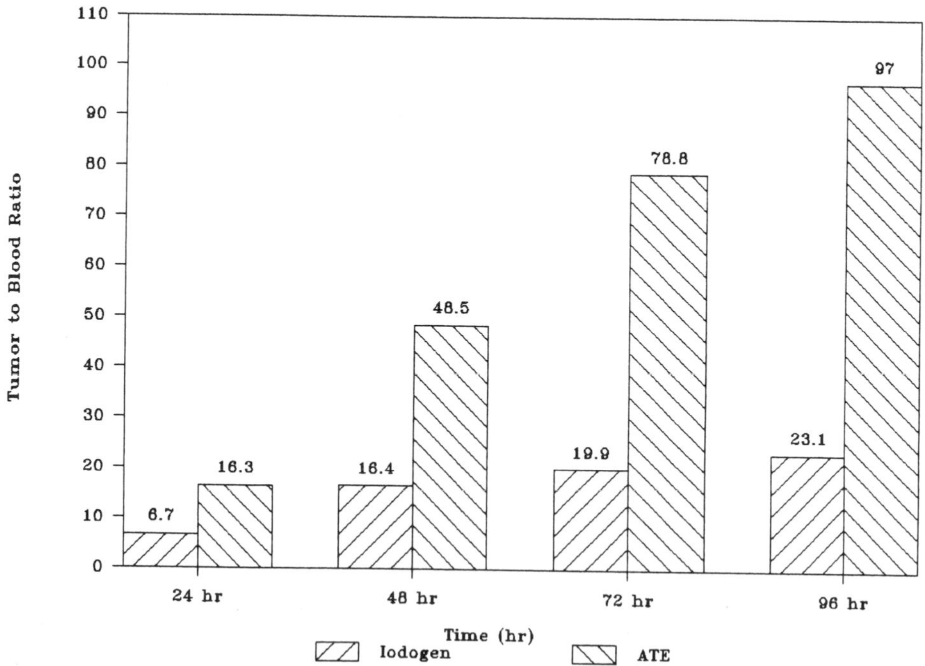

Figure 5. Tumor to blood ratios for OC 125 $F(ab')_2$ antibodies: ATE vs. Iodogen

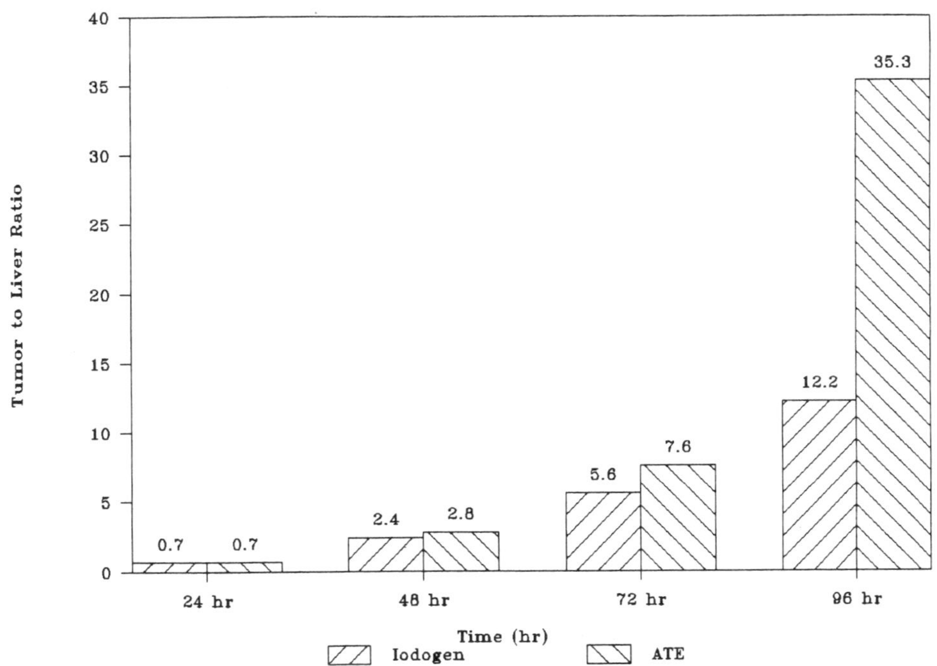

Figure 6. Tumor to liver ratios for OC 125 F(ab')2 antibody: ATE vs. Iodogen

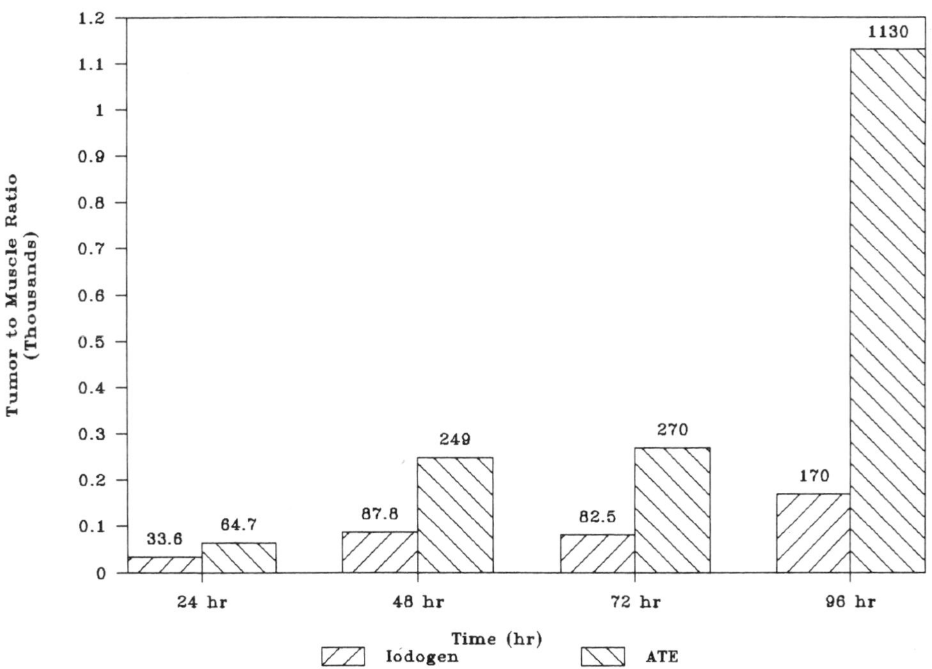

Figure 7. Tumor to muscle ratios for OC 125 F(ab')2 antibody: ATE vs. Iodogen

SUMMARY

Herein, we have reported a new method for the radiohalogenation of proteins via N-succinimidyl 3-(tri-*n*-butylstannyl) benzoate, an activated, tin-containing ester (ATE). This compound could be labeled with either ^{125}I or ^{131}I in greater than 80% yield. Recently, we have also been able to label ATE with ^{211}At in about 60% yield. Adequate separation of radioiodinated ATE from unreacted ATE facilitates its subsequent use as a protein acylation agent. Protein labeling efficiencies of greater than 60% have been achieved routinely, a value about twice that generally observed with the Bolton-Hunter reagent. The higher yields obtained with our method are presumed to be related in part to the use of t-butyl hydroperoxide in chloroform-acetic acid to oxidize the iodine while minimizing the hydrolysis of the N-succidimidyl ester.

When proteins labeled using the ATE reagent were injected into mice, the thyroid uptake of radioiodine was significantly less than that observed with proteins labeled using Iodogen. This was particularly evident for the $F(ab')_2$ fragment of antibody OC 125 where a more than a 100-fold decrease in thyroid uptake was observed. We believe that the decreased dehalogenation of proteins labeled using the ATE reagent is related to the absence of a hydroxyl group ortho to the iodine on the labeled aromatic ring. This not only deactivates the ring towards loss of halogen but also decreases the structural similarity to thyroid hormones for which there are known dehalogenases.

In vitro binding studies suggest that antibodies labeled via ATE retain a high affinity for their corresponding tumor-associated antigens. The increased affinity and greater *in vivo* stability of antibodies labeled using the ATE reagent both probably contribute to the increased tumor to normal tissue ratios observed in paired-label experiments. In conclusion, we believe that these results suggest that use of the ATE reagent is a promising approach for the radiohalogenation of proteins and warrants further development.

ACKNOWLEDGEMENTS

The authors wish to thank Su Suddarth for excellent technical assistance. We also thank Dr. Robert C. Bast for the OC 125 $F(ab')_2$ antibody. This work was supported by Grant CA 42324 from the National Cancer Institute.

REFERENCES

1. J.A. Carrasquillo, Radioimmunoscintigraphy with polyclonal or monoclonal antibodies, in: "Antibodies in Radiodiagnosis and Therapy", M.R. Zalutsky, ed., CRC Press, Boca Raton (in press).

2. H. Sands and B.M. Gallagher, Physiological, pharmacological and immunological aspects of antibody targeting, in: Antibodies in Radiodiagnosis and Therapy", M.R. Zalutsky, ed., CRC Press, Boca Raton (in press).

3. S.E. Halpern, R.O. Dillman, D.F. Witztum, J.F. Shega, P.L. Hagan, W.M. Burrows, J.B. Dillman, M.L. Clutter, R.E. Sobol, J.M. Frincke, R.M. Bartholomew, G.S. David and D.J. Carlo, Radioimmunodetection of melanoma utilizing ^{111}In-96.5 monoclonal antibody: a preliminary report, Radiology 155:493 (1985).

4. J.L. Murray, M.G. Rosenblum, R.E. Sobol, R.M. Bartholomew, C.E. Plager, T.P. Haynie, M.F. Jahns, H.J. Glenn, L.Lamki, R.S. Benjamin, N. Papadopoulus, A.W. Boddie, J.M. Frincke, G.S. David, D.J. Carlo and E.M. Hersh, Radioimmunoimaging in malignant melanoma with ^{111}In-labeled monoclonal antibody 96.5, Cancer Res 45:2376 (1985).

5. J.A. Carrasquillo, P.G. Abrams, R.W. Schroff, A.M. Keenan, A.C. Morgan, K.A. Foon, J.C. Reynolds, P.Perenthesis, M.Horowitz and S.M. Larson, Improved imaging of metastatic melanoma with high dose 9.2.27 In-111 monoclonal antibody, J. Nucl Med. 26:P67 (1985) abstract.

6. D.S. Fairweather, A.R. Bradwell, P.W. Dykes, A.T. Vaughan, S.F. Watson-James and S. Chandler, Improved tumour localisation using indium-111 labeled antibodies, Br. Med. J. 287:167 (1983).

7. M.V. Pimm, A.C. Perkins, N.C. Armitage and R.W. Baldwin, The characteristics of blood-borne radiolabels and the effect of anti-mouse IgG antibodies on localization of radiolabeled monoclonal antibody in cancer patients, J. Nucl. Med. 26:1011 (1985).

8. D.J. Hnatowich, F. Virzi and P.W. Doherty, DTPA-coupled antibodies labeled with yttrium-90, J. Nucl. Med. 26:503 (1985).

9. W.D. Bloomer and S.J. Adelstein, 5-^{125}I-iododeoxyuridine as prototype for radionuclide therapy with Auger emitters, Nature 265:620 (1977).

10. D.F. Hayes, M.R. Zalutsky, W. Kaplan, M. Noska, A. Thor, D. Colcher, and D.W. Kufe, Pharmacokinetics of radiolabeled monoclonal antibody B6.2 in patients with metastatic breast cancer, Cancer Res. 46:3157 (1986).

11. D.C. Sullivan, J.S. Silva, C.E. Cox, D.E. Haagensen, Jr., C.C. Harris, W.H. Briner, and S.A. Wells, Jr., Localization of I-131 labeled goat and primate anti-carcinoembryonic antigen (CEA) antibodies in patients with cancer, Invest. Radiol. 17:350 (1982).

12. P. Dumas, Deshalogenation de divers derives iodes phenoliques chez le rat normal et thyroidectomise, Biochem. Pharmacol. 22:1599 (1973).

13. W. Tong, A. Taurog, and I.L. Chaikoff, The metabolism of 131I-labeled diiodotyrosine, J. Biol. Chem. 207:59 (1954).

14. J.B. Stanbury and M.L. Morris, Deiodination of diiodotyrosine by cell-free systems, J. Biol. Chem. 233:106 (1958).

15. R.C. Smallridge, K.D. Burman, K.E. Ward, L. Wartofsky, R.C. Dimond, F.D. Wright, and K.R. Latham, 3', 5'-diiodothyronine to 3'-monoiodothyronine conversion in the fed and fasted rat: Enzyme characteristics and evidence for two distinct 5'-deiodinases, Endocrinology 108:2336 (1981).

16. J.L. Leonard and I.N. Rosenbert, Subcellular distribution of thyroxine 5'-deiodinase in the rat kidney: A plasma membrane location, Endocrinology 103:274 (1977).

17. M.R. Zalutsky, D. Colcher, W. Kaplan, and D.F. Kufe, Radioiodinated B6.2 monoclonal antibody: Further characterization of a potential radiopharmaceutical for the identification of breast tumors, Int. J. Nucl. Med. Biol. 12:227 (1985).

18. D.S. Wilbur, D.S. Jones, A.R. Fritzberg, and A.C. Morgan, Radioiodination of monoclonal antibodies: Labeling with para-iodophenyl (PIP) derivatives for in vivo stability of the radioiodine label, J. Nucl. Med. 27:959 (1986) abstract.

19. J.L. Goldstein and M.S. Brown, Binding and degradation of low density lipoproteins by cultured human fibroblasts, J. Biol. Chem. 249:5153 (1974).

20. S. Terris and D.F. Steiner, Binding and degradation of ^{125}I-insulin by rat hepatocytes, J. Biol. Chem. 250:8389 (1975).

21. G. Carpenter and S. Cohen, ^{125}I-labeled human epidermal growth factor: Binding, internalization and degradation in human fibroblasts, J. Cell Biol. 71:159 (1976).

22. G.L. Tonnesen, R.N. Hanson and D.E. Seitz, Position-specific radioiodination utilizing an aryltributylstannyl intermediate. Synthesis of [^{125}I]iodotamoxifen, Int. J. Appl. Radiat. Isot. 32:171 (1981).

23. A.E. Bolton and R.M. Hunter, The labelling of proteins to high specific activities by conjugation to a ^{125}I-containing acylating agent, Biochem. J. 133:529 (1973).

24. F.A. Carey and R.J. Sundberg, "Advanced Organic Chemistry", Plenum Press, New York (1984).

25. M.R. Zalutsky and A.S. Narula, A method for the radiohalogenation of proteins resulting in decreased dehalogenation in vivo, Anal. Biochem. (submitted).

26. M.R. Zalutsky and A.S. Narula, Evaluation of a new radioiodinated acylation agent for use in labeling antibodies, Cancer Res. (submitted).

27. R.C. Bast, M. Feeney, H. Lazarus, L.M. Nadler, R.B. Colvin and R.C. Knapp, Reactivity of a monoclonal antibody with human ovarian carcinoma, J. Clin. Invest. 68:1331 (1981).

STUDIES ON A EPITHELIAL/EPITHELIAL MALIGNANCY ASSOCIATED ANTIGEN ASSOCIATED WITH HUMAN ADENOCARCINOMAS

T.F. Bumol, J. Parrish, S.V. DeHerdt, M. E. Spearman, R. Pohland, M.J. Borowitz[1], S.L. Briggs, A.L. Baker, P. Marder, and L.D. Apelgren

Lilly Research Laboratories
Indianapolis, Indiana 46285
[1]Duke University Medical School
Durham, North Carolina 27710

INTRODUCTION

The monoclonal antibody technology has provided the means to explore the malignant cell surface for tumor associated gene products. These molecules, defined as "tumor associated antigens" by appropriate antibodies, could be the basis for possible new developments in cancer diagnosis and therapy. Monoclonal antibodies have not defined tumor specific antigens in human solid tumor but have successfully identified a number of candidate tumor associated gene products in malignancies such as melanoma, lung, breast and colon carcinomas which share varied normal tissue distribution (1-9). These monoclonal antibodies have been the basis of numerous studies in tumor cell biology, tumor immunology, and preclinical and clinical trials for diagnostic imaging and antibody based immunotherapy in man (10-14). Our laboratories have been examining the potential of monoclonal antibodies as vehicles for site-directed oncolytic agent therapy of human solid tumors as monoclonal antibody-drug conjugates. Monoclonal antibody KS1/4, originally developed by immunization of a human lung adenocarcinoma cell line (15), has been selected initially for these studies. This report will demonstrate that the antigen recognized by KS1/4 is broadly distributed among human adenocarcinomas and normal epithelial surfaces and will summarize preclinical studies suggesting that this antigen is a potential target for site-directed therapy with KS1/4-vinca alkaloid conjugates.

MATERIALS AND METHODS

Cell lines utilized in these studies include the P3-UCLA human lung adenocarcinoma cell line (15), the MCF-7 human breast carcinoma cell line obtained from Dr. Ken Hirsch, Lilly Research Laboratories, the HT29 human colon carcinoma cell line and the MDA-231 human breast carcinoma cell line. The KS1/4 hybridoma was maintained in _in vitro_ culture to produce the antibody products described. All cell lines were maintained in DME with 10% fetal calf serum supplemented with glutamine and gentamycin sulfate. In some experiments the 007B subclone of the KS1/4 hybridoma was biosynthetically labelled with S^{35}-methionine utilizing procedures previously established for other cell types (16). All cultures were routinely screened for mycoplasma and other low grade bacterial infections. Nude mice utilized in the described xenograft studies for efficacy and biodistribution experiments were obtained from Charles River and maintained under sterile conditions for all aspects of these studies.

KS1/4 monoclonal antibody was purified by a combination of high performance anion and cation exchange chromatographic steps from concentrated spent media from _in vitro_ tissue culture. The KS1/4-desacetylvinblastine (DAVLB) conjugate was constructed by the combination of the N-hydroxysuccinimide ester of desacetylvinblastine to purified KS1/4 monoclonal antibody utilizing procedures previously described for the construction of vindesine-monoclonal antibody conjugates (17). Conjugation ratios of 4-6 moles of drug/mole of monoclonal antibody were routine.

Tissue and tumor antigenic distribution studies were carried out using a modification (18) of the avidin-biotin technique. Briefly, frozen sections of tissues were cut at 4-6μm onto gelatin coated slides, air dried, and fixed in acetone for five minutes. Following preincubation with 5% horse serum, sections were sequentially incubated with KS1/4, followed by biotinylated horse anti-mouse Ig (Vector Labs, Burlingame, CA.) and a complex of avidin and horseradish peroxidase with washes between steps in phosphate buffered saline, pH 7.2-7.4 containing 1% bovine serum albumin.

Optimal dilutions of all components were determined by "checker-board" titrations. Color was developed using 3,3'-diaminobenzidine and sections were counterstained with hematoxylin.

An additional method utilized in the characterization of the antigen distribution of the KS1/4 monoclonal antibody involved flow cytometry. Fresh viable or paraformaldehyde fixed tumor cells from _in vitro_ culture or isolated peripheral blood components were suspended in 0.1 mls of varying dilutions of KS1/4 and incubated for 30 minutes at 4° C as described previously (29). The cell suspensions were then washed and resuspended in 0.1 ml of $F(ab')_2$ fragments of goat anti-mouse IgG (flourescein conjugated) (Tago, Burlingame, CA) for an additional 30 minutes at 4° C. After two washes in Hank's balanced salt solution containing 1% heat inactivated fetal bovine serum (GIBCO, Grand Island, NY) with 1% sodium azide, the suspensions were resuspended in the same buffer and held on ice until flow analysis.

Prepared cell suspensions were analyzed using an EPICS V flow cytometer (Coulter Electronics Inc., Hialeah, FL.) as previously described (20). Briefly, cells were illuminated with 800 MW of 488 nM coherent light and the forward angle light scatter gated with log green fluorescence signal collected in 256 channel histograms. The mean fluorescence intensity was calculated for each 10,000 cell histogram.

Two variants of a subcutaneously implanted P3-UCLA human lung adenocarcinoma xenograft model were utilized. In the tumor initiation model, P3-UCLA human lung adenocarcinoma cells (10^7 viable cells) were implanted subcutaneously in groups of 8-10 week old 18-22 gram athymic nude mice (Charles River). Intravenous tail vein injections of KS1/4-DAVLB at the doses indicated in the results were utilized in all xenograft immunotherapy experiments. In the tumor initiation model, treatments occurred on days 2,5 and 8 after tumor implantation, a schedule previously determined to eliminate significant antitumor activity in unmodified KS1/4 monoclonal antibody control treatment groups. All doses of KS1/4-DAVLB are expressed in terms of mg/kg with respect to drug content. Tumor mass estimates were determined from tumor volume measurements made with electronic digital calipers (Fred V. Fowler Co., Newton, Ma.) interfaced with a Hewlett-Packard Personal Computer utilizing a previously described formula (21). Data processing for comparative analysis of experimental groups and control groups examining tumor growth suppression was achieved utilizing a program developed by Mr. John Worzalla, Lilly Research Laboratories.

The above described procedure was extended to an established tumor model by allowing the implanted tumors to grow for 14-17 days prior to the initiation of treatment. The treatment schedule utilized for this assay was to administer intravenous doses indicated in the text.

In all of these experiments, careful monitoring of the antigen reactivity of the KS1/4-DAVLB conjugate was achieved prior to *in vivo* use by use of a functional enzyme linked immunoabsobent assay (ELISA) utilizing air dried P3-UCLA target cells and several novel flow cytometric techniques (Marder, P. et al. Manuscript in press, J. Immunol. Methods, 1986).

Biodistribution and tumor localization were analyzed in P3-UCLA human lung xenograft bearing nude mice with ^{3}H-desacetylvinblastine and KS1/4-^{3}H-desacetylvinblastine. These animals were dosed intravenously and sacrificed at the time points indicated in the text followed by dissection and analysis of radioactivity in oxidized tissue samples by liquid scintillation counting. Comparable doses of free drug were administered in parallel control groups to the vinca equivalent dose of KS1/4-DAVLB conjugate administration.

MCF-7 human breast carcinoma cells were implanted in the mammary regions of female nude mice bearing 17-beta-estradiol pellets for biodistribution studies by whole-body autoradiographic technique. Female mice with growing established MCF-7 xenografts were injected with S^{35}-methionine labelled KS1/4 monoclonal antibody and sacrificed at the time points indicated and frozen in a prone position in dry ice/pentane. The animals were maintained at -20° until processed for whole-body autoradiography as previously described in detail (22).

RESULTS

Immunoperoxidase results initially published on the KS1/4 monoclonal antibody (15) suggested that this antigen was highly associated with human adenocarcinomas and had a limited normal tissue distribution. Analysis of a broad range of fresh frozen normal human tissues suggest that the KS1/4 antibody is reactive with epithelial surfaces of various tissues. Tissues exhibiting a strongly positive reaction include the epithelium of the colon, stomach, small intestine and bronchus and alveoli. Tissues with selective reactivity with the KS1/4 monoclonal antibody include the bile ducts of the liver, the distal tubules of the kidney and sweat ducts of the skin. All hematopoietic organs, connective tissue, vessels, and brain tissue were negative for reactivity with KS1/4.

An analysis of tumor reactivity revealed that 13/13 colon tumors 7/7 lung adenocarcinoma tumors and 4/4 epithelial ovarian tumors were very strongly reactive with the KS1/4 monoclonal antibody without exhibiting antigenic heterogeneity. In contrast to these results, 12/13 lung squamous tumors were reactive and 13/13 breast tumors were reactive but with significant variability in the immunoperoxidase staining patterns indicative of antigenic variability in these malignancies. Two examples of this observation are shown in Figures 1 and 2. Figure 1 represents the results of the reactivity of KS1/4 with a breast carcinoma section showing homogenous intense staining while the section in Figure 2 is an example of a breast carcinoma section demonstrating antigenic variability. Flow cytometric analysis of tumor cells suggest similar trends in certain *in vitro* propagated tumors. Figure 3 is a summary of an experiment comparing the reactivity of KS1/4 with four cell lines representing three different types of malignancies. KS1/4 demonstrates high reactivity with the P3-UCLA lung adenocarcinoma cell line and the MCF-7 human breast carcinoma cell line in this analysis. However, a second breast carcinoma cell line, MBA demonstrates little reactivity with the KS1/4 antibody. In other studies not shown here, the KS1/4 antibody has demonstrated homogenous high intensity staining of human lung and HT-29 colon carcinoma shown cell lines but heterogeneous staining of human breast and lung squamous carcinoma cell lines suggesting a parallel antigenic expression in *in vitro* maintained cell lines and fresh human tumor specimens.

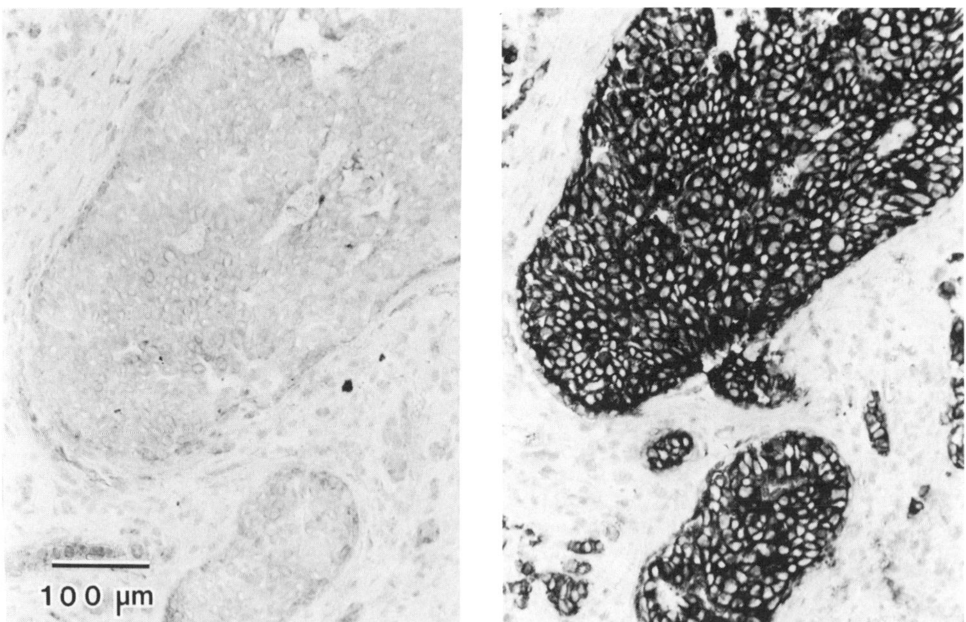

Figure 1: Frozen section of adenocarcinoma of breast stained by immunoperoxidase with control antibody (left panel) and KS1/4 (right panel). Note intense uniform staining of all tumor cells in this case. Sections are counterstained with hematoxylin.

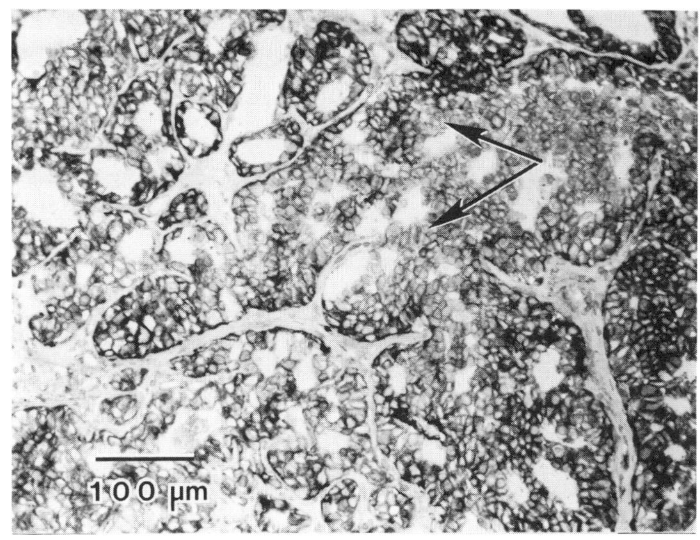

Figure 2: Frozen section of a different case of breast carcinoma from that illustrated in Figure 1, stained by immunoperoxidase with KS1/4. Note variability in the expression of the antigen, some cells staining intensely and other groups of tumor cells demonstrating no staining (arrows). The section is counterstained with hematoxylin.

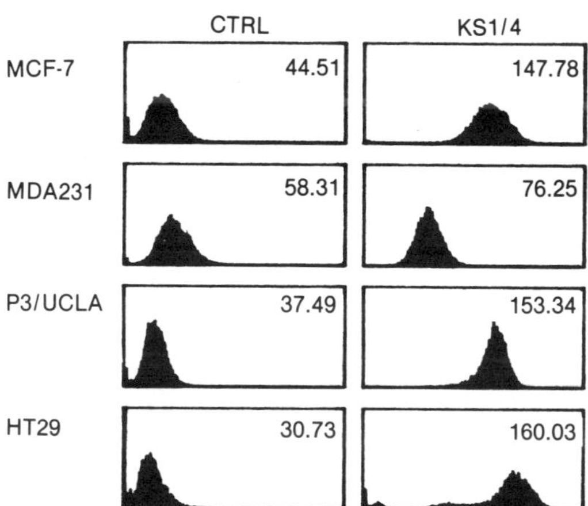

Figure 3: Flow cytometric analysis of the reactivity of the KS1/4 monoclonal antibody with several human solid tumor cell lines. The mean fluorescent intensity is indicated as well as controls which indicate the autofluorescence associated with these cells. Each histogram represents the analysis of 10,000 cells.

Figure 4 is a summary of a xenograft study in which P3-UCLA human lung adenocarcinoma xenografts were allowed to establish for forty eight hours prior to the administration of KS1/4-DAVLB treatment. Three intravenous doses of KS1/4-DAVLB were administered on days 2,5, and 8 at dose levels of 1.0, 2.5, and 10.0 mg/kg vinca alkaloid equivalent. Previous studies (not shown) indicated that this schedule would show the effects of the KS1/4-DAVLB conjugate and not simply the effects of the KS1/4 monoclonal antibody on xenograft growth. Tumor measurements were made on days 14, 21, and 28 after transplantation to monitor the long term effects of this three dose protocol. Tumor growth suppression is observed for all three dose groups at the day 14. But tumors progressed rapidly in the lower dose groups as measured on days 21 and 28. At day 28 long term significant suppression of growth was observed only for the 10 mg/kg dose group. In other experiments, not shown, the 5-10 mg/kg vinca equivalent dose range could affectively suppress the long term growth of the P3-UCLA lung adenocarcinoma xenograft in the model under this minimal dosing schedule. Free drug control groups of vinblastine sulfate at comparable doses did not demonstrate efficacy without significant vinca alkaloid toxicity suggesting that the KS1/4-DAVLB conjugate is significantly less toxic than free drug.

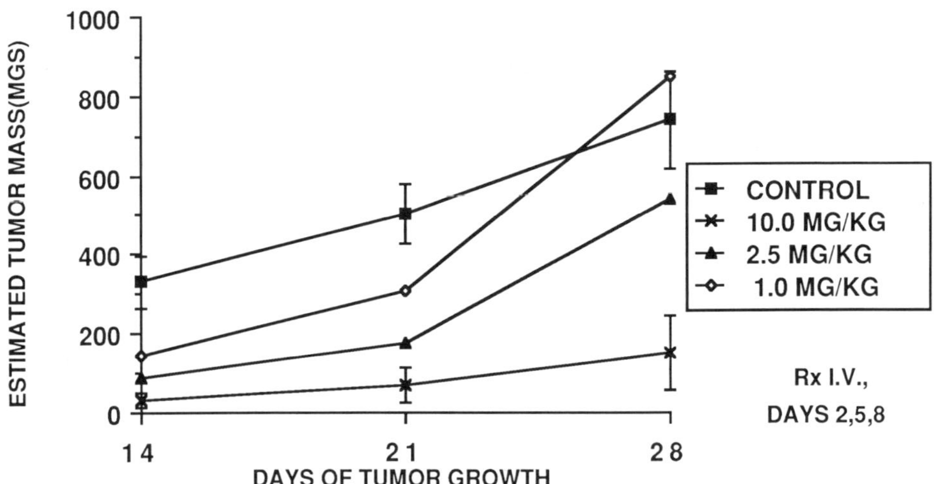

Figure 4: Effects of KS1/4-DAVLB conjugate administration on the P3-UCLA human lung adenocarcinoma xenograft. Tumor masses are plotted versus days of tumor growth. The mean mass of five test animals are compared to a control group of ten animals. Standard errors are plotted on select data points.

Figure 5 represents a similar experiment but on established xenograft tumors of the P3-UCLA human lung adenocarcinoma cell line. In this experiment, xenografts were allowed to grow to approximately a 200 mg size (in a 20-22 gram mouse) prior to the initiating of KS1/4-DAVLB immunotherapy. Four intravenous injections were given on days 16, 18, 22, and 24. Tumor measurements were taken pretest on day 16 and on days 23 and 30. The experiment demonstrates that the tumor growth suppression is dose dependent with optimal tumor growth suppression and regression occurring at the 10.0 and 7.5 mg/kg vinca equivalent dose group. In this experiment, an optimal effect is observed at the 7.5 mg/kg dose group. In other experiments not shown, unmodified monoclonal antibody has no effect on established tumor growth indicating that this effect is conjugate mediated. Treatment with irrelevant myeloma-DAVLB that this effect is antigen mediated. These results suggest that the

KS1/4-DAVLB conjugate can mediate antitumor effects on well established human xenografts. Biodistribution experiments have compared the tissue distribution of free drug administered as desacetylvinblastine (DAVLB) to comparable doses of "conjugated" drug as KS1/4-DAVLB; Figure 6. The maximum concentration of vinca alkaloid radioequivalents was measured immediately after dosing with free DAVLB; others have also reported that the highest concentration of vinca alkaloids in tumor tissue is measured in the first 24 hr. Based upon an average tumor weight of about 450 mg, this concentration accounted for approximately 0.3% of the total administered dosage. However, after dosing with KS1/4-[^{3}H]-DAVLB, the maximum concentration of vinca radioequivalents was observed 96 hr after dosing and accounted for over 5% of the total dosage (based upon an average tumor weight of about 550 mg). Thus, with KS1/4-DAVLB, accumulation of the drug in the tumor was evident. The loss of radiolabel from the tumor tissue proceeded with a half-life (t1/2) of about 145 hr and 84 hr after therapy with KS1/4-DAVLB and free DAVLB, respectively. As a consequence of the higher concentrations and longer t1/2, the total areas under the tissue concentration _vs_ time curve were 3900 and 80.5 vinca alkaloid µg equivalents hr/g after dosing with KS1/4-DAVLB and free DAVLB, respectively. A comparison of the areas under the curve documented that over 1.89 logs more vinca alkaloid equivalents were present in the tumor after therapy with KS1/4-DAVLB when compared with free DAVLB in the nude mouse xenograft model. This study demonstrates that KS1/4-DAVLB affects the accumulation and long residence time of vinca alkaloid species at the xenograft tumor site with a single dose administration. Parallel studies with free drug administration demonstrate significantly less drug at the tumor site with shortened tumor tissue half lives. This study demonstrates that KS1/4-DAVLB can effectively act as a site-directed vehicle to target the vinca alkaloid species to the tumor site. The ultimate success of this effect however will depend on the catabolism of the KS1/4-DAVLB conjugate at the tumor site to liberate appropriately active vinca alkaloid species.

Other tissues which demonstrate significant uptake of the KS1/4-DAVLB conjugate are the liver, lung and splenic tissues. In general, tissues which have significant cellular compartments of reticuloendothelial cells seem to be sites for uptake of the KS1/4-DAVLB conjugate _in vivo_ in the xenograft system. The study also demonstrates that KS1/4-DAVLB does not target organs which are historically possible targets for the toxicity of vinca alkaloids such as bone marrow and nervous tissue, an important difference in distribution mediated by the KS1/4-DAVLB conjugate.

These studies have demonstrated that KS1/4 is an effective targeting agent for the P3-UCLA lung adenocarcinoma xenograft system. Immunoperoxidase and flow cytometric studies indicate that colorectal carcinoma cell systems should be equally good targets for KS1/4-drug conjugates as well. An observation which is borne out in studies with the HT29 human colon carcinoma cell system (shown in figure 3) MCF-7 human breast cancer cells were then examined as a xenograft system for tumor localization by the whole body autoradiography technique. Figure 7 represents a photograph of a autoradiograph taken on thin sections of MCF-7 xenograft bearing nude mice which had been injected with [^{35}S]-labelled KS1/4 monoclonal antibody. This figure demonstrates good tumor localization by the KS1/4 monoclonal antibody of the primary implanted tumor and several metastatic nodules, apparently accelerated in their development by the 17-beta-estradiol treatment.

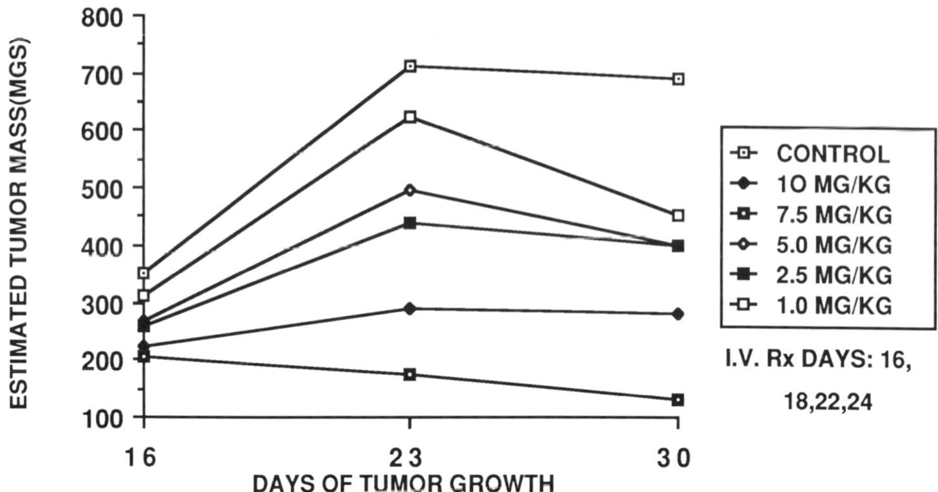

Figure 5: Effects of KS1/4-DAVLB on the growth of established P3-UCLA xenograft tumors. All tumor mass data represent the mean of at least 5 animals/group versus a group of ten control animals. Long term tumor growth suppression or tumor growth plateau is observed for the top two dose groups.

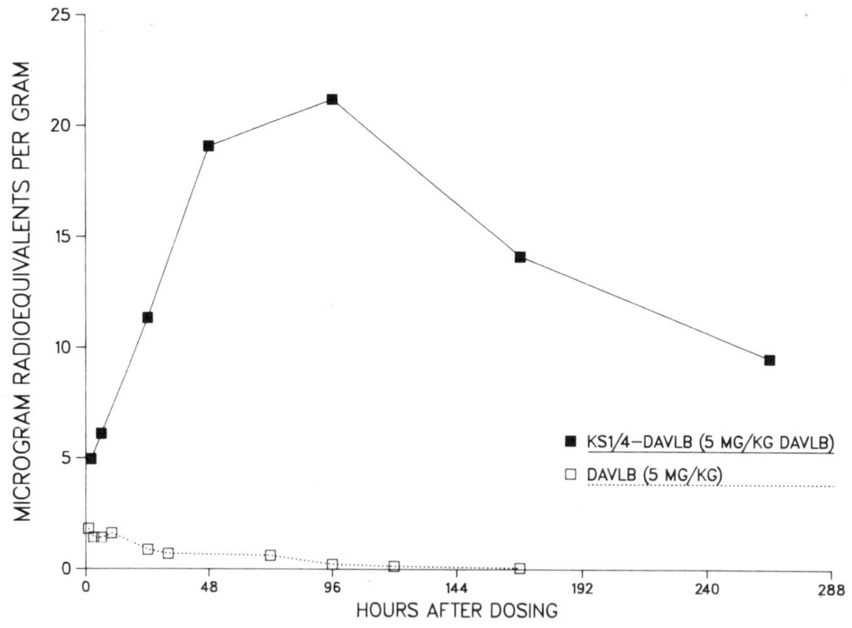

Figure 6. Analysis of the biodistribution to tumor tissue of ^{3}H-DAVLB and KS1/4-^{3}H-DAVLB in P3-UCLA human lung xenograft bearing nude mice. Animals were sacrificed at the time points indicated for both free drug and conjugate treated animals.

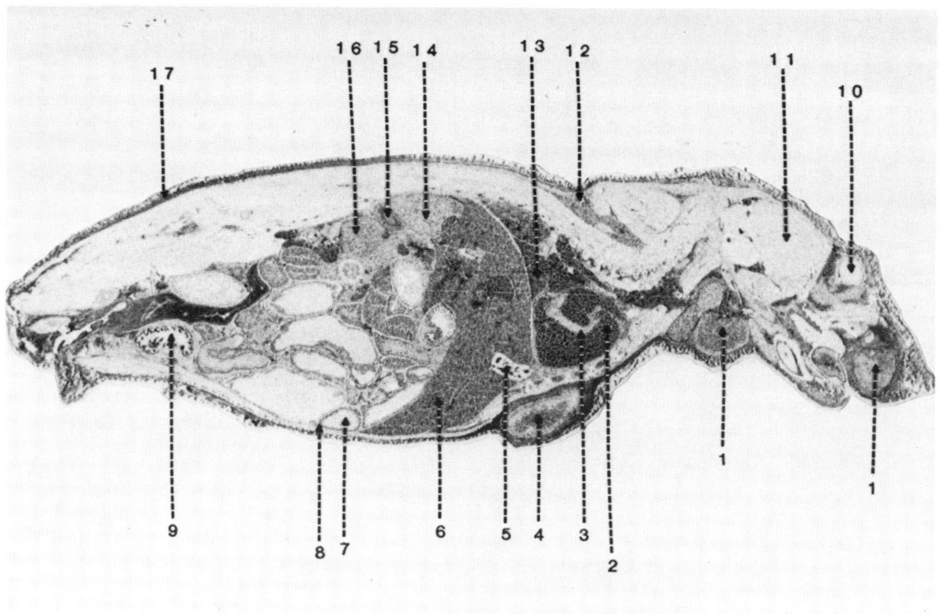

Figure 7: Whole-body autoradiogram of a 20 um section from a nude mouse containing a mammary carcinoma implant (MCF7) killed 48 hours after receiving 8.5 μCi [^{35}S]-KS1/4 by intravenous injection. 2x. (Dark areas correspond to radioactivity). KEY: 1. Metastatic Tumor; 2. Blood, 3. Heart; 4. Implanted Tumor; 5. Gall Bladder; 6. Liver; 7. Intestinal Lumen; 8. Intestinal Wall; 9. Urinary Bladder; 10. Eye; 11. Brain; 12. Brown Fat; 13. Lung; 14. Spleen; 15. Adrenal Gland; 16. Kidney; 17. Skin.

These data demonstrate that KS1/4 will also localize to antigen positive human breast xenografts and identify different tissue metastases. Despite observed human tumor antigenic heterogeneity (Figure 2) in some specimens, conjugates of KS1/4 that may release their drug content in the tumor environment may still be of utility in the treatment of breast carcinoma. Localization of metastatic sites may also be important in certain diagnostic applications.

DISCUSSION

These studies demonstrate that the KS1/4 monoclonal antibody recognizes an antigen associated with normal human epithelial surfaces and related malignancies. This antigen is homogenously expressed in fresh frozen specimens of human lung and colorectal adenocarcinomas but heterogenously expressed in lung squamous carinomas and breast carcinomas. An apparent correlation is observed in this fresh tumor antigenic expression and the antigenic expression of the KS1/4 antigen in human solid tumor cell lines of epithelial origin. This observation allows for the utility of human tumor xenograft models for the evaluation of site-directed therapy strategies with KS1/4-drug conjugates.

KS1/4-DAVLB is a vinca alkaloid-monoclonal antibody conjugate which has demonstrated in vivo efficacy with minimal toxicity on the P3-UCLA human lung adenocarcinoma xenograft system in both low tumor burden tumor initiation models and on established tumors. Biodistribution experiments indicate that the KS1/4-DAVLB conjugates do indeed target drug to the tumor sites in a dramatic fashion as compared to free drug administration. These findings suggest that KS1/4 may be useful as a site-directed targeting vehicle for oncolytic agents.

The normal human tissue distribution of the KS1/4 antigen is not apparent in the preclinical murine models. Innocent bystander tissue toxicology is of course possible in humans where KS1/4 may target drugs to inappropriate sites. Preclinical toxicology models which utilize primates with comparable normal tissue distributions of the target antigen may also be useful in a conjugate's development. Monoclonal antibodies 17-1A and 9.2.27 have significant normal tissue reactivity and have been given to patients in repetitive dosing protocols (22,24,25,26) which suggest that at least naked antibody treatments that may localize to many normal tissues are tolerated.

Additional issues facing the success of a site-directed therapy approach with monoclonal antibody-drug conjugates include: 1.) Potency, 2.) Vascular permeability of tumor sites, and 3.) Immunogenecity of murine proteins in humans. Strategies are evolving to address these issues directly in first and second generation monoclonal antibody-drug conjugates. KS1/4 remains as an excellent candidate for clinical development because of its broad tumor reactivity and high epitope density on major clinical cancers with no existing effective therapies. The utility of antibodies like KS1/4 in malignancies which demonstrate heterogenous expression of the target antigen will await the development of monoclonal antibody "cocktails" which will recognize higher percentages of tumor cells or for therapeutic conjugate strategies that will involve site activated release of a targeted oncolytic agent for diffusion into antigen negative tumor cells.

REFERENCES

1. T. F. Bumol and R. A. Reisfeld, Proc. Natl. Acad. Sci. USA, 79:1245-1249 (1982).
2. D. Colcher, P. Horan Hand, M. Nuti and J. Schlom, Proc. Natl. Acad. Sci., USA 78:3199-3205 (1981).
3. M. Herlyn, Z. Steplewski, D. Herlyn, and H. Koprowski, Proc. Natl. Acad. Sci., USA 76:1438-1442 (1979).
4. R. Muraro, D. Wunderlich, A. Thor, J. Lundy, P. Noguchi, R. Cunningham, and J. Schlom, Cancer Res. 45:5769-5780 (1985).
5. M. J. Bjorn, D. Ring, and A. Frankel, Cancer Res. 45:1214-1221 (1985).
6. D. P. Edwards, K. T. Grzyb, L. G. Dressler, R. E. Mansel, D. T. Zava, G. W. Sledge, Jr., and W. L. McGuire, Cancer Res. 46:1306-1317 (1986).
7. K. E. Hellstrom, I. Hellstrom, and J. P. Brown, Med. Oncol. Tumor Pharmacother. 3:147 (1984).
8. R. A. Reisfeld, J. R. Harper, and T. F. Bumol, Crit. Rev. Immunol. 5:27-53 (1984).
9. S. Kyoizumi, M. Akiyama, N. Kovno, K. Kobuke, M. Hakoda, S. L. Jones, and M. Yamakido, Cancer Res. 45:3274-3281 (1985).
10. R. A. Miller, A. R. Oscroff, P. T. Stratte, and R. Levy, Blood 62:988-995 (1983).
11. H. F. Sears, J. Mattis, D. Herlyn, P. Hayry, B. Atkinson, C. Ernst, Z. Steplewski, and H. Koprowski, Lancet 762-763 (1982).

12. D. L. Shawler, M. C. Miceli, S. B. Wormsley, I. Royston, and R. D. Dillman, Cancer Res. 44:5921-5927 (1984).
13. A. N. Houghton, D. Mintzer, C. Cordon-Cardo, S. Welt, B. Fliegel, S. Vadham, E. Carswell, M. Melamed, H. F. Oetigen, and L. J. Old, Proc. Natl. Acad. Sci. USA 82:1242 (1985).
14. G. E. Goodman, P. Beavmier, I. Hellstrom, B. Fernyhough, and K. E. Hellstrom, J. Clin. Oncol. 3:340-352 (1985).
15. N. M. Varki, R. A. Reisfeld, and L. E. Walker, Cancer Res. 44:681-686 (1984).
16. T. F. Bumol, L. E. Walker, and R. A. Reisfeld, J. Biol. Chem. 259:12733-12741 (1984).
17. G. F. Rowland, C. A. Axton, R. W. Baldwin, J. P. Brown, J. R. F Corvalan, M. J. Embleton, V. A. Gore, P. Hellstrom, K. E. Hellstrom, E. Jacobs, C. H. Marsden, M. V. Pimm, R. G. Simmonds, and W. Smith, Cancer Immunol. Immunother. 19:1-7 (1985).
18. M. J. Borowitz, B. P. Croker, and R. S. Metzgar, Am. J. Clin. Pathol. 79:387-391 (1983).
19. P. Marder, L. D. Apelgren, and T. F. Bumol, J. Immunol. Methods, in press (1986).
20. P. Marder, and J. R. Schmidtke, Immunpharmacology 6:155-163 (1983).
21. J. C. Anderson, R. A. Fugmann, R. L. Stolfi, and D. S. Martin, Cancer Res. 34:1916-1920 (1974).
22. H. F. Sears, D. Herlyn, Z. Sleplewski, and M. Koprowski, Can. Res. 45:5910-5913 (1980).
23. S. Ullberg, Science Tools, The LKB Instrument Journal, 2-29 (1977).
24. H. Koprowski, D. Herlyn, M. Lubeck, E. DeFrietas, and H. F. Sears, Proc. Natl. Acad. Sci. USA 81:216-219 (1984).
25. C. Giradet, V. Angelo, A. Schmidt-Kessen, S. Magaly, S. Carrel, and J. Mach, J. Immunol. 136:1497-1503 (1986).
26. H. G. Gottlinger, I. Funke, J. P. Johnson, J. M. Gokel, and G. Reithmuller, Int. J. of Cancer 38:47-53 (1986).

A SERUM TEST FOR THE DIAGNOSIS AND MONITORING THE PROGRESS OF BREAST CANCER

Steven Stacker[1], Nigel Sacks[1], Christoper Thompson[1], Cheng Smart[2], Robert Burton[2], Jim Bishop[3], Jeff Golder[4], Xing Pei-xiang[1], and Ian F.C. KcKenzie[1]

[1]Research Centre for Cancer and Transplantation University of Melbourne, Parkville, Australia
[2]Discipline of Surgical Sciences, University of Newcastle, Newcastle, Australia
[3]The Cancer Institute, Melbourne, Australia
[4]Australian Med-Research Industries, St. Leonards, N.S.W., Australia

INTRODUCTION

The use of monoclonal antibodies which react predominantly with human breast cancer raises the possibility of performing a simple serum test to diagnose the presence of cancer and to follow fluctuating levels and correlate these with the progress of the disease. In this way antibodies to carcinoma of the colon, such as to CEA and CA-19.9, have proven to be of some value in the monitoring, if not the diagnosis of this disease[1,2] and CA 125 and OM1 have also been used for similar purposes in patients with carcinoma of the ovary[3,4]. Other, or the same antibodies have been used to diagnose carcinoma of the pancreas[2,5]. The advantages of a serum test are clear - sample collection is simple, antibody based tests are easy to perform and the results are measured objectively, compared to a subjective clinical examination and mammography. A serum test can therefore be useful, both for the early diagnosis of disease, perhaps in screening programs, and also for the frequent monitoring of patients with advanced disease, especially those with tumours not amenable to clinical examination. With this in mind we present our studies on the use of 3E-1.2 monoclonal antibody to detect an antigen in serum - mammary serum antigen (MSA) and report on the testing of a large normal population and patients with breast cancer and other diseases. The paper represents an extension of the work originally presented at the First International Workshop[6].

MATERIALS AND METHODS

Monoclonal Antibodies

The IgM monoclonal antibody 3E-1.2 was raised against a fresh human carcinoma of the breast and has been fully characterised on human tissue by the immunoperoxidase technique[7]. Control antibodies used were HMFG-2 (reactive with HMFG - human milk fat globule membrane), 696 (anti-mouse Thy-1.2), 3B11C8 (anti-human lung cancer), 5C1 (anti-human colorectal cancer) and HuLy-m8 (anti-human CD8)- all produced in our laboratory.

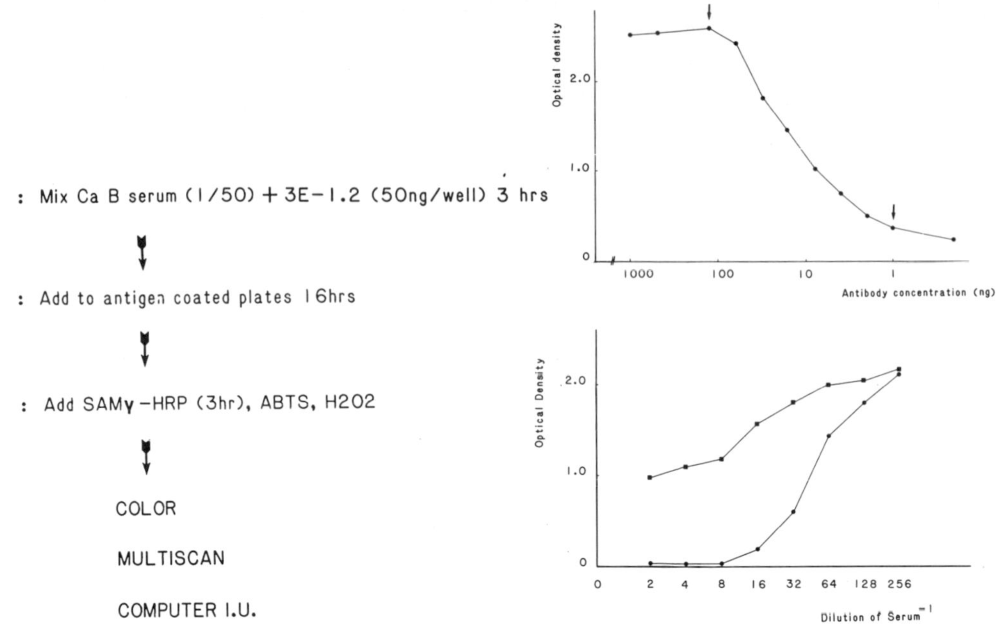

Figure 1. (A) Flow diagram of the ELISA test used to detect MSA; (B) standard antibody curve used to detect I.U.; (C) titration of inhibition obtained with normal (■) and breast serum (•).

Serum Assay

The serum test is shown in Figure 1. Crude extracts of $3E1^+$ tissues (fresh carcinoma, cell lines or kidney) were prepared and fixed to the wells of a microplate using glutaraldehyde. The plates were then incubated, washed with buffer and treated with 1% BSA (bovine serum albumin) at room temperature. In a separate plate, also coated with BSA to prevent non-specific adhesion, patients serum (dilution of 1:50) was incubated with purified monoclonal 3E-1.2 antibody (50ng per well) for 3 hours at room temperature and 50μl of this mixture was then transferred to the antigen coated plates. After an overnight incubation at 4^oC, the plates were washed with buffer (PBS/0.5% Tween 20) and incubated with 50μl of sheep anti-mouse immunoglobulin conjugated to horse radish peroxidase. After removal of excess antibody colour was developed using 50μl of 0.03% ABTS and 0.02% of hydrogen peroxidase in 0.1M citrate buffer pH 4.0. The plates were read in an ELISA plate reader at a wave length of 405 nm and the results fed directly into a computer for analysis using two programs: "Cellisa", used to analyse and store data; and "Decoder", a program designed to convert optical density readings to inhibitory units (I.U.).

Biochemical Procedures

Radiolabelling (^{125}I) of semi-purified MSA and biosynthetic labelling with ^{35}S-methionine of the in vitro cell line BT-20 were performed as previously described[8]. SDS PAGE analysis of immunoprecipitated preparations were performed by vertical slab gel electrophoresis[9]; "Western" transfer of gels were performed by standard techniques[10], except that the transfer conditions were 30 volts for 20 hours to facilitate transfer of high molecular weight species; standard molecular weight proteins were myosin = 20,000, β-galactosidase = 116,000, phosphorylase B = 92,500 and bovine serum albumin = 67,000 daltons. Nitrocellulose membranes containing transferred proteins were immunoblotted with tissue culture supernatants of appropriate hybridomas. Development was achieved using a sheep anti-mouse peroxidase conjugate with a substrate of 4-chloro-napthol/H_2O_2. HMFGM was prepared as previously described[11] and coated to PVC plates using carbonate-bicarbonate buffer (pH 9.6) at approximately 2μg/well. Tissue culture supernatants were reacted with the solid phase antigen and the subsequent binding quantitated using a peroxidase/ABTS EIA system[6]. A solid phase immunoprecipitation technique was performed as described[12].

RESULTS

Chemistry of the Mammary Serum Antigen (MSA)

Initial attempts to define the chemical nature of the antigen detected by the 3E-1.2 antibody have proven to be difficult as cell lines are surface 3E-1.2$^-$, and few have the cytoplasm reacting. Biosynthetic labelling of positive cell lines revealed no specific bands after immunoprecipitation and SDS PAGE analysis of ^{35}S-methionine labelled cell lysates. In retrospect, this was probably due to the highly glycosylated nature of this protein. However the antigen has been isolated in a water soluble form from the serum of breast cancer patients using affinity chromatography with the 3E1.2 antibody and wheat germ agglutination. Gel filtration chromatography shows MSA to be a molecule of high molecular weight (approx. 10^6). On subsequent SDS-PAGE and western blotting analysis, this large component resolves into molecules of approx. 350,000 (Fig. 2).

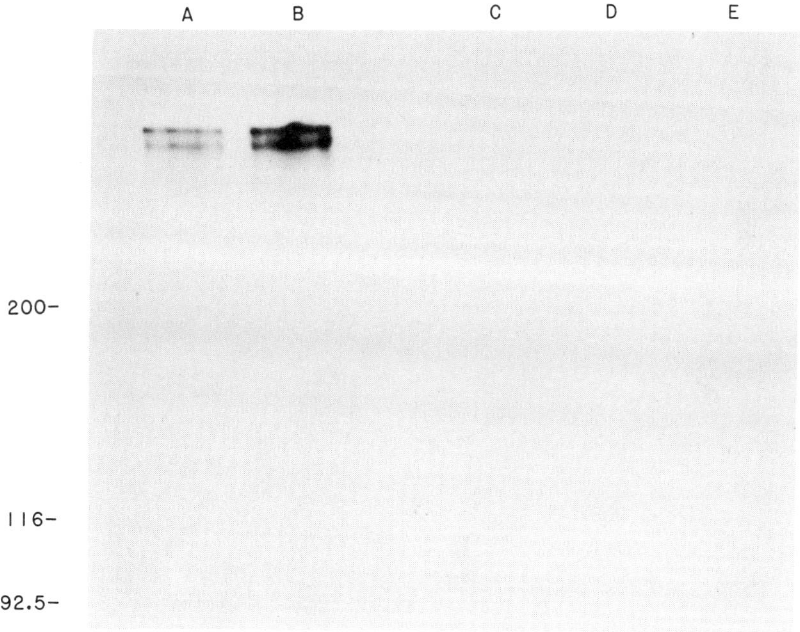

Figure 2. Analysis of radiolabelled MSA from the serum of a patient with breast cancer on SDS PAGE (5%) using a solid phase immunoprecipitation technique. The labelled MSA has been precipitated with the following antibodies:- (A) 3E-1.2 (sample reduced), (B) 3E-1.2 (sample unreduced), (C) 3B11C8, (D) 5C1 and (E) HuLy-m8.

This species is variably represented by up to two distinct bands or a heterogenous smear in different individuals. It is of interest that different individuals have slightly different sized bands indicating a polymorphism of this molecule, but there is no data available on the nature of this polymorphism. Of interest has been the finding that there are also molecules of lower molecular weight, e.g. 80,000 in the serum, but these have only been found in about 20% of the patients' serum investigated so far. Although there are some similarities between the properties of the $3E\text{-}1^+$ molecule and high molecular weight components present on the human milk fat globule membrane (HMFGM), the two are clearly different. This is demonstrated by: (a) the difference in tissue difference of 3E-1.2 and monoclonal antibodies directed to HMFGM; (b) the biochemical features are different; (c) 3E-1.2 monoclonal antibody does not react with HMFG either in an ELISA (Fig. 3) or on a Western blot (data not shown); and (d) $3E\text{-}1^+$ does not react with fresh human milk either by ELISA or immunoblotting.

Comments on the Elisa test

The inhibition enzyme immunoassay (EIA) works reproducibly in our laboratory and has been established in a number of other laboratories. The enzyme conjugate allows rapid reading of the test and coupled with the computer gives a direct readout of inhibition units. A drawback of the test is that it is run over 24 hours and uses a second antibody-conjugate rather than a two-site assay, as the 3E-1.2 antibody detects only one epitope on the MSA molecule (unpublished data). However we have recently obtained some promising results on the direct conjugation of horse radish peroxidase to the 3E-1.2 antibody, allowing shortening of the test with modification for mass production and general use.

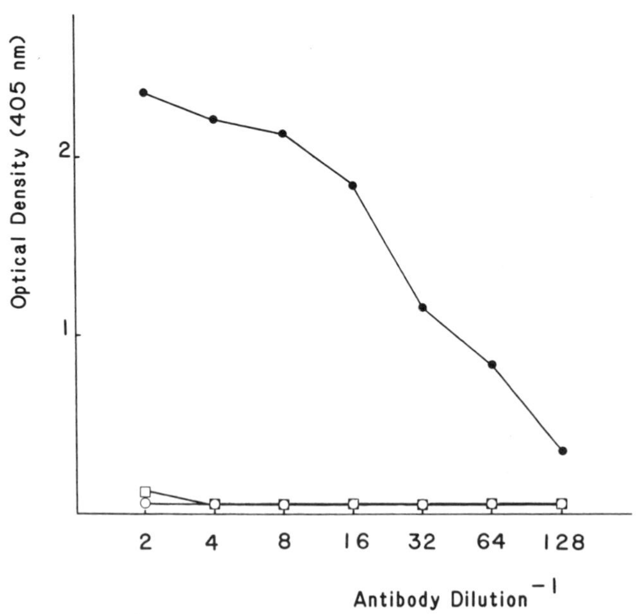

Figure 3. Binding of monoclonal antibodies to HMFG by a solid phase enzyme immunoassay. The monoclonal antibodies are $HMFG_2$ (closed circles), 3E-1.2 (open circles) and HuLy-m8 (open squares).

Table 1. MSA Levels in Normal, Benign and Malignant Tumours in the Breast

Patients/Disease	No.	Mean ± S.E.	% Above 300 I.U.
Normals: All	2400	125±89	1.9
Males	1350	116±90[a]	
Females	1050	130±88[a]	
Smokers	10	165±40	20
Pregnant	30	137±25	13
Benign Disease of Breast			
Fibroadenoma	40	157±26	18
Ca. Breast			
Stage I	15	478±142	53
Stage II	28	703±117	75
Stage III	21	836±281	71
Stage IV	142	3861±322	87
Ca. Breast in remission (no evidence of disease)	109	344±61	18
Other Cancers			
Colon	26	719±383	19
Pancreas	103	371±208	18
Lymphoma	28	152±33	18
Lung	12	373±235	8
Other Diseases			
Pancreatitis	7	947±434	43
Cirrhosis	13	1091±309	62
Hepatitis	14	378±93	57
Other Diseases	500	–	16

[a]Values are mean ± standard deviation

MSA Levels in Normal Individuals (Table 1, Figures 4 and 5)

A large number of samples were examined from normal blood donors appearing at the Red Cross Blood Transfusion Services in both Melbourne and Newcastle (Australia). These were not selected and consisted of individuals of both sexes; MSA levels were slightly higher in females, pregnant females and smokers (Table 1). This is of interest as it indicates that $3E\text{-}1.2^+$ tissues present in females (e.g. breast and endocervix) probably have a small contribution to the total MSA level seen in the normal population. For convenience we selected 300 IU as an arbitary cut off level between normal and abnormal MSA levels – being approximately the value obtained from the mean normal level + 2 standard deviations. When this is used, <2% of normal individuals have MSA levels >300 IU. Of those individuals who were available for further investigation, all had repeat MSA determinations and 9/17 had elevated levels. These individuals were carefully questioned and examined and none had evidence of breast disease or any other disease at the time. None-the-less they are being examined at regular intervals to determine whether occult disease accounts for the raised MSA level.

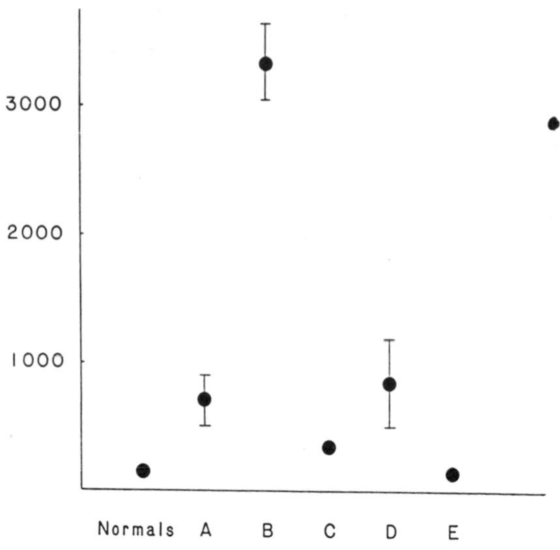

Figure 4. Diagram of the data of Table 1. Vertical axis = MSA I.U. Horizontal axis, A (Stage I and II), (B) Stage III and IV, (C) NED, (D) Stable and active disease and (E) benign disease of the breast.

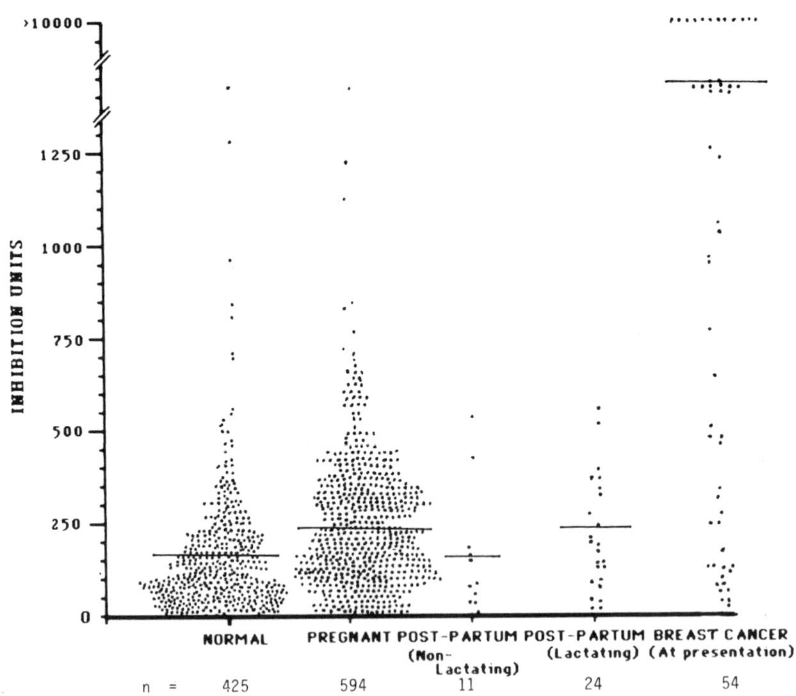

Figure 5. MSA levels in normal, pregnant and post-partum females and those with breast cancer. These tests were performed in a different centre (CYS & RCB) than those of Table 1, Figure 4.

In a totally separate study performed in another Centre (by CYS & RCB) the normal values were similar (n = 425) and the mean levels in pregnancy (n = 594) were clearly higher (Figure 5). The MSA levels were also slightly higher post-partum, especially in lactating females (n = 25) (Figure 5).

MSA Levels in Breast Cancer (Table 1, Figure 4)

Stages I and II: MSA levels are clearly raised in 53-75% of individuals with Stage I and II breast cancer. A proportion of patients with Stage I tumours would be missed if MSA was the only method used for diagnosing the presence of breast cancer. At this time we have no information on the differences between the Stage I lesions with an abnormal MSA level and those with a normal MSA level. In Stage II disease a higher number of positives (MSA > 300IU) were found (75%).

Stages III and IV: Elevated MSA levels were detected in >90% of patients with advanced breast cancer. These patients, on average, had levels much higher than the normal population and those with localized breast cancer. Some very high levels (10,000 IU) have been found in patients with Stage IV disease, although paradoxically, the occasional patient is found with widespread disease but with a normal MSA level. Presumably these patients have a poorly differentiated tumour which no longer produces MSA; we have yet to confirm this by biopsy from patients. In Figure 5 (last column) are the MSA results on 54 patients of whom 37 (=70%) had high levels; however some of these patients had been treated and MSA levels may have fallen (see below).

Correlation of Stages of Disease and MSA Levels

There is clearly an increase in MSA level as the disease extends (Table 1, Figure 4), and there is a relationship between the level of MSA and the stage of disease. However at this time while the numbers are still small we have elected not to give a range of MSA levels for each stage.

MSA Levels in Patients Previously with Breast Cancer but Presently with no Clinical Evidence of Disease (NED)

In patients who previously had breast cancer which had either been removed by surgery or treated with radiotherapy/chemotherapy and were now considered to be clinically in remission, or at least to have no clinical evidence of disease (NED), the MSA levels were clearly lower than those with Stage I-IV disease, although the mean level was higher than that found in normal patients (Table 1). Overall 20% of patients with NED had high levels and at present we are carefully following these patients to determine if those with NED and high MSA levels are more likely to develop recurrence than those with NED and normal MSA levels. These observations will provide a good basis for the monitoring of disease (see below).

It was clear that patients with breast cancer had elevated levels of MSA when compared with normal individuals, and there was an acceptable level of false positives in the normal population (<2%), and of false negative levels in the various stages of breast cancer. It was therefore important to determine how specific was an elevated MSA level for breast cancer.

MSA Levels in Benign Disease of the Breast

MSA levels were determined in 40 patients with a range of benign breast diseases (Table 1, Figure 4). Few patients (18%) had elevated MSA levels, the mean (157±26) being only slightly elevated compared to that seen in the normal population. Raised levels were seen in patients with fibroadenoma, gynaecomastia, cystic hyperplasia and benign mammary dysplasia, although a considerable numbers of patients with these conditions gave normal MSA levels. If this group is used as a base for screening then a cut off level of 400 IU (2.5% raised, means that over 50% of localized breast cancer could be detected by this method).

MSA Levels with Other Tumours and in Other Diseases

A variety of non-breast tumours were examined (Table 1) and most tumours did not give rise to raised MSA levels. About 17% of these malignancies gave elevated MSA levels compared to the normal population. As lung and pancreatic tissue are 3E-1.2$^+$ then the values seen in these diseases are not surprising; however, colon and lymphoma cells were negative for 3E-1.2 indicating a probable source of the MSA molecules in these subjects.

MSA Levels in Non-Malignant Diseases

A variety of other non-malignant diseases were examined. Firstly, 500 samples were obtained from a routine pathology department, obtaining samples from all patients passing through the hospital. Of these 16% had MSA >300 and this 16% included some patients with Ca breast. It was clear that normal levels of MSA occur in a whole range of different diseases. Secondly, 230 samples were obtained and three diseases gave rise to high MSA levels: pancreatitis, hepatitis and cirrhosis (not shown). Pancreatic tissue is 3E-1.2$^+$, which probably explains why this material appears in the serum (it would be of particular interest to determine the molecular form of the MSA antigen in this disease). However, liver tissue is 3E-1.2$^-$ and it is puzzling why the MSA levels are raised in hepatitis and cirrhosis, other than the possibility that the MSA may be metabolized in the liver and faulty catabolism and secretion could falsely raise the MSA levels. Thus it seems that raised MSA levels, apart from a few diseases including some tumours are reasonably specific for breast cancer. It therefore remains to determine the value of the test for monitoring the progress of the disease in response to therapy and for early diagnosis.

The use of MSA Measurements in the Monitoring of the Progress of the Disease (Figure 6)

Forty patients were examined at intervals over a period of up to six months and the MSA levels and their clinical status independently assessed.

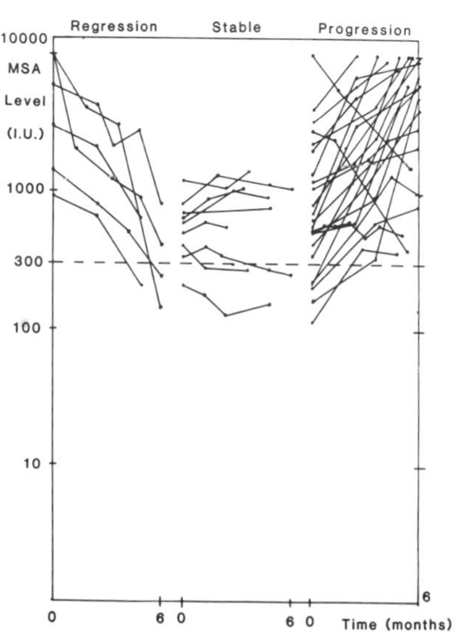

Figure 6. Correlation of MSA levels and clinical course in patients regressing, stable or progressing (Assessed clinically). Several bleeds were taken over a six month period and MSA measured.

The trend was clear, in that patients with progressive disease had rises in their MSA levels, those with stable disease maintained their MSA levels, and those with some degree of remission had a fall in the MSA level. The test is therefore considered to be of value for monitoring the progress of disease and should prove to be useful for the management of patients, assessing responses to established and new drug therapy, and for determining the prognosis.

Comparison of MSA and CEA Levels in Breast Cancer

CEA levels have been considered in some studies[13-15] to be of value in diagnosing and monitoring the progress of breast cancer. We have therefore compared the levels of MSA and CEA in breast cancer (Table 2). Of the samples examined, 41/78 were considered positive for MSA (>300 IU). In this study there were 12 patients with Stage I disease of which 75% had raised MSA levels.

Table 2. Comparison of MSA and CEA as Markers for Breast Cancer

Group	Number Tested	MSA (% >300IU)	CEA (%>2.5 ng/ml)
Breast Cancer			
Stage I	12	75	8
Stage II	9	89	56
Stage IV			
Bone	25	95	60
Liver	6	100	50
Multiple	16	89	82
Lung	10	100	40
TOTALS	78	94%	52%

Comparison of MSA and CA-15.3 Levels in Breast Cancer (Table 3)

In addition to the MSA test, another test, CA-15.3, has recently been described for the detection of serum antigens in breast cancer[16,17]. This test differs from MSA in that it is based on the detection of circulating HMFG protein, and therefore detects a different product to MSA. It was of interest to determine the comparitive sensitivity of the two assays and whether the two, used together, would be of greater benefit that each test used alone.

Table 3. Comparison of 3E-1.2 and CA-15.3 in Breast Cancer

Group	Number Tested	MSA (% >300 IU)	CA-15.3 (%>30IU/ml)
No Evidence of Disease	4	0	0
Pre Mastectomy (Localised)	19	58	21
Advanced Active Cancer[a]	31	84	77

[a] Includes patients with Stage III and IV breast cancer

In the small number of patients studied thus far MSA levels are raised in more patients with Stage I and Stage II disease than detected by the CA-15.3 assay. However, in advanced breast cancer (Stage IV) both tests detected a similar proportion of patients. It was of interest to show that some stage IV patients were $MSA^{-}CA^{-}15.3^{+}$ and $MSA^{+}CA^{-}15.3^{-}$. This observation clearly shows that different products are being detected in the two assays and implies that the two tests used together could be of some value, although in advanced Stage IV disease the measurement of serum antigen is not really necessary for diagnosis as the progress of the disease is only too readily obvious to the clinician.

DISCUSSION

MSA levels are raised in breast cancer and appear to be of value in monitoring the progress of the disease. Indeed, in several cities in Australia the test is now being used routinely on a service basis for this very purpose. The MSA levels are raised in the great majority of patients with Stage III and IV disease and in most (>75%) of patients with Stage I and II disease (Table 1, Figures 4 and 5). In addition the levels show a relationship with the stage of the disease, and fluctuate, depending on the status of the disease (Figure 6). In addition, MSA testing appears to be more sensitive than either CEA (Table 2) or CA-15.3 (Table 3) - particularly in localized disease; this difference is less in more advanced disease.

There are still a number of questions to be answered, e.g. to determine why MSA levels are negative in some patients with advanced disease; why the levels are raised in cirrhosis and why there is a proportion (approx. 25%) of patients with Stage I disease who are MSA^{-}. Whether the production of MSA in Stage I is merely a reflection of the size of the tumour and if the test were more sensitive then the Stage I detection would be improved is not clear at present. Nor whether Stage I patients who are MSA^{+} do in fact have more than local disease, which is not apparent at the time of staging. A number of these patients are currently being observed and these questions can be answered.

Whether MSA levels would be useful in a screening program remains to be seen. However, at this time with the false negative rate at approximately 30-40% in Stage I patients, we would not suggest that the MSA serum test be the only test performed; careful clinical observation, mammography and MSA determinations may together lead to improved diagnosis.

SUMMARY

Monoclonal antibody 3E-1.2 detects a serum antigen, mammary serum antigen (MSA). It is a high molecular weight glycoprotein and appears to be distinct from other high molecular weight molecules originating from breast tissue such as HMFG. The level of MSA in normal individuals (3,000 tested in two cities) was 125 IU with no great difference between males and females. The levels were substantially raised in breast cancer, with 53-75% of Stage I (in two separate studies) to more than 90% in Stage IV having levels of > 300 IU. There was a relationship between MSA level and the stage of disease and furthermore MSA levels fluctuated according to the disease status of the patient, i.e. MSA levels could be used for monitoring progress of the disease and response to therapy. MSA levels are substantially better than CEA for the detection of breast cancer and are also better than the existing CA-15.3 assay. MSA determinations appear to be particularly useful for the monitoring of breast cancer and may be a useful aid in diagnosis.

REFERENCES

1. P. Dhar, T. Moore, M. Zamcheck and H.Z. Zupchick, Carcinoembryonic antigen (CEA) in colonic cancer : use in pre-operative and post-operative diagnosis and prognosis, JAMA 221:31-35 (1972).
2. J. Magnani, Z. Steplewski, H. Koprowski and V. Ginsberg, Identification of the gastrointestinal and pancreatic cancer - associated antigen detected by monoclonal antibody 19-9 in the sera of patients as a mucin. Cancer Res. 43:5489-5492 (1983).
3. R.C. Bast, T.L. Klug, E. St. John, E. Jenison, J.M. Nilhoff, H. Lazaraus, R.S. Berkowitz, T. Leavitt, T. Griffiths, L. Parker, V.R. Zurawski and R.C. Knapp, A radioimmunoassay using a monoclonal antibody to monitor the course of epithelial ovarian cancer, N. Engl. J. Med. 309:883-887 (1983).
4. T.A. DeKretser, H.J. Thorne, D.J. Jacobs and D.G. Jose, The sebaceous gland antigen defined by the OM-1 monoclonal antibody is expressed at high density on the surface of ovarian carcinoma cells, Eur. J. Cancer and Clinical Oncology 9:1019-1035 (1985).
5. R.S. Metzgar, N. Rodriguez, O.J. Finn, M.S. Lan, V.N. Daasch, P.D. Fernsten, W.C. Meyers, W.F. Sindelar, R.S. Sandler and H.F. Seiglar, Detection of a pancreatic cancer-associated antigen (DU-PAN-2 antigen) in the serum and ascites of patients with adenocarcinoma, Proc. Natl. Acad. Sci. USA 81:5242-5246 (1985).
6. S.A. Stacker, C.H. Thompson, M. Lichtenstein, M. Leyden, N. Salehi, J. Andrews and I.F.C. McKenzie, Detection of breast cancer using the monoclonal antibody 3E-1.2. in "Proc. Int. Workshop on Monoclonal Antibodies and Breast Cancer", pp. 233-247 (1985).
7. S.A. Stacker, C.H. Thompson, C. Riglar and I.F.C. McKenzie, A new breast carcinoma antigen defined by a monoclonal antibody, J. Natl. Cancer Inst. 75:801-811 (1985).
8. C.H. Thompson, S.L. Jones, E. Phil and I.F.C. McKenzie, Monoclonal antibodies to human colon and colorectal carcinoma, Br. J. Cancer 47:595-605 (1983).
9. U.K. Laemmli, Clevage of structural proteins during the assembly of the head of bacteriophage T4, Nature 227:680 (1970).
10. H. Towbin, T. Staehelin and J. Gordon, Elecrophoretic transfer of proteins from polyacrylamide gels to nitrocellulose sheets : procedure and some applications, Proc. Natl. Acad. Sci. USA 76:4350-4354 (1979).
11. R.L. Cerianni, K.E. Thompson, J.A. Peterson and S. Abraham, Surface differentiation antigens on human mammary epithelial antigens in breast cancer, Proc. Natl. Acad. Sci. USA 74:582 (1977).
12. I.D. Walker, B.J. Murray, P.M. Hogarth, A. Kelso and I.F.C. McKenzie. Comparison of thymic and peripheral T cell Ly-2/3 antigens, Eur. J. Immunol. 14:906-910 (1984).
13. L.M. Ahleman, H.J. Stabb and F.A. Anderer, Serial CEA determinations as an aid in post-operative therapy management of patients with early breast cancer, Biomedicine 32:194 (1980).
14. J.F. Chatal, F. Chupin and G. Ricolleau, Use of serial carcinoembryonic antigen assays in detecting relapses in breast cancer involving high risk of metastases, Eur. J. Cancer 17:233 (1981).
15. H.C. Falkson, J.J. Van Der Watt and M.A. Protugal, Carcinoembryonic antigen in patients with breast cancer : An adjuvant tool to monitor response and therapy, Cancer. 42:1308 (1978).
16. J. Hilkens, J. Hilgers, F. Bijs, P.H. Hageman, D. Schol, G. Doornewaard, G. and J. Van Der Tweel, Monoclonal Antibodies against human milk fat globule membranes useful in carcinoma research, in "Protides of the Biological fluids", H. Peters, ed., Pergamon Press, Oxford (1984).
17. D. Kufe, G. Inghiramni, M. Abe, D. Hayes, H. Justi-Wheeler and J. Schlom, Differential reactivity of a novel monoclonal antibody (DF3) while human malignant versus benign breast tumours, Hybridoma 3:230-232 (1984).

EXPERIMENTAL THERAPY OF BREAST CANCER WITH ANTI-BREAST EPITHELIAL RADIOIMMUNOCONJUGATES

Roberto L. Ceriani and Edward W. Blank

John Muir Cancer & Aging Research Institute
2055 N. Broadway
Walnut Creek, CA 94596 U.S.A.

INTRODUCTION

Therapy of breast cancer with monoclonal antibodies (MoAbs) conjugated or unconjugated faces serious challenges not only for researchers to obtain MoAbs adequate to bring the desired conjugate to the tumors and spare other organs, but also to create MoAbs that could act in an unconjugated form. Of the latter type, those that will participate in antibody dependent cell mediated and complement dependent cytotoxicity are desired.

On the other hand, when considering the use of conjugates of MoAbs several are the possibilities that need to be taken into account. First of all, the type of conjugate to be used will depend on the antigenic makeup of the tumor primarily (radioisotope conjugates for high heterogeneity and toxin conjugates for low heterogeneity) and secondarily on the conjugation process (easiness of conjugation and non-denaturing procedures). The most popular conjugates at the present moment are those involving toxins, radioactive isotopes and the standard chemotherapeutic drugs.

Other than the problems of conjugation and subsequent preservation of antibody specificity to which most of the interest has been put to date, the thorough study of the target tumor and the pharmacokinetics of the conjugate in circulation should be of great importance in the determination of which conjugate is used. In the case that an immunotoxin conjugate is used, the prevalence, that is the number of cells that carry the antigen in the population is of utmost importance. Heterogeneity of cellular expression of the antigen could well produce a good number of cells with low levels, or, perhaps, with no levels of the antigen in question, permitting thus their escape from therapy. In contrast, in the case of radioconjugates, heterogeneity plays a minor role while level of antigen expression and turnover time of the antigen on the cells is relevant. It is obvious that the amount of antigen on the target cells will condition the amount of radioconjugate that will bind. Anchoring of the conjugated MoAb to the tumor will depend on the cellular concentration of the antigen and where it is present (cell surface or cytoplasm). Further, binding of the conjugated antibody can be aided by antigenic deposits surrounding the tumor cells which are their source. Antigenic detection by immunoperoxidase on histological sections has shown in our laboratory (unpublished results), that in the case of certain cell surface antigens, clouds of such antigens surround and accumulate around breast epithelial cancer cells thus permitting binding of larger amounts of immunoconjugates in tissues in close proximity to tumor cells.

The other parameter, the cellular turnover time of the antigen to be target of the therapy, is also important (1). The amount of time that the radioactively tagged antibody remains on the tumor cell and thus has a chance to irradiate a cell and its surrounding cohorts, is directly related to the antigenic turnover time. This residence time of the bound antibody is of importance to establish appropriate dosimetry and also in the choice of the appropriate unstable isotope to be bound to the MoAb.

To all these considerations it has to be added that there are plenty of unresolved problems in the ability to scale up the production of appropriate antibodies without contaminating hybrid antibody populations and in the pharmacokinetics of tumor targetting. In the latter, depending on the conjugates to be used, not only the specificity of the antibody will affect the biodistribution, but a further liability is the propensity of most of the conjugates to lose their tagging agent which then accumulates in different organs such as liver or kidney, as is the case for certain radioisotopes used as conjugates [e.g., transchelation of ^{111}In-DTPA-MoAb to transferrin (2)].

In another domain, the control of phenotypic expression of the antigens to be target of the therapy is an area of little research of yet (3), however, it could possibly render an important contribution to the ability of these MoAbs to bind and destroy breast cancer cells. Procedures to increase antigenic expression on tumor cells and to increase prevalence or the number of cells expressing the antigen (thus reducing heterogeneity) is a most hoped for goal.

Several attempts are found in the literature of the use of unconjugated MoAbs in the therapy of breast cancer, among them two reports deal with the ability of an unconjugated anti-breast epithelial antibody in arresting growth of human breast tumors grafted in nude mice. The first one of these reports describes the use of anti-breast epithelial cell surface mucin-directed MoAb that arrest the growth of xenografts in nude mice (4). As reported by these authors also (5), the action of this MoAb (called by the ductal carcinoma antigen) is correlated to the phenotypic expresion of the corresponding antigen.

We also have reported the use of four different unconjugated MoAbs directed against breast epithelium in producing similar arrests of human breast tumor growth in nude mice and at times their erradication (1,6). These MoAbs had higher tumoricidal ability when injected simultaneously or in "cocktail" form. A consistent feature was the escape of the human breast tumors under antibody attack and their continued growth in spite of the sustained presence of the "cocktail" of MoAbs, as we demonstrated by immunohistopathology (6). The cellular basis for this phenomenon was the loss of antigenic expression of those breast tumor cells that managed to avoid tumoricidal action by the MoAbs. The appearance of such variant populations is connected to the inherent heterogeneity of tumor tissues which demonstrate their ability to produce cellular variants that are immune to antibody attack (7,8). This avoidance of antibody binding by some tumor cells that results in survival after tumoricidal therapy can be overcome by the use of radioactive conjugates of such antibodies, which will irradiate the cell they bind to and those other cells in its surroundings in proportion to the energy and the ionizing potential of the radioactive particle released.

In addition, in our hands, immunotoxin conjugates were also useful in destroying human breast cells in culture and tumors in vivo. Diptheria toxin chain-A conjugates of MoAb Mc5 proved effective in inhibiting the growth of MCF-7 breast carcinoma cells in vitro (9). In other experimentation, abrin-A chain conjugates of MoAb Mc5 arrested significantly the growth of transplantable human breast tumor MX-1 grafted in nude mice, although without producing prolonged tumor growth arrest or its erradication (10).

In this paper we present experimental evidence of the tumoricidal effectiveness for breast tumors of radioiodinated MoAbs generated against human milk fat globule membrane. The efficiency of tumor destruction is demonstrated for the use of single MoAbs but more so for their mixtures (or "cocktails").

MATERIALS AND METHODS

Tagged BALB/c nu/nu mice were used for tumor transplantation, and were obtained from Life Sciences (St. Petersburg, FL). They were fed Purina Mouse Chow 5015 and acidified water pH 2.5, while kept in isolation in sterile cages and bedding. After radioconjugate injection they were placed in separate cages and the bedding changed more frequently.

The transplantable human tumors MX-1, a human breast carcinoma derived from a primary breast tumor, MX-2, a human breast carcinoma derived from the human breast cell line MDA-MB-231 originally from a pleural effusion, HIG-G, a human breast carcinoma derived from a metastatic carcinoma in a male, LX-1, a human lung carcinoma, derived from a metastatic lung carcinoma and CX-1, a colon adenocarcinoma from the colon carcinoma cell line HT-29 were obtained from the EG&G Mason Research Institute. MX-1A is a fast growing transplantable human breast tumor derived from MX-1. Nude mice were transplanted through a flank incision midway between the front and hind legs with 2-3 mm^3 pieces of each tumor which were pushed just before the hips as already described (1). To obtain the volumes, the width, length, and height of the tumor were measured. The three dimensions were then multiplied and the result divided by 2.

Iodinations were carried out with either ^{125}I (17 Ci/mg), Amersham Corporation (Arlington Heights, IL) or ^{131}I (8-12 Ci/mg), NEN Research Products (Boston, MA). MoAbs were iodinated via the chloramine-T method (11), 0.5 mg/ml at MoAb concentrations of 4-10 mg/ml. Samples were counted in a gamma counter, Multi-Prias 4, Packard Corporation (Downers Grove, IL).

For biodistribution and immunotherapy experiments i.p. injection of the labelled compound were administered to nude mice carrying tumors which were placed in separate cages fed and provided acidified water as usual. For tumor and organ uptake measurements the mice were sacrificed by cervical dislocation, the tumors and organs dissected, weighed and their radioactivity counted. The latter was then related to initial dose once it was expressed per gram of tumor or given tissue.

Hybridomas of the MoAbs used to produce ascites were injected into 2, 6, 10, 14 - tetramethylpentadecane primed BALB/c mice with either Mc1, Mc3, Mc5 or Mc8. The ascites was sterilely removed and purified through a hydroxylapatite prep column 2.5 cm X 5.0 cm, Biorad (Richmond, CA). The purified fraction of MoAb was concentrated with a CX-30 Immersible Millipore (Bedford, MA) and filtered for sterility through a 0.2 μ cellulose acetate filter, Millipore (Bedford, MA).

RESULTS

In experimental immunotherapy unconjugated MoAbs Mc1, Mc3, Mc5, Mc8 and their mixtures, otherwise called "cocktails", were effective in arresting the growth of human breast tumors implanted in nude mice (1, 6). The arrest of growth of established human breast tumors was significant and resulted from repeated injections of a considerable amount of these MoAbs. The arrest of human breast tumor growth obtained eventually terminated and slow growth of the tumor continued in spite of repeated unconjugated MoAb injections. Encouraged by these results we decided to further our immunotherapy studies with the use of radioiodinated conjugates of these MoAbs and their mixtures.

For this purpose MoAbs were labelled with ^{125}I by the chloramine-T method (11), as well as normal mouse serum IgG which was used as a control. In table 1 distribution studies are shown where human breast tumors MX-1, HIG-G, and MX-2, human colon tumor CX-1 and human lung tumor LX-1 were used. Once the human tumors were implanted and established in nude mice, the host mice were injected with approximately 0.5 μCi of each of the antibodies, 0.5 μCi of a "cocktail" composed of equal parts of each of the already mentioned antibodies, or with 0.5 μCi of radioiodinated normal mouse serum IgG. All animals were given injections of 2 mg of potassium iodide 2 hours before tracer administration. As it can be seen in table 1 the MoAbs distributed at 24 hours throughout the organism and bound at high levels the human breast tumors, and in some instances the liver. This secondary undesirable liver binding could have been the result of binding of the radioconjugate to Fc receptors or to hepatic glycoprotein receptors and/or dehalogenation of the radioconjugate and subsequent excretion of the ^{125}I through the biliary tract. Appreciable incorporation can be seen in the breast tumors which in several occasions, as was the case with the "cocktail", accumulated approximately 5% of the total injected dose per gram of tissue. Viewed from another vantage point, the latter mixture accumulated at least 10 times more than did normal serum IgG on the breast tumors, supporting the prediction that concentration of irradiating unstable isotope on breast tumors could be achieved by this methodology.

Table 1. Tissue distribution at 24 hours of radiolabelled MoAbs in nude mice carrying human breast tumors.

	Mc1	Mc3	Mc5	Mc8	Cocktail[c]	Normal Serum IGg
MX-1[a]	0.99±0.13[d]	4.90±1.00	3.70±0.25	3.62±0.65	5.43±0.72	0.49 ±0.07
HiG-G[a]	2.70±0.87	2.96±1.70	0.35±0.08	ND	ND	ND
MX-2[a]	ND	0.72±0.29	3.02±0.86	ND	ND	ND
CX-1[a]	ND	ND	1.24±0.12	ND	0.39±0.06	1.52 ±1.44
LX-1[a]	ND	0.48±0.02	1.28±0.61	ND	ND	ND
Spleen[b]	0.56±0.45	0±0	0.25±0.14	0.27±0.24	0±0	0.06 ±0.04
Kidney[b]	0.34±0.20	0.51±0.17	0±0	2.49±0.61	0±0	0.03 ±0.02
Liver[b]	1.55±0.19	0.81±0.21	0.79±0.35	3.78±1.14	1.09±0.26	0.17 ±0.02
Muscle[b]	0.18±0.26	0.34±0.11	0.85±0.25	0.36±0.26	0.33±0.06	0.32 ±0.10
Brain[b]	0.30±0.12	0.79±0.06	0.31±0.15	0.26±0.11	0.13±0.01	0.004±0.003

a MX-1, MX-2, and HiG-G are human breast tumors. CX-1 is a human colon tumor and LX-1, a human lung tumor. All are transplantable in nude mice.

b Tissues removed from the host nude mice.

c The "cocktail" was composed of equal amounts of Mc1, Mc3, Mc5 and Mc8.

d Results are expressed as mean ± SE.

In table 2 the distribution of this MoAb tagged with ^{125}I in nude mice carrying non-breast human tumors can be seen. Approximately 5.0 µCi of each radioiodinated antibody were injected this time in nude mice carrying the human colon tumor CX-1. It can be clearly seen that after three days there was no specific accumulation of any of the antibodies in any organ of the mice or on the breast tumors, except the higher binding shown by Mc3 to CX-1, which represents an added range of specificity of the MoAb. Results shown in tables 1 and 2 gave support to the proposal of trying experimental immunotherapy of human breast tumors in nude mice with each of the radioiodinated MoAbs Mc1, Mc3, Mc5, Mc8 and with a "cocktail" composed of equal parts of each of them.

Table 2. Tissue distribution at 72 hours of radiolabelled MoAbs in nude mice carrying human colon tumors.

	Mc1	Mc3	Mc5	Mc8
Blood	1.21 ± 0.15[a]	8.84 ± 0.94	7.19 ± 1.33	1.71 ± 0.37
Skin	0.32 ± 0.05	2.06 ± 0.22	1.47 ± 0.17	0.48 ± 0.08
CX-1[b]	0.77 ± 0.08	6.83 ± 0.87	3.77 ± 0.41	1.02 ± 0.16
Brain	0.04 ± 0.01	0.45 ± 0.11	0.36 ± 0.11	0.12 ± 0.01
Spleen	0.27 ± 0.04	1.56 ± 0.21	1.51 ± 0.31	0.40 ± 0.01
Kidney	0.35 ± 0.05	2.38 ± 0.34	1.91 ± 0.35	0.59 ± 0.08
Liver	0.42 ± 0.05	2.64 ± 0.28	1.98 ± 0.28	0.70 ± 0.10
Lung	0.48 ± 0.04	3.63 ± 0.61	2.72 ± 0.47	0.79 ± 0.12
Stomach	0.26 ± 0.05	1.25 ± 0.27	1.15 ± 0.31	0.55 ± 0.07
Intestine	0.22 ± 0.03	1.22 ± 0.26	0.82 ± 0.13	0.36 ± 0.05
Bone	0.13 ± 0.02	0.69 ± 0.07	0.78 ± 0.14	0.18 ± 0.05
Muscle	0.13 ± 0.03	0.95 ± 0.12	0.59 ± 0.08	0.19 ± 0.02

a Results are expressed as mean ± SE.

b CX-1 is a human colon carcinoma.

To test for the ability of each of these MoAbs, in radioiodinated form, to destroy human breast tumors, ^{131}I-conjugates of Mc1 labelled at a specific acitivity of 9.48 mCi/mg, Mc3 at 11.62 mCi/mg and Mc8 at 6.42 mCi/mg were injected at day 0 in doses of 500 µCi per tumor host mouse, Figure 1. All three MoAbs managed to reduce tumor size within 4 days. Reductions of close to 50% in tumor mass were effected by the three antibodies, however, at day 12 only MoAb Mc3 could hold the tumors at half their original size, while those treated with MoAbs Mc1 and Mc8 had already started regrowth at a pace slightly slower than that of the uninjected control. At day 16 the untreated control had increased 160% its original volume, while the tumors injected with Mc1 and Mc8 had grown approximately 70% and 10% their original volume. In contrast those injected with Mc3 still experienced a decrease of 40% from the original tumor volume.

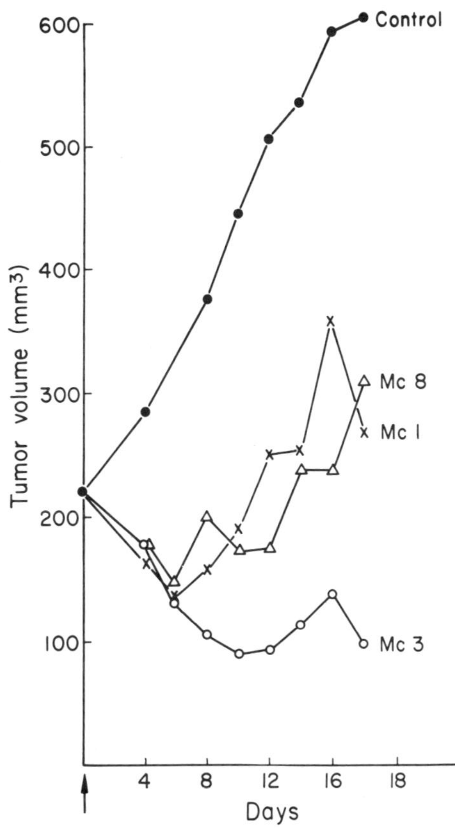

Figure 1. Tumor growth after injection at day 0 of ^{131}I-labelled MoAbs Mc1, Mc3 and Mc8 into nude mice carrying as an established transplantable tumor human breast carcinoma MX-1. Control represents tumor growth in uninjected nude mice.

A similar experiment was conducted with MoAb Mc5 where 500 µCi of ^{131}I-labelled Mc5 with a specific activity of 6.68 mCi/mg were injected in nude mice carrying transplantable human breast tumor MX-1. As it can be seen in Figure 2 ^{131}I-Mc5 diminished tumor size by approximately 40% at day 6, but from there on the tumor gradually grew back to its original volume by day 16. In contrast, those tumors injected with 500 µCi of radioiodinated normal mouse serum immunoglobulin with a specific activity of 4.34 mCi/mg grew unimpeded, as much as the uninjected control. By day 20 both the uninjected control and the normal mouse serum IgG had approximately 300% their initial volume. From all the experiments above it can be clearly seen that these MoAbs were effective in human breast tumor destruction, ranging from 40-60% at days 6-10, followed by regrowth of the tumor at a lesser or a higher rate, depending on the MoAb(s) injected (Figure 2).

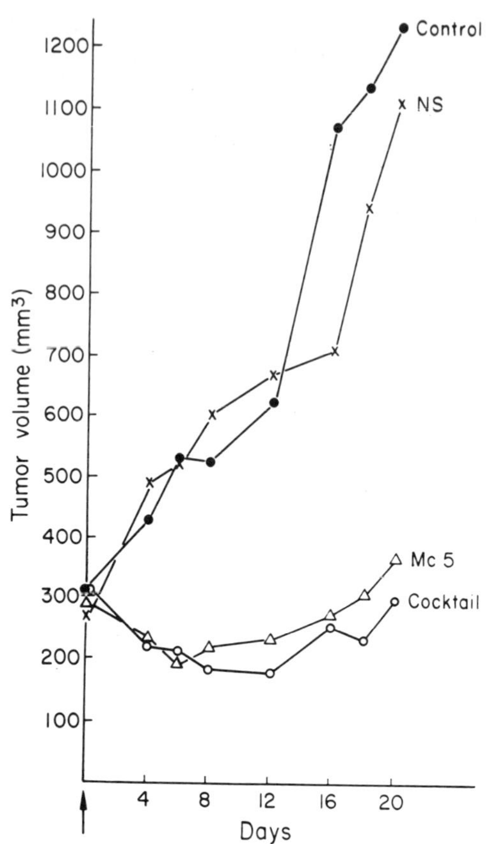

Figure 2. Tumor growth after injection at day 0 of ^{131}I-labelled MoAb Mc5, normal mouse serum IgG and a "cocktail" composed of equal parts of MoAbs Mc1, Mc3, Mc5 and Mc8 into nude mice carrying as an established transplantable tumor human breast carcinoma MX-1. Control represents tumor growth in uninjected nude mice.

In Figure 2 we have also a group that was injected at day 0 with 500 μCi of ^{131}I-labelled "cocktail" of the above mentioned MoAbs, at a specific activity of 5.25 mCi/mg. The "cocktail" was highly effective in destroying tumor cells, as evidenced by a decrease in tumor volume of close to 50% in 12 days after the injection of radioconjugates. After that, a slow regrowth of the tumor ensued at a rate which was much slower than that of the controls. The arrest of growth of the human breast tumor was of longer duration and more significant with the use of the "cocktail" of MoAbs. At 20 days the tumors treated with the radioiodinated "cocktail" had hardly regained their volume of day 0, the day of the original therapeutic radioconjugate injection.

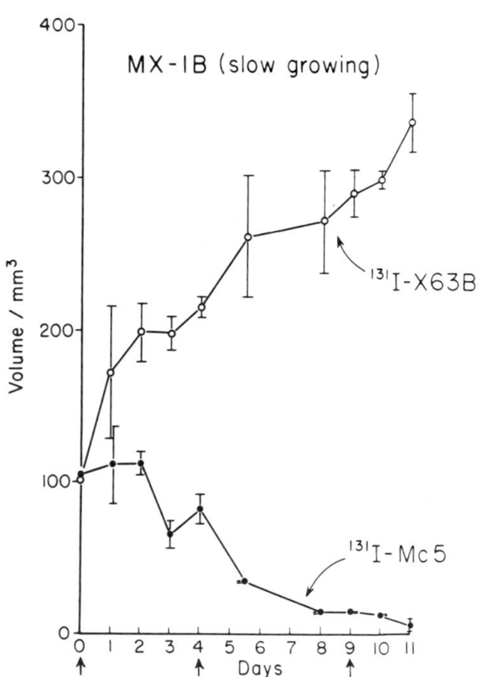

Figure 3. Tumor growth after injections at day 0, 4 and 9 of ^{131}I-labelled MoAb Mc5 and secreted myeloma IgG of mouse myeloma X63B (the parent cell line of the hybridoma secreting MoAb Mc5) into nude mice carrying as an established transplantable tumor slow-growing human breast carcinoma MX-1. Results are expressed as mean ± SE.

Since MoAb Mc5 diminished tumor volume up to 40% at day 6 after injection, repeated injections of 500 μCi doses of MoAb Mc5 were used. Three different radioiodinations that yielded conjugates with specific activities of 4.96, 5.98, and 4.32 mCi/mg of HPLC purified MoAb Mc5, were injected into nude mice carrying transplantable human breast tumor MX-1. Simultaneously HPLC purified normal mouse serum IgG was labelled and injected on three occasions in doses of 500 μCi and at specific activities of 3.92, 4.79, and 5.79 mCi/mg. Each respective preparation of MoAb Mc5 and normal mouse immunoglobulin was injected at day 0, 4 and 9. As it can be seen in Figure 3 tumor volume was sharply decreased by the first injection and continued to decline in volume after the second as well as after the third. The growth of the normal immunoglobulin injected human breast tumor continued unimpeded. It should be pointed out that the mice in both groups injected with the radiolabelled MoAbs showed high toxicity and a loss of 25% of the body weight and eventual demise (Figure 3). However, tumor growth continued in the group of nude mice injected with radioiodinated X63B immunoglobulin while tumor growth was drastically arrested in those mice injected with radioiodinated Mc5.

Figure 4 shows a paired symmetrical experiment, where 500 μCi of labelled MoAb Mc5 with specific activities of 4.96, 5.98, and 4.32 mCi/mg respectively were injected at day 0, 4 and 9 to nude mice carrying fast growing human breast tumor MX-1A. Five hundred μCi of normal mouse immunoglobulin identical to that used in the previous experiment with MX-1 human mammary tumor (Figure 3) were injected also at days 0, 4 and 9. As it can be seen in Figure 4 the group injected with normal immunoglobulin grew very fast and unimpeded for 11 days, achieving 11 times the volume of the original tumor. In that same time the MoAb injected tumors remained at approximately 20% their original volume. High toxicity as well as significant loss of body weight was noticed in both the control group, X63B-injected, and the one injected with radioiodinated Mc5, both having high mortality.

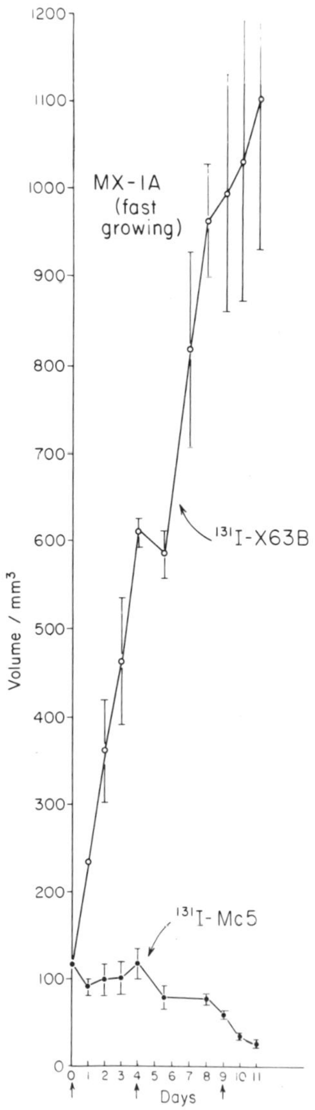

Figure 4. Tumor growth after injections at days 0, 4 and 9 of ^{131}I-labelled MoAb Mc5 and secreted myeloma IgG of mouse myeloma X63B (the parent cell line of the hybridoma secreting MoAb Mc5) into nude mice carrying an established transplantable tumor fast-growing human breast carcinoma MX-1A. Results are expressed as mean ± SE.

In view of the high toxicity of three repeated injection of 500 µCi of MoAb Mc5 one injection of a "cocktail" of MoAbs Mc1, Mc3, Mc5 and Mc8 was used. The "cocktail" of MoAbs had a specific activity of 7.13 mCi/mg, Figure 5. This sole injection of 500 µCi of the "cocktail" of MoAbs managed to slow down appreciably the growth of this human breast tumor. So much, that after 71 days the group injected with radioiodinated MoAbs carried tumors which were approximately 5.5 times their original size of 72 mm^3 while the uninjected control carried tumors 56 times their original size, Figure 5.

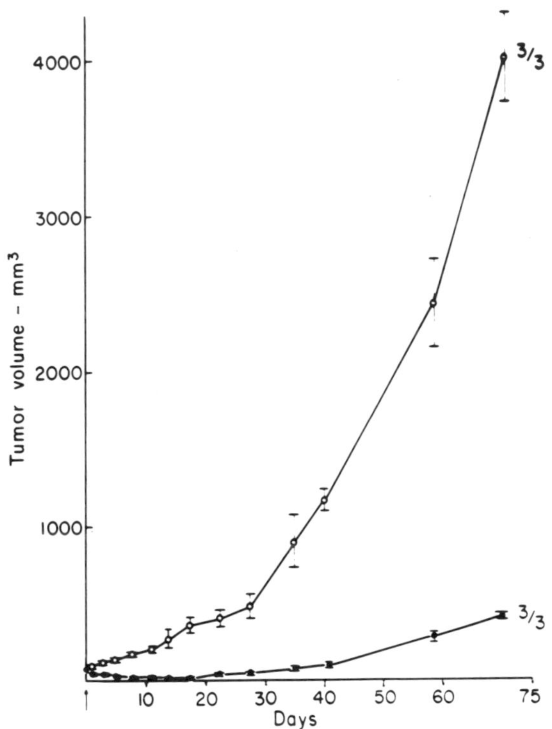

Figure 5. Tumor growth after injection at day 0 of ^{131}I-labelled "cocktail" composed of equal parts of MoAbs Mc1, Mc3, Mc5 and Mc8 into nude mice carrying as established transplantable tumors human breast carcinoma MX-1. Control represents tumor growth in uninjected nude mice. Ratio shows survivors at day 71 over number of nude mice in the same group at day 0. Results are expressed as mean ± SE.

As shown before (Figures 3 and 4), sequential injections at short intervals with 500 µCi of radioiodinated MoAb Mc5 was shown to be very toxic to the experimental animals. For this reason an experiment was planned whereby 500 µCi of the MoAb "cocktail" were injected at day 0 and at day 35, thus allowing for enough time for recovery from the radiation damage of the host mice. As it can be seen in Figure 6 the uninjected control and the control injected with normal mouse immunoglobulin continued to grow unobstructed for a period of 90 days reaching a volume of approximately 45 times that of the original tumor volume of 270 mm^3 in this period of time. In contrast the human breast tumors growing in nude mice injected with two doses of 500 μCi of MoAb "cocktail" at days 0 and 35 had only increased the tumor size by approximately 6 times in 90 days. In this experiment two items are to be remarked, first there was a strong arrest of tumor growth for a prolonged period of time after the injection of two doses of 500 μCi of radiolabelled "cocktail" of MoAbs, in this case with no appreciable toxic effect to the host. Second, after each of the injections demonstrable tumor destruction occured pointing out the fact that a second injection continued to be effective in human breast tumor cell destruction.

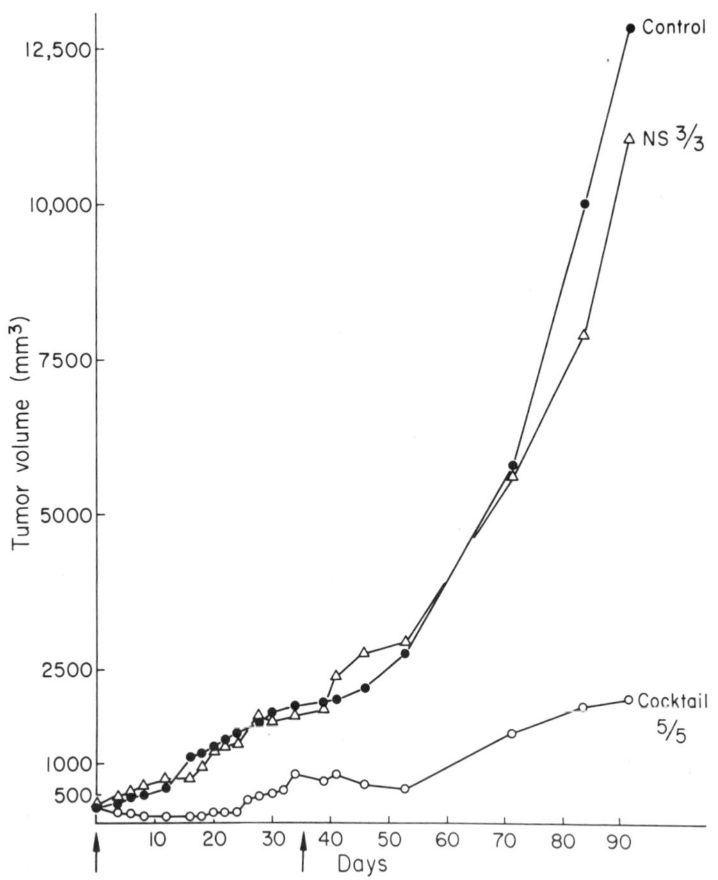

Figure 6. Tumor growth after injections at days 0 and 35 of ^{131}I-labelled normal mouse serum IgG and "cocktail" composed of MoAbs Mc1, Mc3, Mc5 and Mc8 into nude mice carrying as established transplantable tumors human breast carcinoma MX-1. Control represents tumor growth in uninjected nude mice. Ratio shows survivors at day 90 over number of nude mice in the same group at day 0.

DISCUSSION

^{131}I-conjugated MoAbs show to be effective in breast tumor destruction at low toxic levels. In addition their use in the form of a mixture or "cocktail" shows to be even more effective when compared to the injection of radioconjugates of a single MoAb. Single doses of the latter of up to 500 µCi destroyed tumor masses without apparent toxicity in most cases. This tumor destruction could be reenacted by a second similar injection after a period of time without apparent toxicity, prolonging the interference with tumor growth for more than 80 days. It is noteworthy that levels of circulating breast epithelial antigens are found in the host while this therapy was administered as we have already reported (12).

The benefit of the "cocktail" approach is clearly proven by these experiments, as it was also the case in experimental immunotherapy of human breast tumors with unconjugated MoAbs (1,6). A much longer effective time of tumor growth arrest is shown for the "cocktail" than for single antibodies. A further advantage for the use of a "cocktail" of MoAbs is seen in that many of these MoAbs do cross react with other tissues in the organism so a "cocktail" will permit the use of lower concentrations of each of the independant antibodies with a total maximum effect. By providing a mixture of MoAbs it could also be argued that most likely the targeting on the tumor is more uniform when compared to the use of one or only two MoAbs, since the "cocktail" will possibly cover all carcinoma cells of the tumor or most of them. In addition, it is very important to note that the surrounding tissues are saturated with antigen released by the tumors that might well anchor some of these MoAbs tagged with the radioiodine, and, therefore, irradiate proximate breast epithelial tumor cells.

The dose chosen for testing efficacity of breast tumor therapy with the MoAbs radioconjugates (500 µCi) seemed to be tumoricidal as a consequence of its tumor binding as shown by the fact that a similar dose of a radioconjugate composed of normal mouse IgG was not effective (even when compared to the uninjected control) and also did not seem to have appreciable toxic effects to the host (Figures 2 and 6).

The distribution studies show that, at least against a nude mouse background, the human breast tumors concentrate far above any of the other tissues the tagged anti-breast MoAbs, thus giving grounds to the successful therapeutic response reported, with low toxicity. Furthermore, for Mc5 and for the bound "cocktail" of MoAbs the turnover on and around the tumor cells is rather slow and can be calculated to be in the order of four to six days for bound Mc5 and bound "cocktail" (unpublished results). Considering the increased percent of dose binding, at an equal amount of IgG with the former "cocktail" of MoAbs when compared to single MoAbs the better results obtained in terms of therapy are not surprising. It is also noteworthy that high accumulations of radiolabelled MoAbs can be seen on breast tumors while radiolabelled normal mouse serum IgG bound at very low levels, again supporting the fact that tumoricidal effects are not systemic as a result of the dose of radioactivity injected, but local as the result of the binding of the radioconjugates.

Maximum response after a dose of ^{131}I-labelled-MoAbs is usually obtained at day 6 after injection. For that reason repeated doses were administered to the slow growing and the fast growing tumors at day 0, 4 and 9. As a result of these injections a complete destruction of almost all tumor tissue can be obtained even in fast growing tumors, Figures 3 and 4. Obviously, repeated doses as these shown here will have to be evaluated against their toxic effects, thus requiring single doses or appropriate recovery periods in between each injection. In fact, repeated doses with appropriate time intervals are very effective in restraining the growth of these breast tumors for prolonged times while displaying low toxicity to the host (Figure 6), giving an indication of how this therapy could be of use in the breast cancer patient.

The tumor volume measurements that quantitate the attack of MoAbs on the tumor are substantiated by the large histological destruction of the tumors that could be visualized in the histopathological sections (not shown). Almost all epithelial cells are destroyed and the remaining mass of the tumor is occupied by collagenous infiltrative tissue. Thus, it can be firmly stated that the action of these MoAbs is by direct destruction of the breast epithelial cells contained in the tumor. A further point to be made, is that residual volumes of breast tumors after the present therapy could be deceiving and could only represent scar and necrotic tissue remaining after carcinoma cell destruction by the radioiodinated MoAbs.

Most breast tumors survived the present therapy and eventually growth reoccurred in a percentage of them but, however, they had a much slower regrowth rate than the original tumor indicating that a subpopulation, possibly with lower replicative capacity survived the irradiation effects, or perhaps, that local tumor conditions, such as proliferation of vascular and support cells, could have been affected.

It should also be mentioned that tumor attack by MoAb radioconjugates in an immunodeficient host could well be very different from that occurring in an immunocompetent host. It could be possible that attack of the tumor by the conjugated MoAbs could be aided in a substantial way by the host reaction to the tumor and the disturbances created by the conjugate attack on it.

This latter potentiation of the attack of the MoAbs on the tumor by the host immune response could also be optimized by modifying tumor conditions propitiatory to immunotherapy. One example of the latter improvements are shown in this study. The slowing down of the speed of growth of the tumor under MoAb conjugate attack, as we show, could be of value since slower tumors respond best to this therapy than faster growing ones. In the same line of thinking, manipulation of the tumor phenotype to increase antigen expression and prevelance also fall in this category. Hormonal or growth factor stimulation of breast epithelial antigenic synthesis could well represent an increase of targeting for radioconjugated MoAbs.

REFERENCES

1. M. Sasaki, J.A. Peterson, and R.L. Ceriani. Monoclonal antibodies against breast epithelial cell surface antigens in breast cancer therapy. Hybridoma, 2:120 (1983).

2. D.J. Hnatowich, F. Virri, and P.W. Doherty. DTPA-coupled antibodies labelled with yttrium-90. J. Nucl. Med. 26:503 (1985).

3. G.C. Buehring. Effect of hormones and chemicals on expression of milk fat globule antigens by breast cell line MCF-7. In Vitro, 22:50A (1986).

4. P.M. Capone, L.D. Papsidero, G.A. Croghan, and T.M. Chu. Experimental tumoricidal effects of monoclonal antibody against solid tumors. Proc. Natl. Acad. Sci. USA, 80:7328 (1983).

5. P.M. Capone, L.D. Papsidero, and T.M. Chu. Relationship between antigen density and immunotherapeutic response elicited by monoclonal antibodies against solid tumors. J. Natl. Cancer. Inst., 72:673 (1984).

6. R.L. Ceriani, E.W. Blank, and J.A. Peterson. Experimental immunotherapy of human breast carcinomas implanted in nude mice with a mixture of monoclonal antibodies against human milk fat globule components. Cancer Res. 47:532 (1987).

7. J.A. Peterson, R.L. Ceriani, E.W. Blank, and L. Osvaldo. Comparison of rates of phenotypic variability in surface antigen expression in normal and cancerous human breast epithelial cells. Cancer Res., 43:4291 (1983).

8. R.L. Ceriani, J.A. Peterson, and E.W. Blank. Variability in surface antigen expression of human breast epithelial cells cultured from normal breast, normal tissue peripheral to breast carcinomas, and breast carcinomas. Cancer Res., 44:3033 (1984).

9. M. Monaco, J. Mack, M. Dugan, and R.L. Ceriani. Synthesis of monoclonal antibody-toxin conjugates which specifically interact with MCF-7 breast carcinoma cells. Ann. N.Y. Acad. Sci., 464:389 (1986).

10. K.M. Hwang, E.W. Blank, and R.L. Ceriani. Experimental immunotherapy of human breast tumors with conjugated and unconjugated monoclonal antibodies. 8th Annual San Antonio Breast Cancer Symp., Nov. (1985).

11. F.C. Greenwood, W.M. Hunter, and J.I. Glover. The preparation of ^{131}I-labelled human growth hormone of high specific radioactivity. Biochem. J., 89:114 (1963).

12. M. Sasaki, J.A. Peterson, W. Wara, and R.L. Ceriani. Human mammary antigens (HME-Ags) in the circulation of nude mice implanted with breast and non-breast tumors. Cancer, 48:2214 (1981).

ANTIBODY GUIDED DIAGNOSIS AND THERAPY OF PATIENTS WITH BREAST CANCER

Haralambos P. Kalofonos and Agemenmon A. Epenetos

Imperial Cancer Research Fund Oncology Group
Department of Clinical Oncology
Royal Postgraduate Medical School
Hammersmith Hospital and
Imperial Cancer Research Fund
Lincolns Inn Field
P.O. Box 123, London WC2

ABSTRACT

Tumour associated monoclonal antibodies HMFG1 and HMFG2, labelled with iodine-123, and $F(ab')_2$ of HMFG1, labelled with indium-111, were used to detect primary and metastatic breast cancer, by external body scintigraphy, in 13 patients with measurable disease. Tumours became visible in the majority (9 out of 13) of patients. We detected both primary breast cancer and bony and soft tissue metastases. The presence of antibody in the tumours was confirmed by autoradiography and immunoperoxidase staining of surgically removed tissues. 111-In labelled $F(ab')_2$ fragments were superior to whole antibody. We imaged successfully the disease in 5 out of 7 patients, injected with radiolabelled $F(ab')_2$ of HMFG1. 2 patients with negative antibody scans had received prior chemotherapy and were in clinical remission.

Tumour associated monoclonal antibodies HMFG1, HMFG2 and AUA1 radiolabelled with iodine-131, were given intracavitary (intrapleurally and intrapericardially) to patients with malignant serous effusions secondary to breast and other epithelial cancers. Ten out of thirteen effusions (3 pericardial and 7 pleural) in 11 patients, responded completely with no fluid reaccumulation, between 3 and 18 months. No toxicity was encountered.

We conclude that this new method of treatment is nontoxic and effective, resulting in improved quality of life and in some cases, prolongation of survival of patients with breast or other epithelial origin neoplasms.

INTRODUCTION

With the introduction of the hybridoma technique (1), monoclonal antibodies have been produced that react with antigens associated with many types of cancer including carcinoma of the breast, lung, ovary, colon, melanoma, etc. (2). Subsequently radiolabelled monoclonal antibodies have been utilized in patients for tumour localisation by external body scintigraphy and encouraging clinical results have been reported by many workers (3-6). Other potential uses of monoclonal antibodies include the delivery of chemotherapy (7), toxins (8) or radionuclides (9-11) to specifically destroy tumour cells. The use of monoclonal antibodies to target cytotoxic agents has a primary aim to increase the amount of drug localising in tumours and secondary to reduce normal tissue toxicity. This approach requires that the monoclonal antibody localises effectively in the tumour. Therefore cancer therapy with monoclonal antibodies is based on the exploitation of both qualitative and quantitative differences between neoplasm and normal tissue.

In this chapter, we present our experience in the use of tumour associated monoclonal antibodies and $F(ab')_2$ fragments labelled with radionuclides for detection of primary and metastatic breast cancer and intracavitary therapy of malignant serous effusions, secondary to breast or other cancers.

Breast cancer which is the most common malignant neoplasm in the female population is the leading cause of death among women between the ages of 35 and 54 years, and among those in subsequent years, it is second only to heart disease (12). In the majority of women, breast cancer appears to be a systemic disease at the time of initial diagnosis (13). A minority of breast carcinomas are truly localised and are eradicable by local means, but approximately 40 per cent of patients with "operable" breast cancer develop overt recurrences (14). Thus a more sensitive technique is needed for the early detection of disease in order to identify those patients with truly local disease who would be potentially cured by surgery.

Cancer therapy is based on the exploitation of both qualitative and quantitative difference between neoplasm and normal tissue. Ideally, reagents used in cancer treatment should concentrate therapy at tumour sites whilst minimising side-effects on normal tissues. It has been shown that radiolabelled monoclonal antibody can preferentially target sites of active disease (15, 29).

Radioactively labelled antibodies administered intravenously have been, so far, of limited value in the treatment of malignant melanoma and hepatocellular cancer (9, 11, 18). Encouraging results have been obtained when radioactively labelled antibodies were administered intraregionally, either into body cavities (10) or as an arterial infusion for the treatment of some tumours, including brain gliomas (19). Recurrent malignant pleural or pericardial effusion is a frequent problem seen in patients with various forms of cancer particularly of breast, lung or ovarian origin (20-22). External beam radiotherapy, radioactive isotopes, intracavitary tetracycline, bleomycin and alkylating agents have all been used as forms of palliation with some success. Unfortunately, complications such as pain and rigours can occur and also there is reaccumulation of serous fluid in many cases (20-24).

In previous studies of malignant serous effusions, secondary to epithelial origin tumours, we found that neoplastic cells express tumour-associated antigens detected by monoclonal antibodies HMFG1, HMFG2 and AUA1 (25). A new therapeutic method termed "regional antibody guided irradiation" was introduced where two patients, one with malignant pericardial effusion and one with a malignant pleural effusion were treated by intracavity administration of iodine-131-labelled monoclonal antibody HMFG2 with encouraging results (10). This prompted us to perform a larger clinical study in order to extend and confirm our previous preliminary results.

MATERIALS AND METHODS

Monoclonal Antibodies

Mouse monoclonal antibodies HMFG1 and HMFG2, both IgG1, are directed against components of human milk-fat-globule membranes (26, 27). These antibodies react strongly with the lactating breast and also with a range of neoplasms of epithelial origin, particularly adenocarcinomas of breast and ovary. They react weakly with normal non-lactating breast and other epithelial tissues. They are, therefore, not tumour specific, but epithelium specific; because of their high reactivity with carcinomas they can be described as tumour associated antibodies.

AUA1 is a mouse IgG1, immunoglobulin directed against a cell surface determinant that seems to be associated with proliferating cells (28, 29). It reacts strongly with carcinomas of colon, breast and ovary as well as some normal cells, particularly colonic mucosal epithelium.

Radiolabelling

Pure iodine-123 (AERE, Harwell, U.K.) was supplied as "dry" sodium iodide, 15 mCi per container. Iodination involved a modification of the iodogen method (30). The specific activity of labelled antibody ranged from 5 to 8 mCi/mg immunoglobulin. Iodine-131 (Amersham International, UK) was added to antibody and iodination was performed in iodogen tubes. The labelled antibody was separated from free iodine-131 using gel filtration (Sephadex G-50). Specific activity was in the range of 4-8 mCi/mg immunoglobulin. Radiolabelled antibodies were diluted in 1% human serum albumin and filtered through Millipore prior to administration to patients.

Labelling with indium-111 (INSI, Amersham International, UK), involved conjugation with diethylenetriaminepentaacetic acid (DTPA) by means of the cyclic anhydride (31, 32). Unbound indium-111 was separated by means of gel filtration (Sephadex G50). Specific activity was in the range of 3.5 - 6.0 mCi/mg.

Kinetic Studies

Samples of blood and urine were taken regularly to calculate the half life of the radiolabelled antibodies in the circulation and their rate of excretion. Blood was collected in 5 ml EDTA - containing tubes at 0.1 min and 5 min, 2 hr, 4 hr, 12 hr, 2, 3 and 5 days after the injection.

Blood was centrifuged at 1,500 x g for 10 min. Aliquots (1.0 ml) of the plasma (supernatant) and of the pellet were counted. The pellet was previously washed twice with normal saline and centrifuged at 1,500 x g for 10 min. Quantitation of the radioactivity in the pellet and the supernatant was counted in a gamma-well counter.

Protein bound radioactivity in the plasma was assessed by polyacrylamide gel electrophoresis (PAGE) and autoradiography. Blood clearance of the radiolabelled antibodies was calculated, corrected for the decay and plotted against time as a percentage of the injected amount. In vivo kinetics of labelled antibodies were measured by means of serial external body counting, using a large field-of-view camera.

Immunoreactivity of Antibodies. This was tested in an enzyme immunosorbent assay (ELISA) with solid phase antigen. Antibodies were tested at sample concentration of 10 µg/ml and dilutions up to 10^{-6}, in duplicate. A comparison of antibody titres before and after radiolabelling and a direct radioimmunoassay including competition with unlabelled antibody were performed.

Autoradiography. Autoradiographs of fresh-frozen and fixed sections were carried out to demonstrate further the targetting of monoclonal antibodies to tumours and to study their cellular distribution. Autoradiographs were prepared using Ilford K-5 fluid emulsion. After drying in air, sections were exposed for 3 days before being developed, fixed and counterstained with haematoxylin for light microscopy.

Immunoperoxidase Staining. Formalin-fixed and paraffin wax-embedded or fresh-frozen sections of tumours and normal tissues were stained by an indirect two-stage immunoperoxidase procedure and counterstained with haematoxylin. Sections were tested against a range of monoclonal antibodies including AUA1, HMFG1 and HMFG2, and a negative control antibody 11.4.1; this antibody is directed against mouse H-2Kk antigen and does not react with human tissues (33). To demonstrate the presence of injected mouse antibody in tissues a one-stage direct immunoperoxidase technique was used applying rabbit anti-mouse-peroxidase to fresh-frozen sections and counterstaining with haemotoxylin.

Immunocytochemistry. Smears of cells obtained from serous effusions were examined against the selections of antibodies, using an indirect immunoperoxidase reaction (25). The antibody with the highest reactivity was selected for use. Immunocytochemistry was considered to be positive when >50% of neoplastic cells stained with at least one antibody. This was the case with all patients except one.

Antibody Guided Therapy Studies. These were carried out in two parts: In part I, pleural effusions were tapped as near dryness as possible and then 1.0 mCi radiolabelled antibody was administered into the cavity and was "washed in" with 500 ml of normal saline in patients with pleural effusions and 20 ml of normal saline in patients with pericardial effusions. Gamma camera scans were taken daily, from immediately after and up to 7 days after injection to calculate the required amount of radioactivity to deliver a cytotoxic dose.

In part II, a higher dose of iodinated antibody was given and scans from day 7 to day 28 were taken to calculate the delivered dose of radiation. After part II, each patient was kept in a single room until the emitted radiation was at a low level (below 30 mCi).

Dosimetry

For effective treatment the dose of radiation to the target should be high relative to the whole body or other sensitive organs. To calculate these doses it is necessary to know the proportion of the administered activity going to the target and to other relevant organs, the time course of the activity in the target and through the body, and the volume of distribution of the activity in the target. Volumes of the major organs of the body have been tabulated for "reference man" and may be assumed to be sufficiently accurate for most calculations of dosage. Each of these factors can be found only approximately and errors in the final dosimetry calculations are to be expected. Uptakes in the various parts of the body are assessed by quantative imaging aided by blood activity disappearance curves. Conventional imaging of the body does not usually take into account the varing attenuation of the emitted radiation and the varying response of the detector over different sites, so that the picture of count rates that is obtained reflects only the distribution of activity. Scintillation cameras and rectilinear scanners can, however, be calibrated using phantoms and deriving attenuation factors to give results in millicuries. Sequential conventional imaging under the same conditions with recording of the results using a computer system allows a time activity curve to be obtained from any region of interest in the body. When the source is sufficiently well localised the disappearance of activity can be monitored with a collimated probe counter viewing the same site over several successive days. Assessing the volume over which the activity in the tumour is distributed is difficult. Tomographic imaging is necessary for a full three dimensional description of the volume, and, although x-ray computed tomography has been employed, the anatomy described may not correspond to the functioning tissues taking up the activity. Isotope tomography often has too low a resolution for the small volumes encountered. Thus, often only an approximate estimate of volume based on a projected area combined with an assumed thickness is available. In the case of a pleural cavity the unknown thickness may vary from millimetres to centimetres and the final dosimetry estimates will reflect this inaccuracy. The mean dose absorbed to the target and other affected organs is obtained using the method of the Medical Internal Radiation Committee (34). This dose is the product of the cumulated activity (in mCi hours) in the region and the summed products of all the equilibrium dose constants and specific absorbed fractions for the emissions of the radionuclides used. For this work a conventional camera, a rotating tomographic camera interfaced to a nuclear medicine computing system, and a quantative whole body scanning camera with off line computing facilities have all been used at various stages to monitor and image the distributions of activity. A probe counter was also used to obtain time over activity curves for localised sources.

Quality Control. All reagents were produced sterile, and monoclonal antibodies were tested for sterility and pyrogenicity by an independent laboratory (Safepharm Laboratories). Patients gave written informed consent prior to entering the studies. Thyroid uptake of free and realeased iodine was blocked by potassium iodide, 120 mg/day orally, starting 24 hr before the injection and continuing for a week in patients with low activity for imaging studies and for three weeks in patients after therapy. Before intravenous injection of labelled antibodies, patient's skin was tested for hypersensitivity to mouse immunoglobulins. No reactions were recorded.

RESULTS

Imaging Studies

Patients were scanned at the day of injection and subsequently at various intervals, up to 48 hours, in the case of iodine-123 (Table I) and up to 7 days, when indium-111 (Table II) labelled antibodies were administered. Half of the 123-I labelled antibody was cleared from the blood by 13-21.6 hours; the average was 18 hours. 33% of the injected radioactivity was found in the urine by 18 hours.

In vivo kinetics of indium-111-labelled $F(ab')_2$ fragments, were measured by means of external body counting, on a large field-of-view camera, as well as blood sampling at various times. Blood samples were counted and corrected for the decay from the time of injection and plotted against time as a percentage of the injected amount. Blood clearance was biphasic with an early rapid fall in the level of circulating $F(ab')_2$ fragments in the first 2 hours to about 50% of the immediate level ($t_{1/2a}$=2 hr). Subsequently the fall was more gradual ($t_{1/2b}$=42 hr). Figure 1a and 1b show good localisation in a patient with breast cancer metastatic to the right humerus. Figure 1c is a conventional bone scan confirming the abnormality.

TABLE I. Localisation of human tumor with 123-I labelled HMFG1 and HMFG2.

Patient	Age	Extent	Antibody Injected	Dose of Antibody	^{123}I Injected Radioactivity	Therapy at time of antibody Administration	Antibody Scanning Results
1.	45	Chest; Skeleton	HMFG1	100 µg	0.2 mCi	Nil	Abdomen: -ve Skeleton: -ve
2.	57	Breast; Skin; Axillary Adenopathy	HMFG2	180 µg	0.5 mCi	Aninoglu- -tethimide	Chest: -ve
3.	77	Breast; Pelvis and (R) Femur; Liver	HMFG2	100 µg	1.25 mCi	Tamoxifen	Chest: +ve Abdomen: +ve Pelvis: +ve
4.	45	Bilateral recurrent laryngeal nerve paralysis	HMFG2	100 µg	1.6 mCi	Nil	Chest: +ve
5.	75	Chest; Abdomen; Sternum	HMFG1	2 mg	2 mCi	Nil	Chest: +ve Abdomen: +ve Sternum: +ve
6.	68	Liver; Thorocolumbar Spine; Ribs	HMFG2	200 µg	0.2 mCi	Aminoglu- -tethimide	Chest: +ve Abdomen: +ve

TABLE II. Localisation of human tumor with 111-In labelled $F(ab')_2$ HMFG1 fragments.

Patient	Age	Extent	Dose of Antibody	^{111}In Injected Radioactivity	Therapy at time of antibody Administration	Antibody Scanning Results
1.	72	(R) Humerus; (R) Acetabulum; (R) Ribs (8,11) (Mastectomy)	165 µg	35 MBq		(R) Humerus: +ve (R) Acetabulium: +ve (R) Ribs (8,11): +ve
2.	55	Extensive bone metastases: Cervical adenopathy(R)&(L); (Mastetcomy)	220 µg	37 MBq	CR after chemotherapy	Nil
3.	57	Breast (R) Lump; Liver; Skin; Thorocolumbar Spine	160 µg	28 MBq	Chemo; Radiotherapy thoracolumbar spine	Liver: +ve
4.	47	Breast (R) Lump; Axillary adenopathy (R);	195 µg	33 MBq		Breast (R)/up: +ve Adenopathy: +ve
5.	43	Multiple subcutaneous nodules (Mastectomy)	325 µg	70 MBq		Nodules: +ve
6.	54	Skin (Mastectomy)	290 µg	40 MBq		Skin: +ve
7.	56	Bone metastases;	300 µg	40 MBq	CR after chemotherapy	Nil

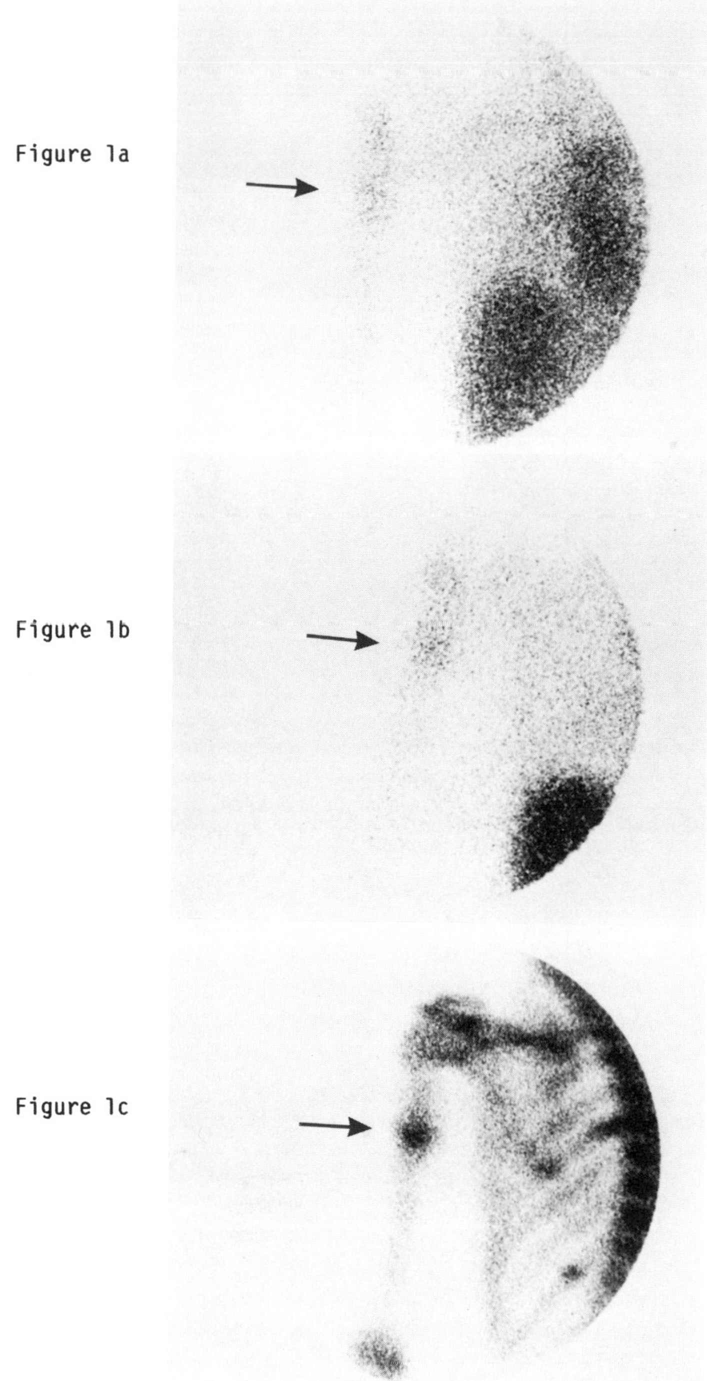

Fig. 1 - This shows an antibody scan (HMFG1 F(ab')2 - 111-In-labelled) taken at 24 hr (figure 1a) and 48 hr (figure 1b) after injection in a patient with breast cancer metastatic to the right humerus (arrows) as confirmed by conventional isotope bone scanning (figure 1c).

Therapy

We studied 11 consecutive and unselected patients, with 13 recurrent pleural or pericardial malignant effusions from a variety of primary tumours resistant to chemotherapy and/or radiotherapy, carried out at the Hammersmith Hospital.

We treated five male and six female, aged 30-73 years (mean age 53 years). Four patients had lung cancer (three adenocarcinoma and one squamous cell carcinoma), three patients had ovarian carcinoma, two patients had breast carcinoma, one patient had carcinoma of the prostate and one patient had pancreatic carcinoma. Three of them had pericardial effusions and nine had pleural effusions. The patient with squamous cell carcinoma of the lung, had both pleural and pericardial effusions and one patient with carcinoma of the ovary, had bilateral effusions. All patients had measurable and persistent disease following previous chemotherapy and/or radiotherapy.

Ten out of thirteen effusions (7 pleural and 3 pericardial) responded favourably to treatment without reaccumulation of fluid, followed up to between three and eighteen months (mean 7 months) after treatment. All three patients with malignant pericardial effusions responded completely to antibody therapy, with no fluid reaccumulation after 3, 12 and 18 months respectively.

Three patients failed to respond to antibody therapy. One of them had an effusion secondary to adenocarcinoma of lung, and he was treated with 46 mCi of iodine-131-labelled AUA1 antibody. Another patient had a large and recurrent effusion secondary to carcinoma of prostate. He was treated empirically with 21 mCi of iodine-131-labelled HMFG2 antibody without prior immunocytochemical analysis (there were insuffient malignant cells in the fluid for immunocytochemistry). It was interesting that when his recurrent effusion was examined immunocytochemically, malignant cells were negative for the presence of HMFG2 antigen. The third patient had a bilateral pleural effusion secondary to an ovarian carcinoma. Left pleural effusion was treated with 30 mCi of a mixture of HMFG2 and AUA1 antibody, and it recurred two months after treatment. Right pleural effusion was treated with 56 mCi of iodine-131-labelled HMFG1 antibody and has not recurred (follow up 6 months). Nine patients were treated with a mixture of HMFG1, HMFG2, and AUA1 monoclonal antibodies. Three out of three pericardial effusions and seven out of ten pleural effusions responded completely.

DISCUSSION

In this chapter, we outline the results obtained using radioactively labelled tumour associated monoclonal antibodies HMFG1, HMFG2, AUA1 and $F(ab')_2$ fragments of HMFG1 for tumour localisation in patients with breast cancer. Furthermore we report a new form of therapy for malignant recurrent pleural and pericardial effusion resistant to conventional forms of therapy.

Using iodine-123 labelled HMFG1 and HMFG2 monoclonal antibodies, we could get specific imaging in four out of six patients with primary and metastatic breast cancer lesions. However, we could not image lesions in the other two patients, even though immunoperoxidase staining of tumour cells was positive for HMFG1 and HMFG2. On the other hand using indium-111 labelled $F(ab')_2$ of HMFG1 we could detect all primary and metastatic, lesions including soft tissues such as skin and subcutaneous nodules. Thus our clinical study confirms preclinical findings of improved localisation with $F(ab')_2$ fragments (40-44). Successful radioimmunolocalisation was achieved without employing any techniques of imaging subtraction and enhancement of visualisation. This may be due to the favourable properties of monoclonal antibodies HMFG2 and HMFG1 and to the use of 111-In and 123-I in preference to 131I for gamma camera imaging (17). The advantages of iodine-123 over -131, as an imaging agent are well known and are due to the high photon yield and the favourable energy, 0.159 MEV, providing accurate imaging and only a slight radiation hazard to patients and staff. However dehalogenation can occur causing uptake of free iodine-123 by thyroid, stomach and other organs. The quality of images could be improved by the use of alternative labels such as indium-111 (32, 35-38).

Disadvantages using indium-111 labelled monoclonal antibodies include higher uptake in the liver and transchelation to transferrin (16, 39) but nevertheless, indium-111 remains one of the most suitable radioisotopes currently available for imaging. (Figure 1).

A natural step from the successful use of radioactively labelled monoclonal antibodies for in vivo diagnosis is their use for targetted therapy. We have previously shown that the IV route of antibody administration leads only to very small uptake by tumour cells (mean value of 0.015% of total injected amount per g of tumour occuring 1 day of postadministration (15) and this is the reason why we explored other routes, such as intracavitary administration (10). In this study we report successful palliation of malignant serous effusions by the intracavity administration of radiolabelled antibodies. The best results were observed in patients with pericardial effusions. This is probably due to the higher doses delivered to pericardium as compared to doses delivered to pleural cavity. It was of interest that in a patient with bilateral pleural effusions the one effusion treated with 30 mCi of activity recurred whilst the other effusion treated with 56 mCi of activity did not recur. Nevertheless in other patients a satisfactory remission was achieved with doses of 30 mCi. Therefore, two contributing factors for the successful outcome of antibody guided-irradiation appear to be a) tumour bulk and b) the delivered dose of iodine-131. From our data it is suggested that for effective therapy, 30 mCi of iodine-131-labelled antibody should be given intrapericardially and 60 mCi intrapleurally. The efficacy of this new method (10 out of 13 responders) appears to be superior to previously reported methods with nonspecific agents such as colloidal radioactive phosphorus, bleomycin or tetracycline (20-23). Nevertheless, our data at present is not conclusive with regard to the superiority of this method over previous techniques. Finally, the fact that in one of the three cases where there was fluid reaccumulation the malignant cells were negative against the administered antibody, indicates that this new method of treatment may act via specific antigen antibody interaction. A randomised study is required to establish conclusively the efficacy and the mode of action of this novel therapeutic approach.

REFERENCES

1. Kohler G. and Milstein C. Continuous cultures of fused cells secreting antibodies of predefined specificity. Nature 256:495-497 (1975).
2. Wright G. Application of monoclonal antibodies to the study of human cancer, in: "Monoclonal Antibodies and Cancer," G.L. Wright, ed., Marcel Dekker, New York, pp 1-31 (1984).
3. Epenetos A.A., Britton K.E., Mather S., et al. Targetting of 123 I-labelled-tumour associated monoclonal antibodies to ovarian, breast and gastrointestinal tumours. Lancet 2:999-1003 (1982).

4. Mach J.P., Buchegger F., Forni M., et al. Use of radiolabelled monoclonal anti-CEA antibodies for the detection of human carcinomas by external photoscanning and tomoscintigraphy. Immunology Today December, 239-249 (1981).
5. Farrands P.A., Perkins A.C., Pimm M.V. et al. Radioimmunodetection of human colorectal cancer by an anti-tumour monoclonal antibody. Lancet 2:397-400 (1982).
6. Larson S.M., Brown J.P., Wright P.W. et al. Imaging of melanoma with I-131-labelled monoclonal antibodies. J. Nucl. Med. 23:123-129 (1983).
7. Baldwin R.W., Pimm V. Antitumour monoclonal antibodies for radioimmunodetection of tumours and drug targeting. Cancer Metastasis Rev. 2:89-106 (1983).
8. Thorpe R.E. and Ross W.C. The preparation and cytotoxic properties of antibody-toxin conjugates. Immuno. Rev. 62, 119 (1982).
9. Order S.E., Klein J.L., Ettinger D. et al. Use of isotopic immunoglobulin in therapy. Cancer Res. 40:3001 (1980).
10. Epenetos A.A., Courtenay-Luck N., Halnan K.E., et al. Antibody guided irradiation of malignant lesions. Lancet 30:1441-1443 (1984).
11. Carrasquilo J.A., Krohn K.A., Beaumier P., et al. Diagnosis of and therapy for solid tumours with radiolabelled antibodies and immune fragments. Cancer Treat. Rep. 68:371-378 (1984).
12. Haskell C.L. Cancer Treatment. Breast Cancer. Ed. C.L. Haskell, W.B. Saunders, pp 137-180 (1985).
13. Fisher B. Laboratory and clinical research in breast cancer. Cancer Res. 40:3863 (1980).
14. Brinkley D., Haybittle J.L. The curability of breast cancer. Lancet ii, 95-97 (1975).
15. Epenetos A.A., Snook, D., Durbin, H. et al. Limitations of radiolabeled monoclonal antibodies for localization of human neoplasms. Cancer Res. 46:3183-3191 (1986).
16. Rainsbury R.M., Ott R.J., Westwood J.H. et al. Location of metastatic breast carcinoma by a monoclonal antibody chelate-labelled with indium-111. Lancet 22:934-938 (1983).
17. Hayes D.F., Zalutsky M.R., Kaplan W. et al. Pharmacokinetics of radiolabelled monoclonal antibody B6.2 in patients with metastatic breast cancer. Cancer Res. 46:3157-3163 (1986).
18. Order S.E., Klein J., Ettinger D., et al. Phase I-II study of radiolabelled antibody integrated in the treatment of primary hepatic malignancies. Int. J. Rad. Oncol. Biol and Physics 6, 703-710 (1980).
19. Epenetos A.A., Courtenay-Luck N., Pickering D., et al. Antibody guided irradiation of brain glioma by arterial infusion of radioactive monoclonal antibody against epidermal growth factor receptor and blood group A antigen. Br. Med. J. 290, 1463-1466 (1985).
20. Anderson C., Philpott G. and Ferguson T., et al. The treatment of malignant pleural effusions. Cancer 33:916 (1974).
21. Wallach H.W. Intrapleural tetracycline for malignant pleural effusions. Chest 68, 50 (1975).
22. Paladine W., Cunningham T., Spoyzo R., et al. Intracavity bleomycin in the management of malignant effusions. Cancer 38:1903 (1976).
23. Strober S., Kloty E., Kuperman and Gossein N. Malignant pleural disease. A radiotherapeutic approach to the problem. JAMA 226, 296 (1973).
24. Osteowski M. and Halsall G. Intracavitary bleomycin in the management of malignant effusions: a multicentre study. Cancer Treat. Rep. 66, 1903 (1982).

25. Epenetos A.A., Canti G., Taylor-Papadimitriou J., et al. Use of two epithelium-specific monoclonal antibodies for diagnosis of malignancy in serous effusions. Lancet ii, 1004-1006 (1982).
26. Arklie J., Taylor-Papadimitriou J., Bodmer W.F., et al. Differentiation antigens expressed by epithelial cells in the lactating breast and also detectable in breast cancers. Int. J. Cancer 28:23-29 (1981).
27. Taylor-Papadimitriou J., Peterson J.A., Arklie J., et al. Monoclonal antibodies to epithelium-specific components of the human milk fat globule membrane. Production and reaction with cells in culture. Int. J. Cancer 28:17-21 (1981).
28. Arklie J. Studies of the human epithelian cell surface using monoclonal antibodies. Ph.D. Dissertation, University of Oxford (1981).
29. Epenetos A.A., Nimmon C.C., Arklie J., et al. Detection of human cancer in an animal model using radiolabelled tumour associated monoclonal antibodies. Br. J. Cancer 46:1-6 (1982).
30. Fraker P.J. and Speck J.C. Protein and cell membrane iodination with sparingly soluble shloramide, 1,3,4,6-tetrachloro-5, 6-diphenylglycouril. Biochem. Biophys. Res. Commun. 80,849 (1978).
31. Hnatowich D.J., Layne W.W., and Childs R.L. The preparation and labelling of DTPA-coupled albumin. Int. J. Appl. Radio. Isot. 33, 327-332 (1982).
32. Hnatowich D.J. et al. Radioactive labelling of antibody: a simple and efficient method. Science 220:613-15 (1983).
33. Oi V.T., Jones P.P., Goding J.W., et al. Current properties of monoclonal antibodies to mouse Ig allotypes, H-2 and Ia antigens. Curr. Topic. Microbiol. Immunol. 81:115-29 (1979).
34. Snyder W.S., Ford M.R., Warner G.G. Estimates of specific absorbed fractions for photon sources uniformly distributed in various organs of a heterogenous phantom. New York; Society of Nuclear Medicine, 1978:5-67. (Medical Internal Radiation Dose (MIRD) pamphlet 5).
35. Scheinberg D.A., Strand M., Gansow O.A., et al. Tumour imaging with radioactive metal chelates conjugated to monoclonal antibodies. Science 215:1511-1513 (1982).
36. Paxton R.J., Jakowatz J.G., Beatty D., et al. High-specific-activity of indium-111 labelled anti-carcinoembryonic antigen monoclonal: improved method for the synthesis of diethylenetriaminopentacetic acid conjugates. Cancer Res. 45:5694-5699 (1985).
37. Epenetos A.A., Hooker G., Durbin H., et al. Indium-111-labelled, monoclonal antibody to placental alkaline phosphatase in the detection of neoplasms of tesis, ovary and cervix. Lancet i, 350-353 (1985).
38. Hnatowich D.J., Griffin T.W., Kosciaczyk D., et al. Pharmacokentics of an indium-111-labelled monoclonal antibody in cancer patients. J. Nucl. Med. 26:849-858 (1985).
39. Sakahara H., Endo K., Nakashima T., et al. Effect of DTPA conjugation on the antigen binding activity and biodistribution of monoclonal antibodies against α-fetoprotein. J. Nucl. Med. 26:750-755 (1985).
40. Wahl R.L., Parker C.W., and Philpott G.W., et al. Improved radioimaging and tumour localisation with monoclonal F(ab')2 fragments. J. Nucl. Med. 24, 316-325 (1983).
41. Fawwaz R.A., Wang T.S.T., Eastbrook K.A., et al. Immunoreactivity and biodistribution of indium-111-labelled monoclonal antibody to human high molecular weight-melanoma associated antigen. J. Nucl. Med. 26:488-492 (1985).

42. Harwood P.J., Boden J., Pedley R.B., et al. Comparative tumour localisation of antibody fragments and intact IgG in nude mice bearing a CEA-producing human colon tumour xenograft. _Eur. J. Cancer Clin. Oncology_ 21, 1512-1522 (1985).
43. Colcher D., Zalutsky M., Kaplan W., et al. Radiolocalization of human mammary tumours in athymic mice by monoclonal antibody. _Cancer Res._ 43:736-742 (1983).
44. Buchegger F., Haskell C.M., Schreyer M., et al. Radiolabelled fragments of monoclonal antibodies against carcinoembryonic antigen for localization of human colon carcinoma grafted into nude mice. _J. Exp. Med._ 158, 413-427 (1983).

CONTRIBUTORS

R. Agresti, Istituto Nazionale Tumori, Via Venezian 1, Milan, Italy

S. Andreola, Istituto Nazionale Tumori, Via Venezian 1, Milan, Italy

L.D. Apelgren, Lilly Research Laboratories, Lilly Corporate Center, Indianapolis, Indiana 46285

A.L. Baker, Lilly Research Laboratories, Lilly Corporate Center, Indianapolis, Indiana 46285

H. Battifora, M.D., City of Hope National Medical Center, 1500 East Duarte Road, Duarte, California 91010

J. Bishop, The Cancer Institute, Melbourne, Australia

E.W. Blank, John Muir Cancer & Aging Research Institute, 2055 N. Broadway, Walnut Creek, California 94596

M.J. Borowitz, Duke University Medical School, Durham, North Carolina 27710

S.L. Briggs, Lilly Research Laboratories, Lilly Corporate Center, Indianapolis, Indiana 46285

T.F. Bumol, Lilly Research Laboratories, Lilly Corporate Center, Indianapolis, Indiana 46285

J. Burchell, Imperial Cancer Research Fund, P.O. Box 123, Lincoln's Inn Fields, London WC2A 3PX, U.K.

R. Burton, Discipline of Surgical Sciences, University of Newcastle, Newcastle, Australia

N. Cascinelli, Istituto Nazionale Tumori, Via Venezian 1, Milan, Italy

G. Cattoretti, Istituto Nazionale Tumori, Via Venezian 1, Milan, Italy

V. Cavailles, Unite d'Endocrinologie Cellulaire et Moleculaire (U148) INSERM, 60 rue de Navacelles, 34100 Montpellier, France

R.L. Ceriani, John Muir Cancer & Aging Research Institute, 2055 N. Broadway, Walnut Creek, California 94596

M.I. Colnaghi, Istituto Nazionale Tumori, Via Venezian 1, Milan, Italy

R.J. Cote, Memorial Sloan-Kettering Cancer Center, 1275 York Avenue, New York, New York 10021

M.G. Da Dalt, Istituto Nazionale Tumori, Via Venezian 1, Milan, Italy

S.V. DeHerdt, Lilly Research Laboratories, Lilly Corporate Center, Indianapolis, Indiana 46285

C.M. DeRose, Arthur Purdy Stout Laboratory of Surgical Pathology and Department of Surgery, College of Physicians and Surgeons, Columbia University, New York, New York 10032

M. Del Vecchio, Istituto Nazionale Tumori, Via Venezian 1, Milan, Italy

D. Derocq, Unite d'Endocrinologie Cellulaire et Moleculaire (U148) INSERM, 60 rue de Navacelles, 34100 Montpellier, France

G. Di Fronzo, Istituto Nazionale Tumori, Via Venezian 1, Milan, Italy

A.S. Dion, Institute of Molecular Genetics, Center for Molecular Medicine and Immunology, One Bruce Street, Newark, New Jersey 07103

L.G. Dressler, Department of Medicine/Oncology, University of Texas Health Science Center at San Antonio, 7703 Floyd Curl Drive, San Antonio, Texas 78284

D.P. Edwards, Department of Pathology, University of Colorado Health Sciences Center, 4200 East Ninth Avenue, Denver, Colorado 80262

D. El-Ashry, University of Colorado Health Sciences Center, 4200 East Ninth Avenue, Denver, Colorado 80262

A.A. Epenetos, Imperial Cancer Research Fund Oncology Group, Department of Clinical Oncology, Royal Postgraduate Medical School, Hammersmith Hospital and Imperial Cancer Research Fund, Lincoln's Inn Field, P.O. Box 123, London WC2A 3PX, U.K.

P.A. Estes, University of Colorado Health Sciences Center, 4200 East Ninth Avenue, Denver, Colorado 80262

J.L. Flowers, Duke University Medical Center, Durham, North Carolina 27710

G. Freiss, Unite d'Endocrinologie Cellulaire et Moleculaire (U148) INSERM, 60 rue de Navacelles, 34100 Montpellier, France

S.A.W. Fuqua, Department of Medicine/Oncology, University of Texas Health Science Center at San Antonio, 7703 Floyd Curl Drive, San Antonio, Texas 78284

M. Garcia, Unite d'Endocrinologie Cellulaire et Moleculaire (U148) INSERM, 60 rue de Navacelles, 34100 Montpellier, France

S. Gendler, Imperial Cancer Research Fund, P.O. Box 123, Lincoln's Inn Fields, London WC2A 3PX, U.K.

E. Gero, The Netherlands Cancer Institute, Antoni van Leeuwenhoekhuis, Division of Tumor Biology, Plesmanlaan 121, 1066 CX Amsterdam, The Netherlands; National Cancer Institute, Oncopathological Research Institute, Budapest, Hungary; Present Address: Centocor, Inc., 244 Great Valley Parkway, Malvern, Pennsylvania 19355

J. Golder, Australian Med-Research Industries, St. Leonards, N.S.W., Australia

G.L. Greene, The Ben May Institute and Department of Pathology, The University of Chicago, 5841 S. Maryland Avenue, Chicago, Illinois 60637

A.B. Griffiths, Imperial Cancer Research Fund, P.O. Box 123, Lincoln's Inn Fields, London WC2A 3PX, U.K.

D.V. Habif, Arthur Purdy Stout Laboratory of Surgical Pathology and Department of Surgery, College of Physicians and Surgeons, Columbia University, New York, New York 10032

Ph. Hageman, The Netherlands Cancer Institute, Antoni van Leeuwenhoekhuis, Division of Tumor Biology, Plesmanlaan 121, 1066 CX Amsterdam, The Netherlands

J. Hilgers, The Netherlands Cancer Institute, Antoni van Leeuwenhoekhuis, Division of Tumor Biology, Plesmanlaan 121, 1066 CX Amsterdam, The Netherlands

J. Hilkens, The Netherlands Cancer Institute, Antoni van Leeuwenhoekhuis, Division of Tumor Biology, Plesmanlaan 121, 1066 CX Amsterdam, The Netherlands

A.N. Houghton, Memorial Sloan-Kettering Cancer Center, 1275 York Avenue, New York, New York 10021

M. Ishida, McGill Cancer Centre, McIntyre Medical Sciences Building, 3655 Drummond, Montreal, PQ H3G IY6, Canada

H.P. Kalofonos, Imperial Cancer Research Fund Oncology Group, Department of Clinical Oncology, Royal Postgraduate Medical School, Hammersmith Hospital and Imperial Cancer Research Fund, Lincoln's Inn Field, P.O. Box 123, London WC2A 3PX, U.K.

S. Khalaf, Laboratoire de Biochimie Cellulaire Hormonale, Faculte de Medecine, Montpellier, France

L.B. Kinsel, Duke University Medical Center, Durham, North Carolina 27710

J. Konrath, The University of Chicago, Chicago, Illinois

J. Lawler-Heavner, University of Colorado Health Sciences Center, 4200 East Ninth Avenue, Denver, Colorado 80262

G.S. Leight, Duke University Medical Center, Durham, North Carolina 27710

P.P. Major, McGill Cancer Centre, McIntyre Medical Sciences Building, 3655 Drummond, Montreal, PQ H3G IY6, Canada

P. Marder, Lilly Research Laboratories, Lilly Corporate Center, Indianapolis, Indiana 46285

T. Maudelonde, Laboratoire de Biochimie Cellulaire Hormonale, Faculte de Medecine, Montpellier, France

K.S. McCarty, Duke University Medical Center, Durham, North Carolina 27710

W.L. McGuire, Department of Medicine/Oncology, University of Texas Health Science Center at San Antonio, 7703 Floyd Curl Drive, San Antonio, Texas 78284

I.F.C. McKenzie, Research Centre for Cancer and Transplantation, University of Melbourne, Parkville, Australia

S. Menard, Istituto Nazionale Tumori, Via Venezian 1, Milan, Italy

D.M. Morrissey, Memorial Sloan-Kettering Cancer Center, 1275 York Avenue, New York, New York 10021

A.S. Narula, Department of Radiology, Duke University Medical Center, Durham, North Carolina 27710

H.F. Oettgen, Memorial Sloan-Kettering Cancer Center, 1275 York Avenue, New York, New York 10021

L.J. Old, Memorial Sloan-Kettering Cancer Center, 1275 York Avenue, New York, New York 10021

L. Ozzello, Arthur Purdy Stout Laboratory of Surgical Pathology and Department of Surgery, College of Physicians and Surgeons, Columbia University, New York, New York 10032

F. Paolucci, Clin Midy Sanofi, Rue du Pr Joseph Blayac, 34082 Montpellier, France

J. Parrish, Lilly Research Laboratories, Lilly Corporate Center, Indianapolis, Indiana 46285

B. Pau, Clin Midy Sanofi, Rue du Pr Joseph Blayac, 34082 Montpellier, France

X. Pei-xiang, Research Centre for Cancer and Transplantation, University of Melbourne, Parkville, Australia

J.A. Peterson, John Muir Cancer & Aging Research Institute, 2055 N. Broadway, Walnut Creek, California 94596

R. Pohland, Lilly Research Laboratories, Lilly Corporate Center, Indianapolis, Indiana 46285

M.F. Press, The Ben May Institute and Department of Pathology, The University of Chicago, 5841 S. Maryland Avenue, Chicago, Illinois 60637

F. Rilke, Istituto Nazionale Tumori, Via Venezian 1, Milan, Italy

H. Rochefort, Unite d'Endocrinologie Cellulaire et Moleculaire (U148) INSERM, 60 rue de Navacelles, 34100 Montpellier, France, Laboratoire de Biochimie Cellulaire Hormonale, Faculte de Medecine, Montpellier, France

H. Rogier, Clin Midy Sanofi, Rue du Pr Joseph Blayac, 34082 Montpellier, France

N. Sacks, Research Centre for Cancer and Transplantation, University of Melbourne, Parkville, Australia

G. Salazar, Unite d'Endocrinologie Cellulaire et Moleculaire (U148) INSERM, 60 rue de Navacelles, 34100 Montpellier, France

F.A. Salinas, Advanced Therapeutics Department, Cancer Control Agency of British Columbia, and Department of Pathology, University of British Columbia, Vancouver, B.C. V5Z 4E6, Canada

C. Smart, Discipline of Surgical Sciences, University of Newcastle, Newcastle, Australia

M.E. Spearman, Lilly Research Laboratories, Lilly Corporate Center, Indianapolis, Indiana 46285

S. Stacker, Research Centre for Cancer and Transplantation, University of Melbourne, Parkville, Australia

E. Suba, University of Colorado Health Sciences Center, 4200 East Ninth Avenue, Denver, Colorado 80262

J. Sugar, National Cancer Institute, Oncopathological Research Institute, Budapest, Hungary

J. Taylor-Papadimitriou, Imperial Cancer Research Fund, P.O. Box 123, Lincoln's Inn Fields, London WC2A 3PX, U.K.

C. Thompson, Research Centre for Cancer and Transplantation, University of Melbourne, Parkville, Australia

L. Verderio, Istituto Nazionale Tumori, Via Venezian 1, Milan, Italy

M.R. Zalutsky, Department of Radiology, Duke University Medical Center, Durham, North Carolina 27710

INDEX